STRUCTURE OF THE HUMAN BRAIN A Photographic Atlas

THIRD EDITION

STEPHEN J. DeARMOND, M.D., Ph.D.

Associate Professor
Department of Pathology (Neuropathology)
University of California, San Francisco

MADELINE M. FUSCO, Ph.D.

Professor
Department of Anatomical Sciences
State University of New York at Stony Brook

MAYNARD M. DEWEY, Ph.D.

Professor and Chairman
Department of Anatomical Sciences
State University of New York at Stony Brook

NEW YORK OXFORD · OXFORD UNIVERSITY PRESS · 1989

Oxford University Press

Oxford New York Toronto
Delhi Bombay Calcutta Madras Karachi
Petaling Jaya Singapore Hong Kong Tokyo
Nairobi Dar es Salaam Cape Town
Melbourne Auckland

and associated companies in
Berlin Ibadan

Published by Oxford University Press, Inc.
198 Madison Avenue, New York, New York 10016-4314

Oxford is a registered trademark of Oxford University Press

Library of Congress Cataloging-in-Publication Data
DeArmond, Stephen J.
Structure of the human brain.
Includes index.
1. Brain—Atlases. I. Fusco, Madeline M.
II. Dewey, Maynard M. III. Title. [DNLM: 1. Central
Nervous System—anatomy & histology—atlases.
WL 17 D285s]
QM455.D4 1989   611'.81   88-19551
ISBN 978-0-19-504357-0

25 26 27

Printed in China

CONTENTS

ACKNOWLEDGMENTS

Before all others, we would like to thank Jeffrey House, Vice President and Executive Editor of Science and Medicine, of Oxford University Press in New York. It is largely through his efforts and gentle prodding that this edition of the Atlas was completed. The first edition came about under his guidance 20 years ago. He has become a good and close friend since then and there is no question that his professionalism and attention to details are largely responsible for the quality of the publication and its success. Dr. Jack deGroot of the University of California at San Francisco must also be thanked, not only for providing the high quality MRI and CT scans which appear in this edition, but also for his cheerful encouragement and advice. Dr. Marian Diamond of the University of California at Berkeley played a pivotal role because she gave us the reassurance and assistance we needed to add a section devoted to the chemoarchitecture of the human brain. Dr. John Pearson of New York University Medical Center, an expert in the immunohistochemical localization of neurotransmitters in human brain, graciously found the time during a particularly difficult year to send us the now classical photomicrographs of neurons immunostained with tyrosine hydroxylase antibodies. Those photographs bring a reality to the drawings in the chemoarchitectural section. We want to acknowledge the technical skills of Ms Warnitta Montgomery in the Neuropathology Unit at the University of California at San Francisco for performing the many neurohistological stains on sections of the brain stem and diencephalon which were used to help define the borders of reticular formation nuclei. We also want to thank Mr. Walter Denn of Biomed Arts Associates, Inc. in San Francisco for his contribution to maintaining high quality reproductions in the Atlas through the tedious job of masking and airbrushing the background on the new photographs of the coronal sections of the gross brain. We must also thank Dr. Bernadette Naughton DeArmond and Jennifer DeArmond for their help once again with the preparation of the index. Finally, it is necessary to acknowledge K. Spirit, an embodiment of truth, caring, and hope which we have seen in many, but unfortunately not in all, of our students' and colleagues' eyes and without which science and medicine are meaningless.

INTRODUCTION

This edition of *The Structure of the Human Brain* was produced for two reasons. First, in the more than two decades since the first edition was begun, there have been major advances in the localization of neurotransmitters and neuromodulators in the nervous system by means of histochemical and immunohistochemical methods. Second, advances in neuroradiologic imaging techniques, magnetic resonance imaging and computerized tomography in particular, have made it imperative that medical students as well as clinicians develop a clear understanding of the gross anatomy of the brain.

For these reasons we have made three changes in this edition. First, eleven full coronal sections of the gross brain with attached brain stem (1.3× magnification) have been added to match the plane now routinely displayed by advanced clinical imaging techniques. These planes are also preferred by neuropathologists because they make it possible to analyze pathological changes in relationship to the

vascular territories and watershed regions of the brain. The new section of the book complements the horizontal sections of the gross brain that were added to the second edition. Second, we added a unique new section, "Chemoarchitectural-Neuroanatomic Relationships in the Human CNS," which correlates the location of adrenalin, noradrenalin, dopamine, serotonin, and acetylcholine containing nerve cell bodies and pathways with classically defined neuroanatomical structures and boundaries. Third, to complement the new chemoarchitectural section and emphasize current concepts in neurotransmitter anatomy of the brain, we updated illustrations throughout the book to define structures with new-found importance such as the basal forebrain cholinergic system and reticular nuclei of the brain stem.

The main goal of all three editions of the Atlas has been to display as clearly as possible both the commonly discussed, clinically important nuclei and

pathways for the beginning student of neuroanatomy as well as some of the more esoteric CNS structures. The latter are often mentioned in passing in neuroanatomy courses and textbooks and are of relevance to more advanced students and to researchers and clinicians. However, there has been an occasional complaint that we have labeled too many structures in the Atlas. Thus, we issue the following warning to overzealous beginning students of neuroanatomy: *Select structures to learn as needed. Attempts to memorize all of the information contained in this book may be detrimental to your mental health.* Indeed, learning neuroanatomy is analogous to learning a language or geography; it is a slow process of building inch by inch and learning by repetition.

We believe that one of the unique features of this Atlas has been the care given to presenting the highest quality photographs and accurate matching diagrams. To preserve resolution during enlargement and reproduction, most of the photomicrographs were made from 8 × 10 inch negatives and the remaining photomicrographs and photographs of the gross brain were made from 4 × 5 inch negatives. Each negative was painstakingly painted wtih an opaquing medium to eliminate irrelevant, confusing background and to clearly define the borders of central nervous system structures. The first edition alone took six years to complete for these reasons.

This will probably not be the last edition of this Atlas. In the coming years we will need to modify our current figures and add additional information as new data become available and as the functional and/or clinical significance of chemical-structural relationships are unraveled. To those colleagues of ours who have questioned whether there is anything new in neuroanatomy which could be added to a classical-type atlas of the nervous system, we would say that the structure of the human brain has only begun to be illustrated.

University of California   S.J.D.
San Francisco

State University of New York   M.M.F.
at Stony Brook   M.M.D.
January 1989

THE GROSS BRAIN AND SPINAL CORD

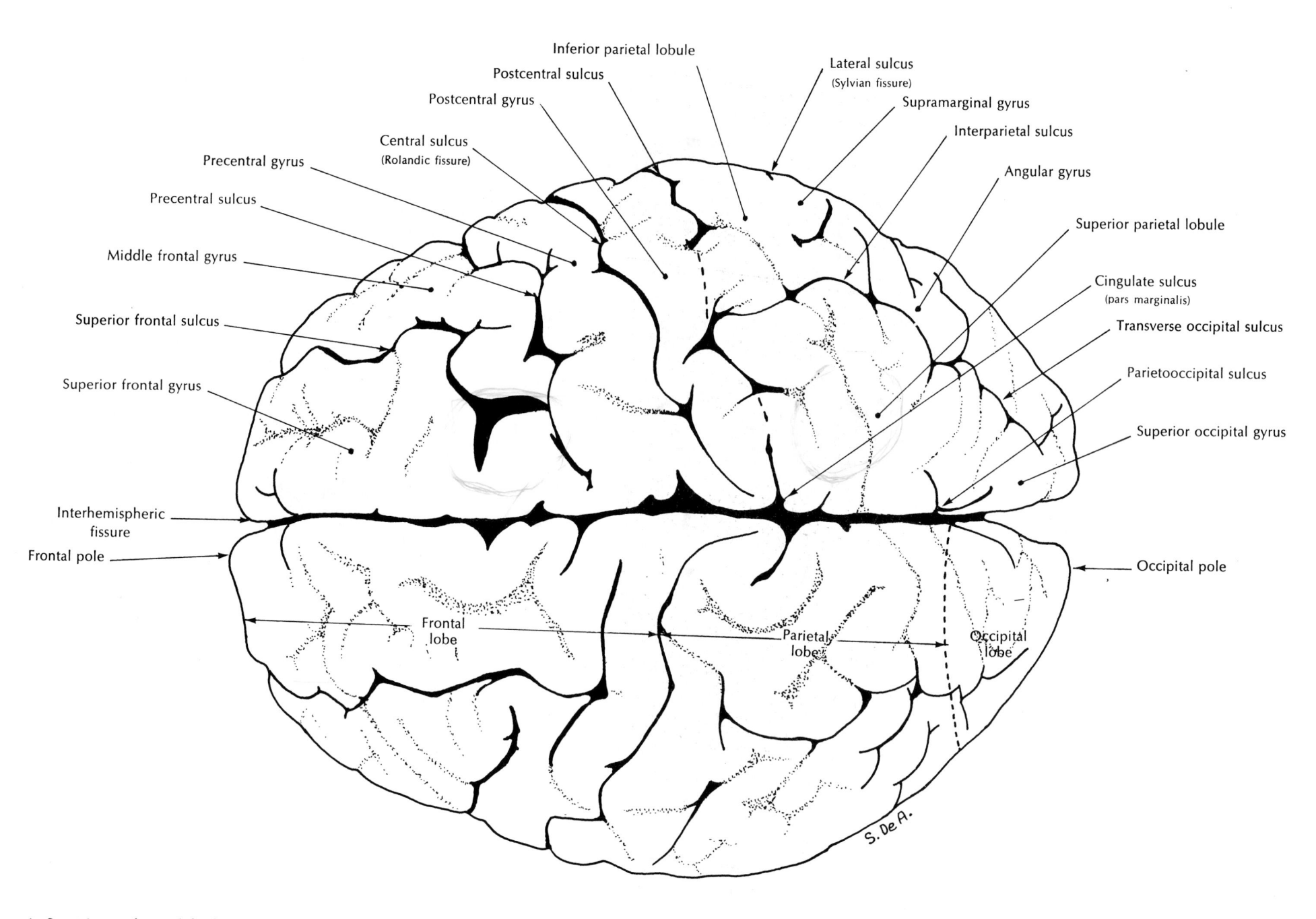

Inferior parietal lobule

Postcentral sulcus

Postcentral gyrus

Lateral sulcus
(Sylvian fissure)

Supramarginal gyrus

Central sulcus
(Rolandic fissure)

Interparietal sulcus

Precentral gyrus

Angular gyrus

Precentral sulcus

Superior parietal lobule

Middle frontal gyrus

Cingulate sulcus
(pars marginalis)

Superior frontal sulcus

Transverse occipital sulcus

Superior frontal gyrus

Parietooccipital sulcus

Superior occipital gyrus

Interhemispheric
fissure

Frontal pole

Occipital pole

Frontal
lobe

Parietal
lobe

Occipital
lobe

S. De A.

Figure 1. Superior surface of the brain—actual size

2

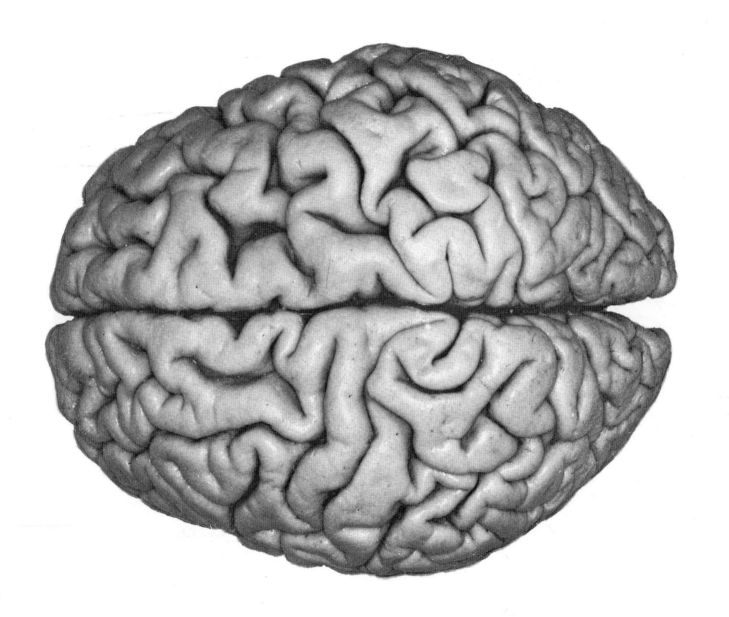

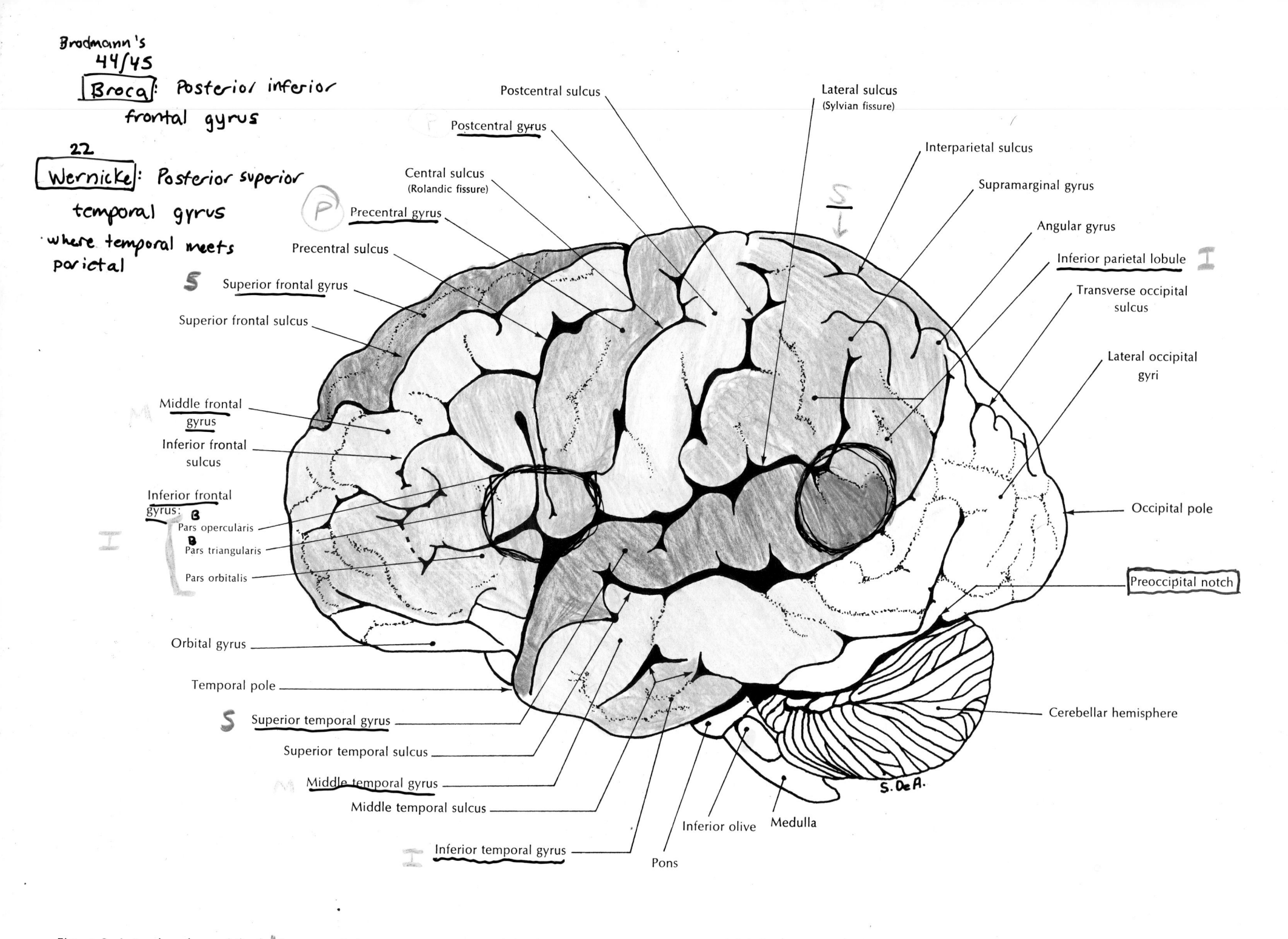

Brodmann's
44/45
Broca: Posterior inferior frontal gyrus

22
Wernicke: Posterior superior temporal gyrus
where temporal meets parietal

Postcentral sulcus

Postcentral gyrus

Central sulcus
(Rolandic fissure)

Precentral gyrus

Precentral sulcus

Superior frontal gyrus

Superior frontal sulcus

Middle frontal gyrus

Inferior frontal sulcus

Inferior frontal gyrus:

Pars opercularis

Pars triangularis

Pars orbitalis

Orbital gyrus

Temporal pole

Superior temporal gyrus

Superior temporal sulcus

Middle temporal gyrus

Middle temporal sulcus

Inferior temporal gyrus

Lateral sulcus
(Sylvian fissure)

Interparietal sulcus

Supramarginal gyrus

Angular gyrus

Inferior parietal lobule

Transverse occipital sulcus

Lateral occipital gyri

Occipital pole

Preoccipital notch

Cerebellar hemisphere

S. De A.

Inferior olive   Medulla

Pons

Figure 2. Lateral surface of the brain—actual size

4

Frontal: reward, attn, short term memory, planning, motivation (executive fxning)
· 1° motor cortex
· Broca

Temporal: auditory/visual processing
· hippocampus
· wernicke

Parietal: integrates sensory (mapping)
· 1° sensory cortex

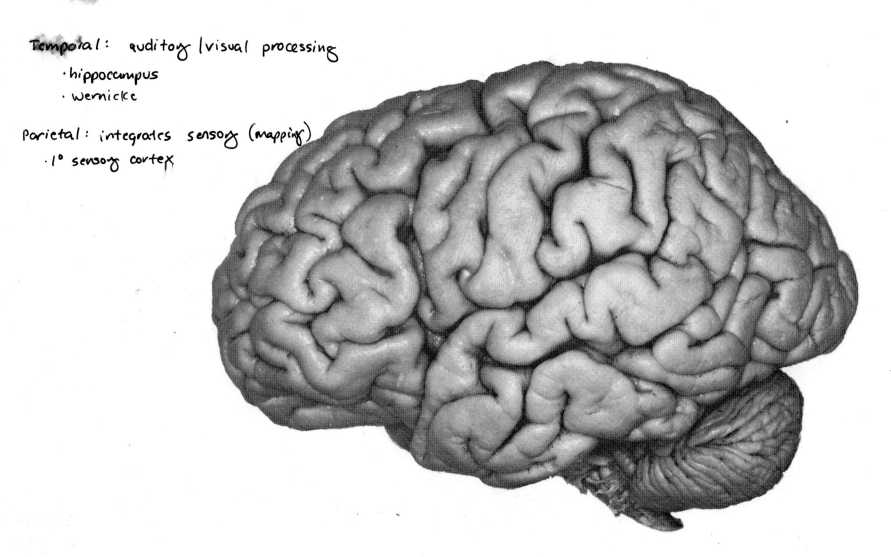

Uncus: ant extremity of parahippocampal gyrus

SMELL

· Uncinate Fit (seizure) → hallucinations of horrible odors

· Herniation: ↑P in cranium
→ eyes: blown, down & out

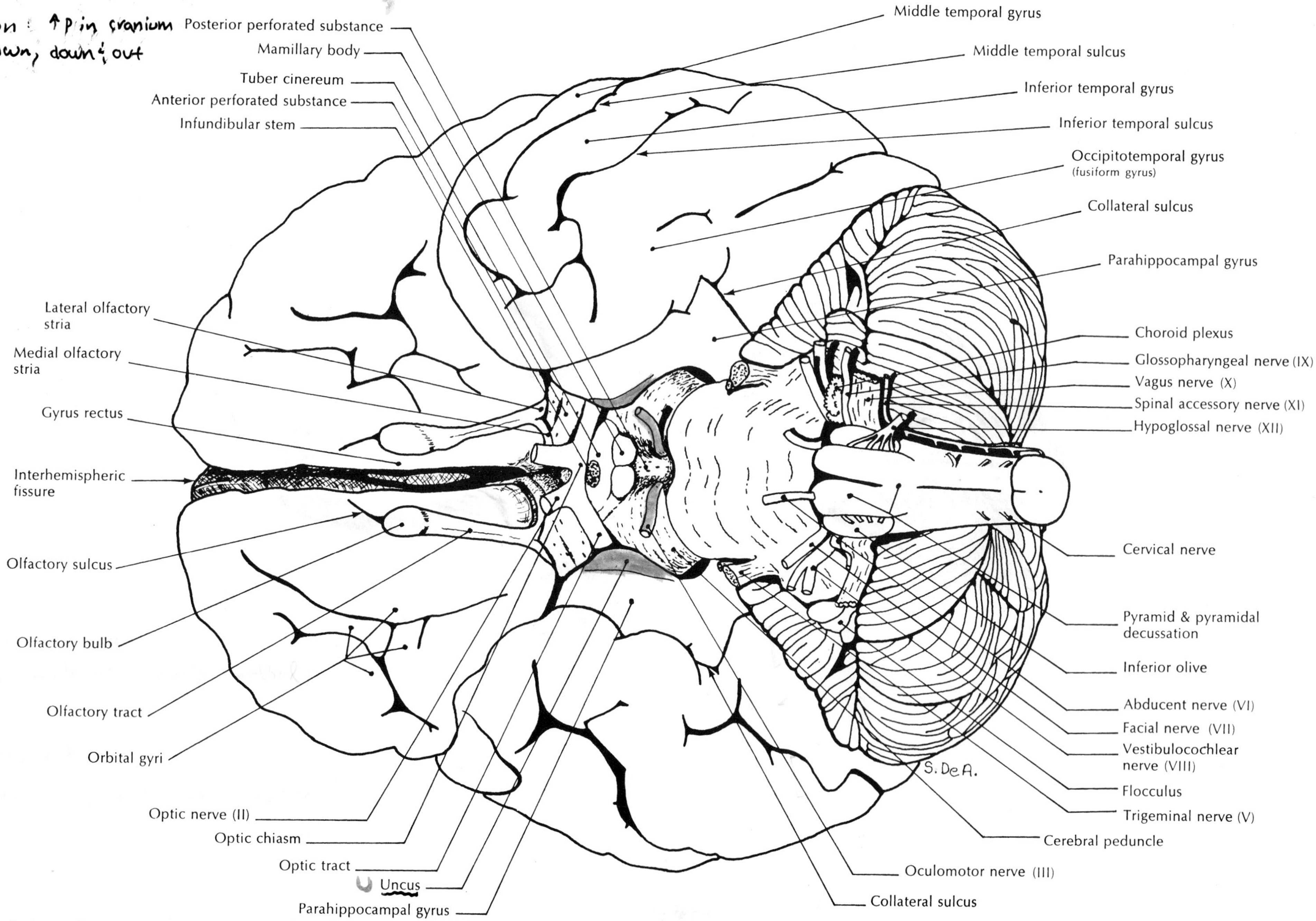

Posterior perforated substance

Mamillary body

Tuber cinereum

Anterior perforated substance

Infundibular stem

Middle temporal gyrus

Middle temporal sulcus

Inferior temporal gyrus

Inferior temporal sulcus

Occipitotemporal gyrus
(fusiform gyrus)

Collateral sulcus

Parahippocampal gyrus

Choroid plexus

Glossopharyngeal nerve (IX)

Vagus nerve (X)

Spinal accessory nerve (XI)

Hypoglossal nerve (XII)

Lateral olfactory stria

Medial olfactory stria

Gyrus rectus

Interhemispheric fissure

Olfactory sulcus

Olfactory bulb

Olfactory tract

Orbital gyri

Cervical nerve

Pyramid & pyramidal decussation

Inferior olive

Abducent nerve (VI)

Facial nerve (VII)

Vestibulocochlear nerve (VIII)

Flocculus

Trigeminal nerve (V)

Cerebral peduncle

Optic nerve (II)

Optic chiasm

Optic tract

Uncus

Parahippocampal gyrus

Oculomotor nerve (III)

Collateral sulcus

S. De A.

Figure 3. Inferior surface of the brain—actual size

6

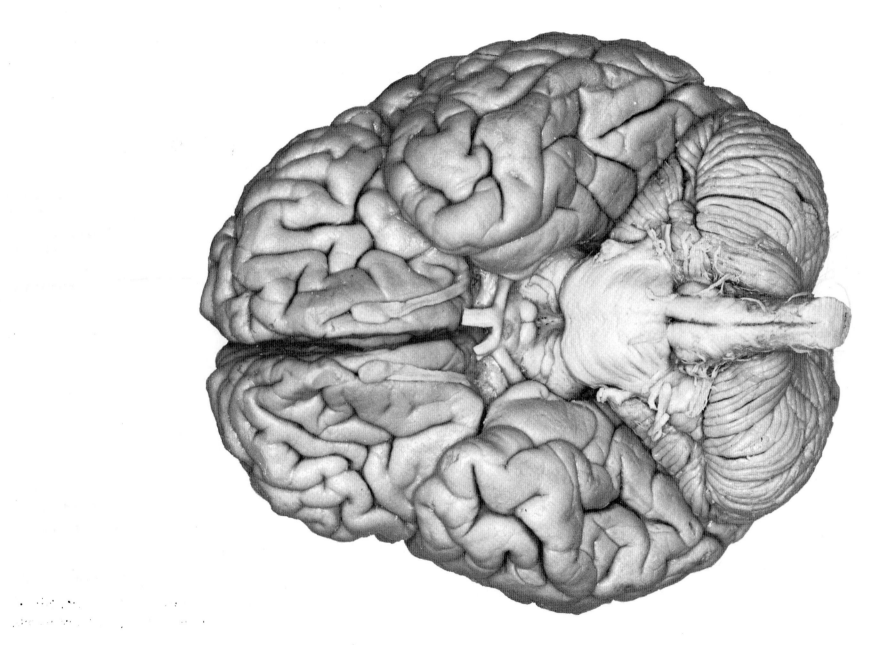

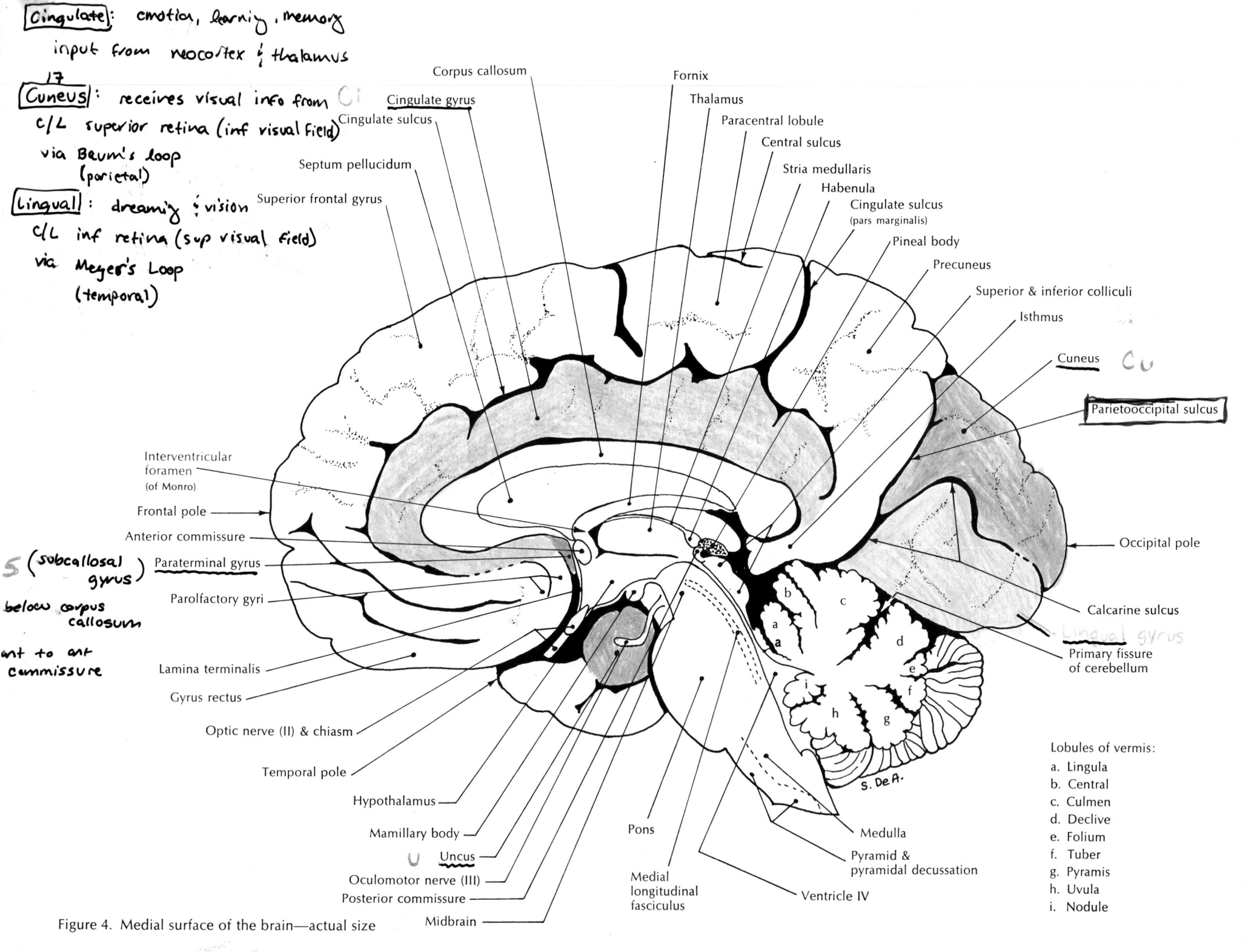

Cingulate: emotion, learning, memory
input from neocortex & thalamus

Cuneus: receives visual info from 17
c/L superior retina (inf visual field)
via Beum's loop
(parietal)

Lingual: dreaming & vision
c/L inf retina (sup visual field)
via Meyer's Loop
(temporal)

S (subcallosal gyrus)
below corpus callosum
ant to ant commissure

Corpus callosum
Cingulate gyrus
Cingulate sulcus
Septum pellucidum
Superior frontal gyrus

Fornix
Thalamus
Paracentral lobule
Central sulcus
Stria medullaris
Habenula
Cingulate sulcus
(pars marginalis)
Pineal body
Precuneus
Superior & inferior colliculi
Isthmus
Cuneus
Parietooccipital sulcus

Interventricular foramen
(of Monro)
Frontal pole
Anterior commissure
Parerminal gyrus
Parolfactory gyri
Lamina terminalis
Gyrus rectus
Optic nerve (II) & chiasm
Temporal pole
Hypothalamus
Mamillary body
Uncus
Oculomotor nerve (III)
Posterior commissure
Midbrain

Occipital pole
Calcarine sulcus
Lingual gyrus
Primary fissure
of cerebellum

Pons
Medial longitudinal fasciculus
Medulla
Pyramid & pyramidal decussation
Ventricle IV

Lobules of vermis:
a. Lingula
b. Central
c. Culmen
d. Declive
e. Folium
f. Tuber
g. Pyramis
h. Uvula
i. Nodule

Figure 4. Medial surface of the brain—actual size

8

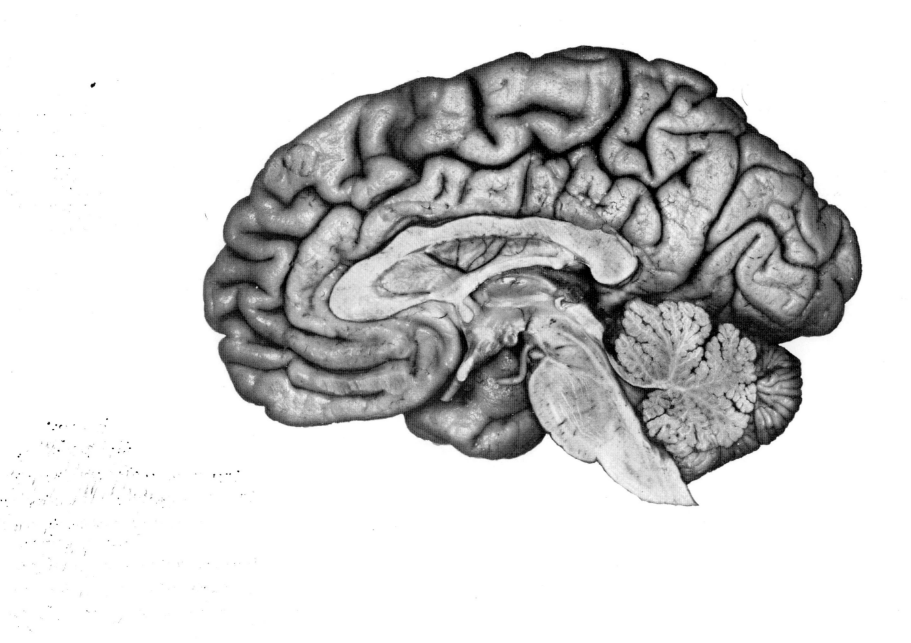

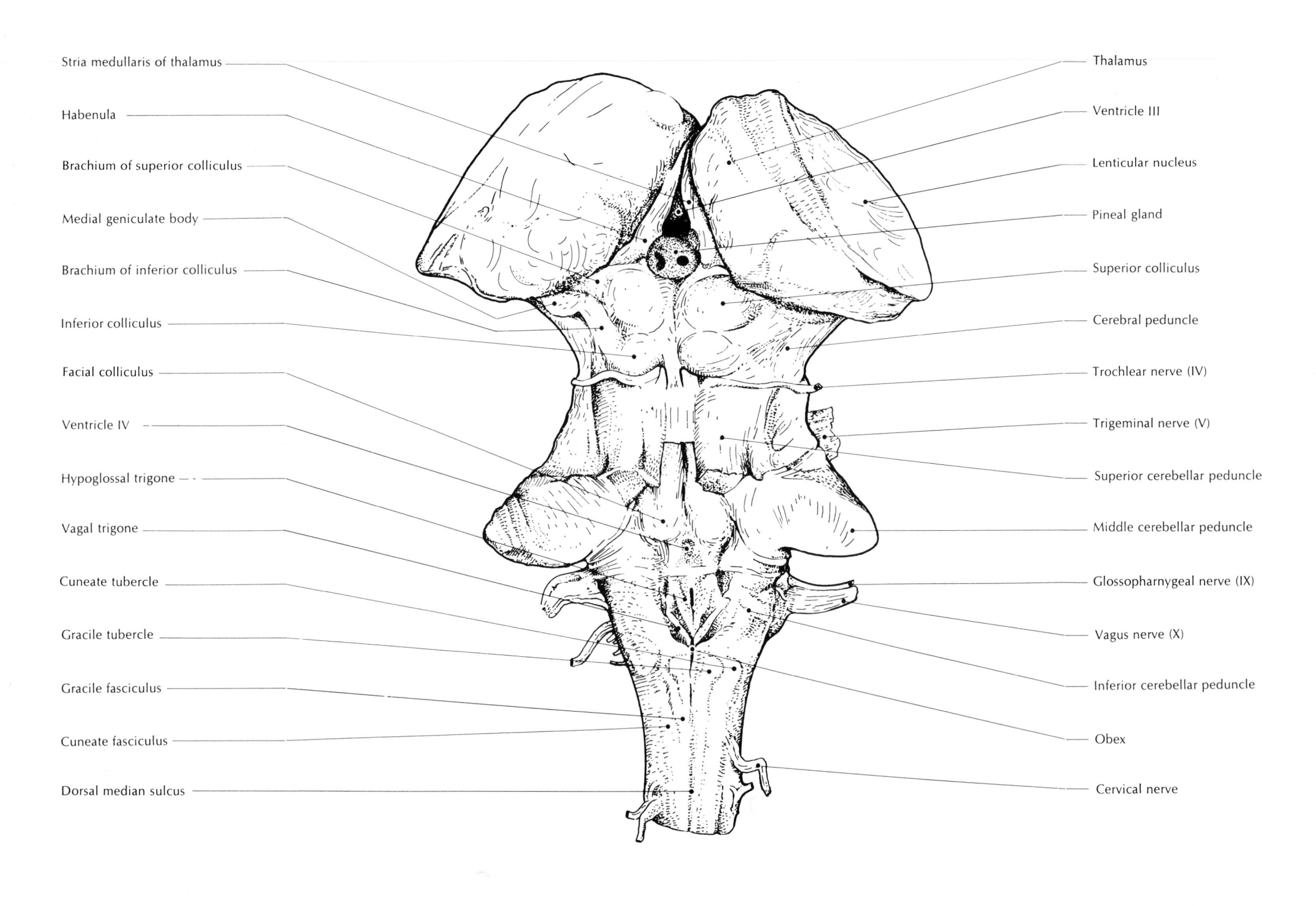

Stria medullaris of thalamus

Habenula

Brachium of superior colliculus

Medial geniculate body

Brachium of inferior colliculus

Inferior colliculus

Facial colliculus

Ventricle IV

Hypoglossal trigone

Vagal trigone

Cuneate tubercle

Gracile tubercle

Gracile fasciculus

Cuneate fasciculus

Dorsal median sulcus

Thalamus

Ventricle III

Lenticular nucleus

Pineal gland

Superior colliculus

Cerebral peduncle

Trochlear nerve (IV)

Trigeminal nerve (V)

Superior cerebellar peduncle

Middle cerebellar peduncle

Glossopharnygeal nerve (IX)

Vagus nerve (X)

Inferior cerebellar peduncle

Obex

Cervical nerve

Figure 5. Dorsal surface of the brain stem—1.5X

10

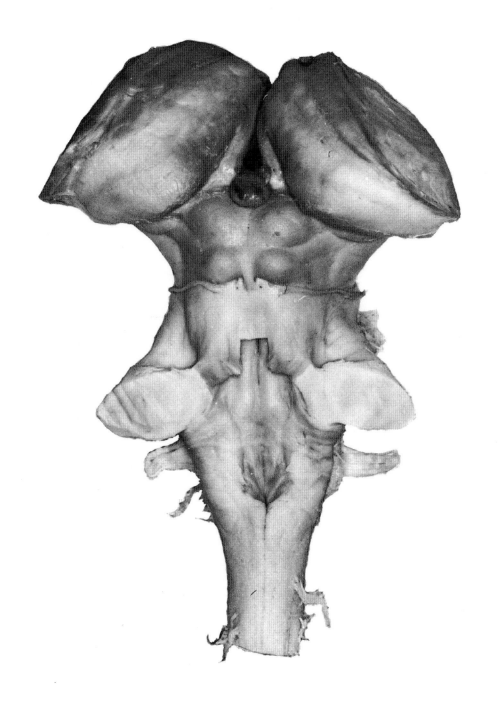

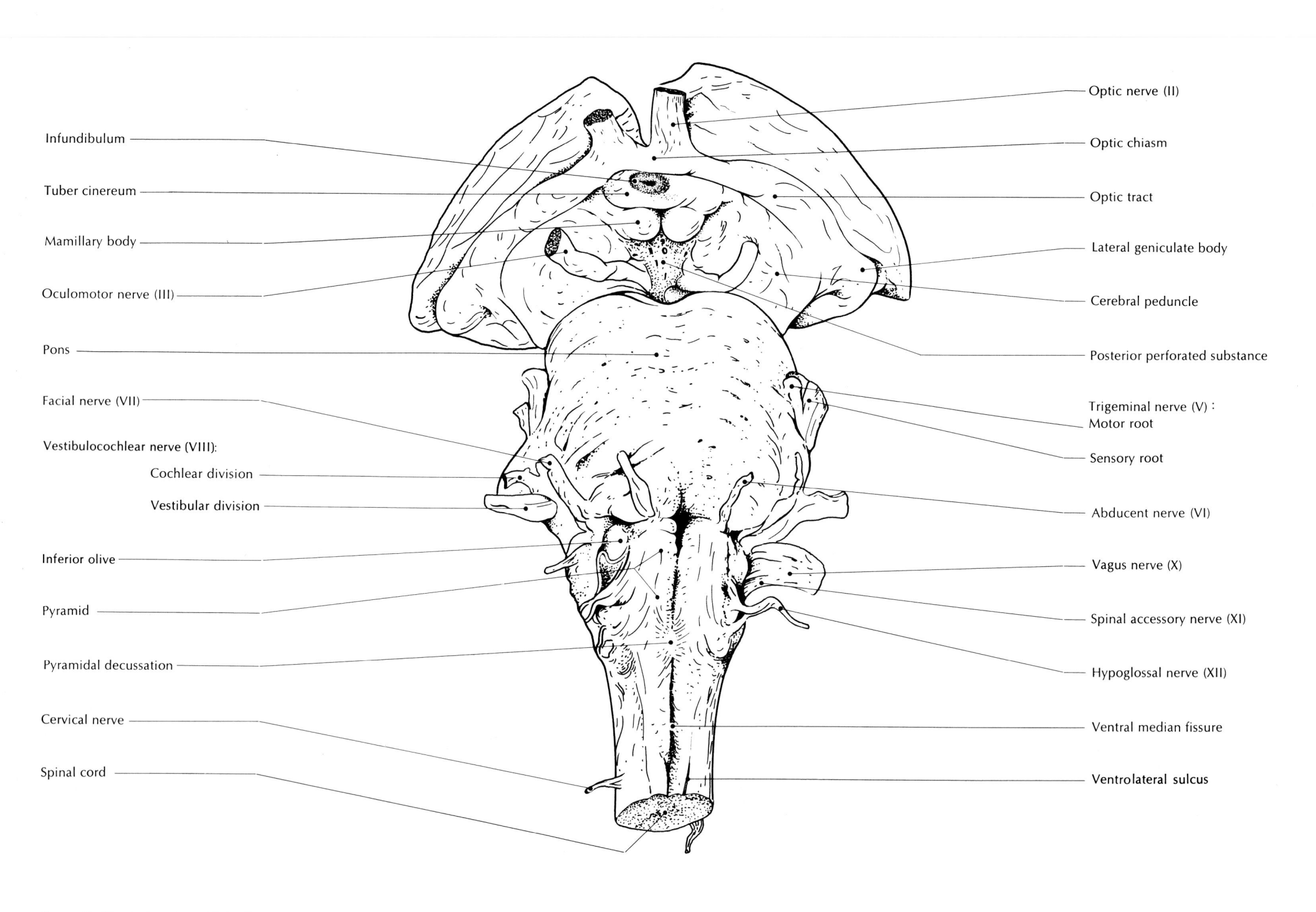

Optic nerve (II)

Infundibulum

Optic chiasm

Tuber cinereum

Optic tract

Mamillary body

Lateral geniculate body

Oculomotor nerve (III)

Cerebral peduncle

Pons

Posterior perforated substance

Facial nerve (VII)

Trigeminal nerve (V):
Motor root

Vestibulocochlear nerve (VIII):

Sensory root

Cochlear division

Vestibular division

Abducent nerve (VI)

Inferior olive

Vagus nerve (X)

Pyramid

Spinal accessory nerve (XI)

Pyramidal decussation

Hypoglossal nerve (XII)

Cervical nerve

Ventral median fissure

Spinal cord

Ventrolateral sulcus

Figure 6. Ventral surface of the brain stem—1.5X

12

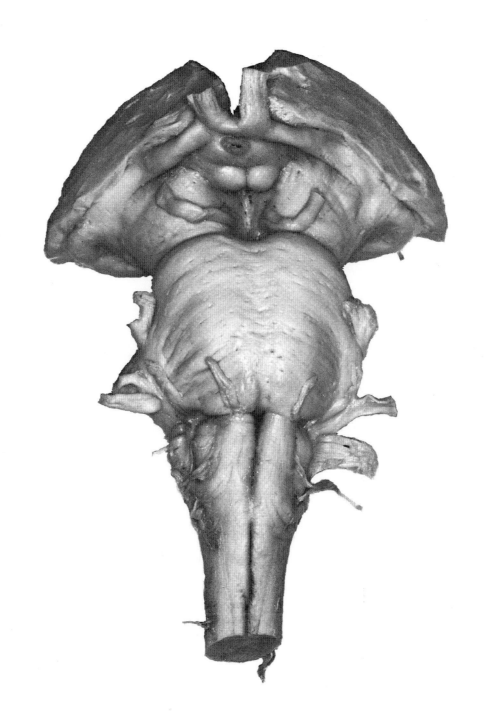

HORIZONTAL SECTIONS OF THE GROSS BRAIN: CORRELATION WITH COMPUTERIZED TOMOGRAPHY AND MAGNETIC RESONANCE IMAGING

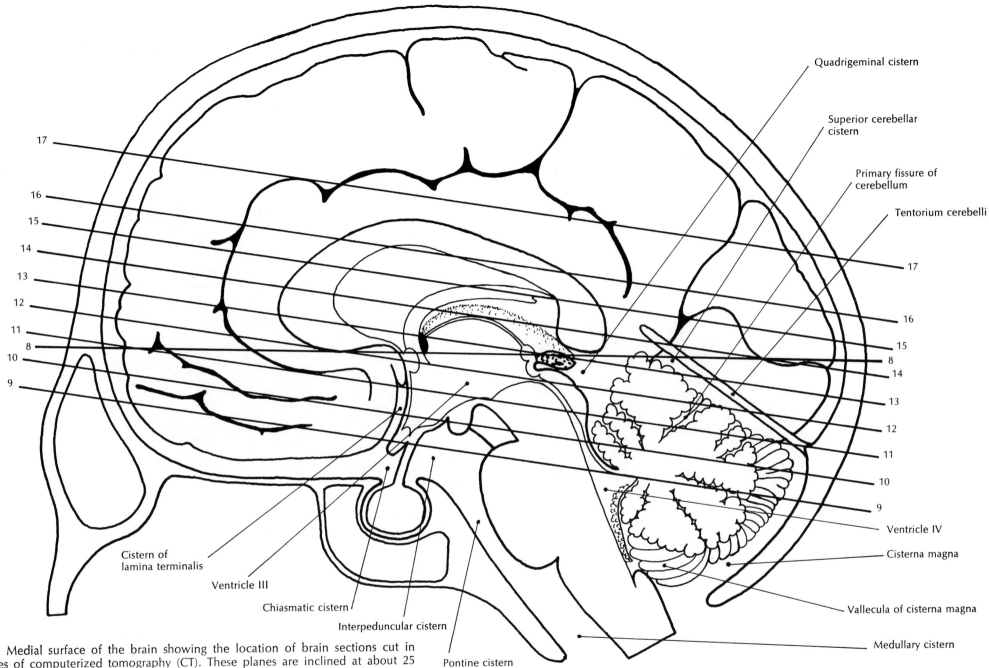

Quadrigeminal cistern

Superior cerebellar cistern

Primary fissure of cerebellum

Tentorium cerebelli

17

16

15

8

14

13

12

11

10

9

Ventricle IV

Cisterna magna

Vallecula of cisterna magna

Medullary cistern

17

16

15

14

13

12

11

8

10

9

Cistern of lamina terminalis

Ventricle III

Chiasmatic cistern

Interpeduncular cistern

Pontine cistern

Figure 7. Medial surface of the brain showing the location of brain sections cut in the planes of computerized tomography (CT). These planes are inclined at about 25 degrees to the traditional horizontal brain section and parallel to the orbital-meatal line, but newer CT scanners and magnetic resonance images are not constrained to these planes. Each brain section is 4 mm thick. Figure numbers indicated

15

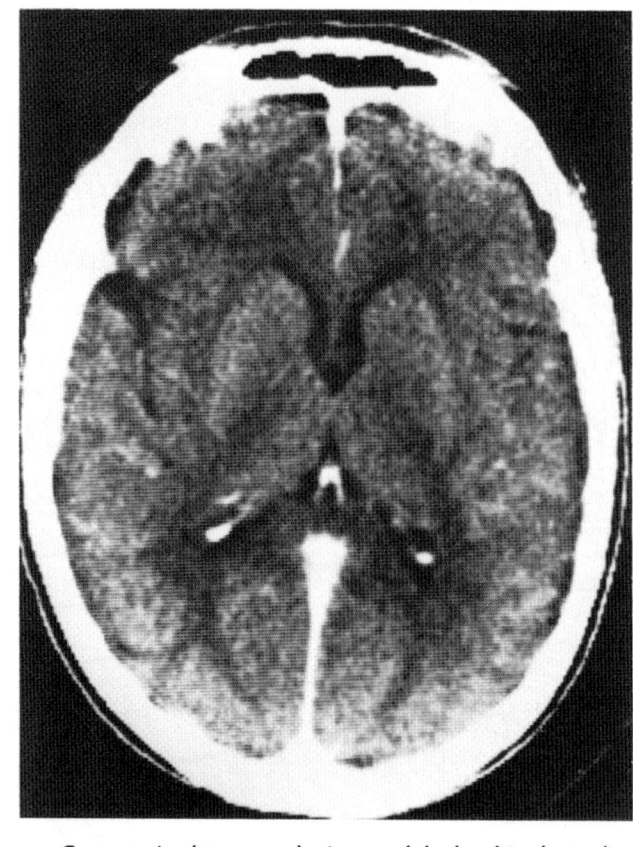

a. Computerized tomography image of the head in the traditional horizontal plane

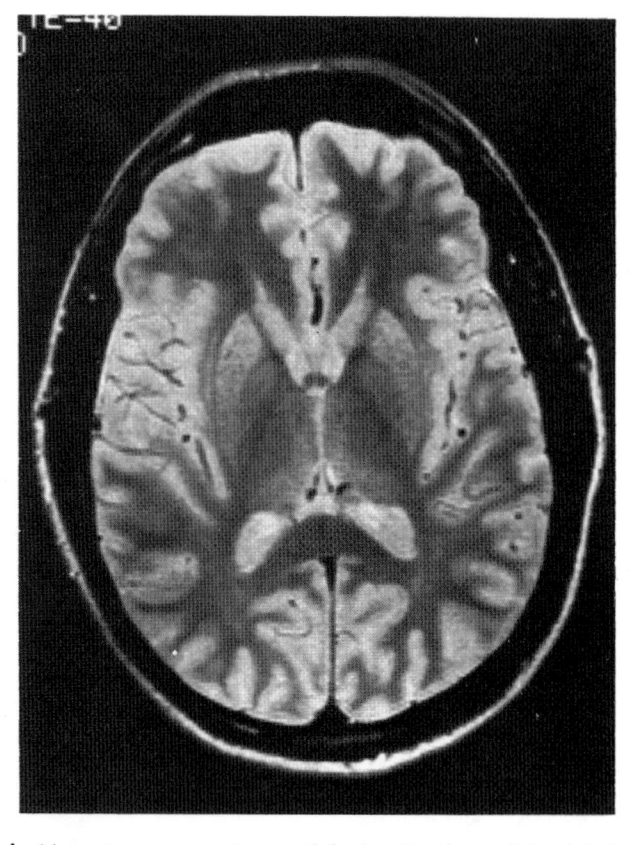

b. Magnetic resonance image of the head in the traditional horizontal plane

16

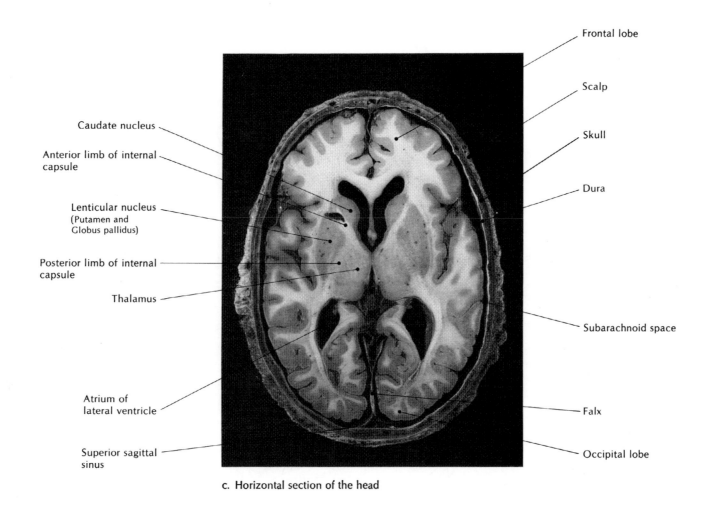

Caudate nucleus

Anterior limb of internal capsule

Lenticular nucleus (Putamen and Globus pallidus)

Posterior limb of internal capsule

Thalamus

Atrium of lateral ventricle

Superior sagittal sinus

Frontal lobe

Scalp

Skull

Dura

Subarachnoid space

Falx

Occipital lobe

c. Horizontal section of the head

Figure 8. Comparison of computerized tomography and magnetic resonance images of brain, skull, and scalp with a whole section of the head in the same plane. For further details, the following references will be helpful:

1. de Groot, J. *Correlative Neuroanatomy of Computed Tomography and Magnetic Resonance Imaging*. Lea and Febiger, Philadelphia, 1984.
2. de Groot, J., Chusid, J. G. Imaging of the brain. In: *Correlative Neuroanatomy*. Appleton & Lange, East Norwalk, CT, 1988.
3. Mills, C. M., de Groot, J., Posin, J. P. *Magnetic Resonance Imaging Atlas of Head and Spine*. Lea and Febiger, Philadelphia, 1988.

17

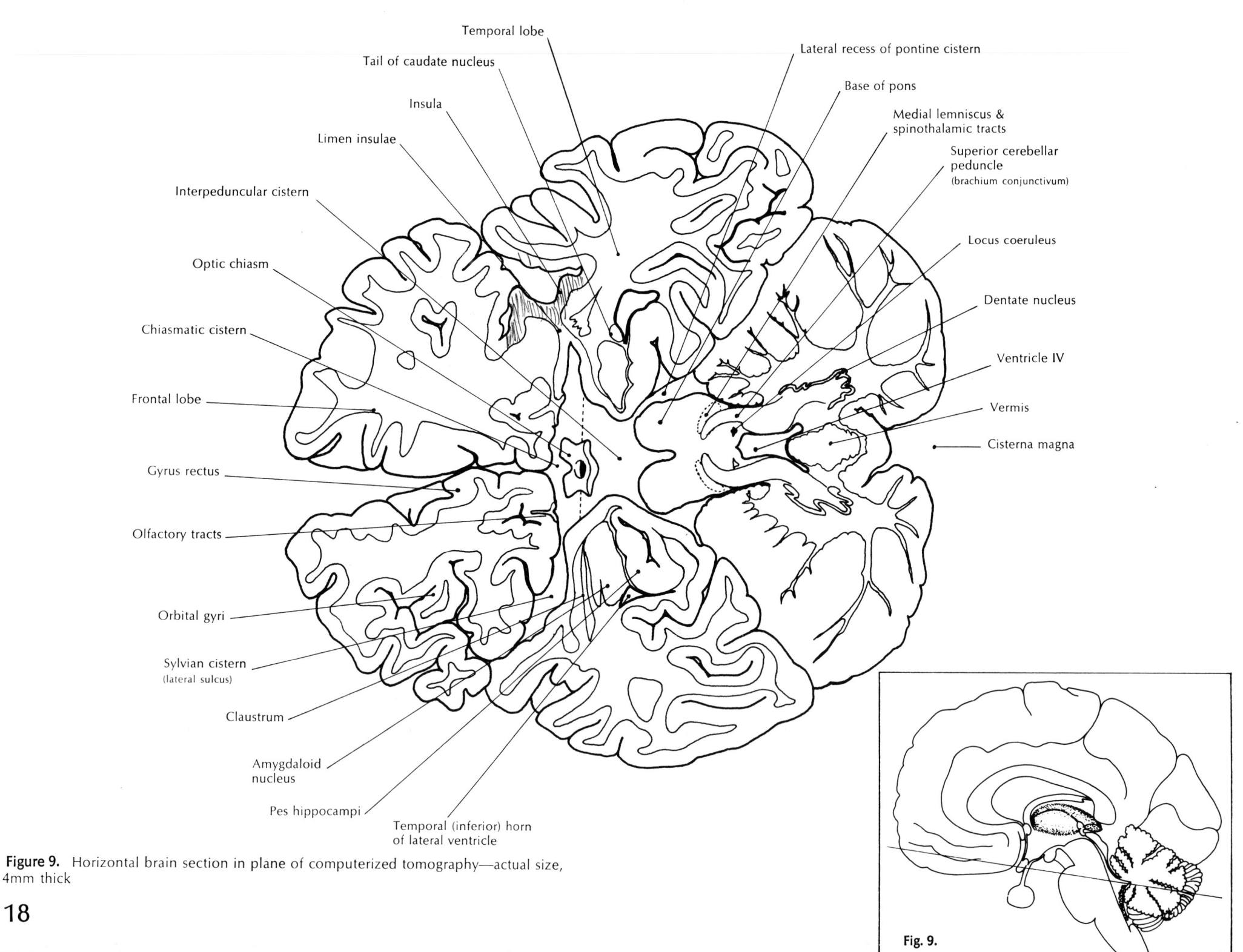

Temporal lobe

Tail of caudate nucleus

Insula

Limen insulae

Interpeduncular cistern

Optic chiasm

Chiasmatic cistern

Frontal lobe

Gyrus rectus

Olfactory tracts

Orbital gyri

Sylvian cistern
(lateral sulcus)

Claustrum

Amygdaloid
nucleus

Pes hippocampi

Temporal (inferior) horn
of lateral ventricle

Lateral recess of pontine cistern

Base of pons

Medial lemniscus &
spinothalamic tracts

Superior cerebellar
peduncle
(brachium conjunctivum)

Locus coeruleus

Dentate nucleus

Ventricle IV

Vermis

Cisterna magna

Figure 9. Horizontal brain section in plane of computerized tomography—actual size, 4mm thick

18

Fig. 9.

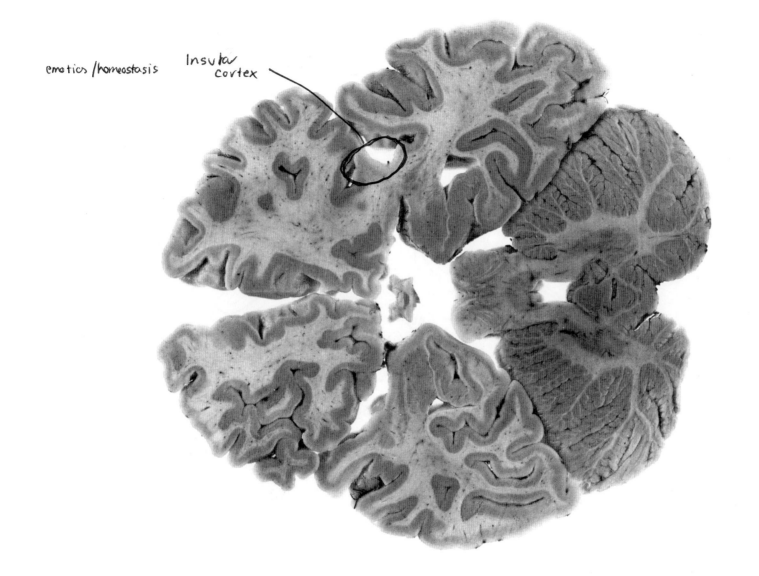

emotics/homeostasis   Insular
                       cortex

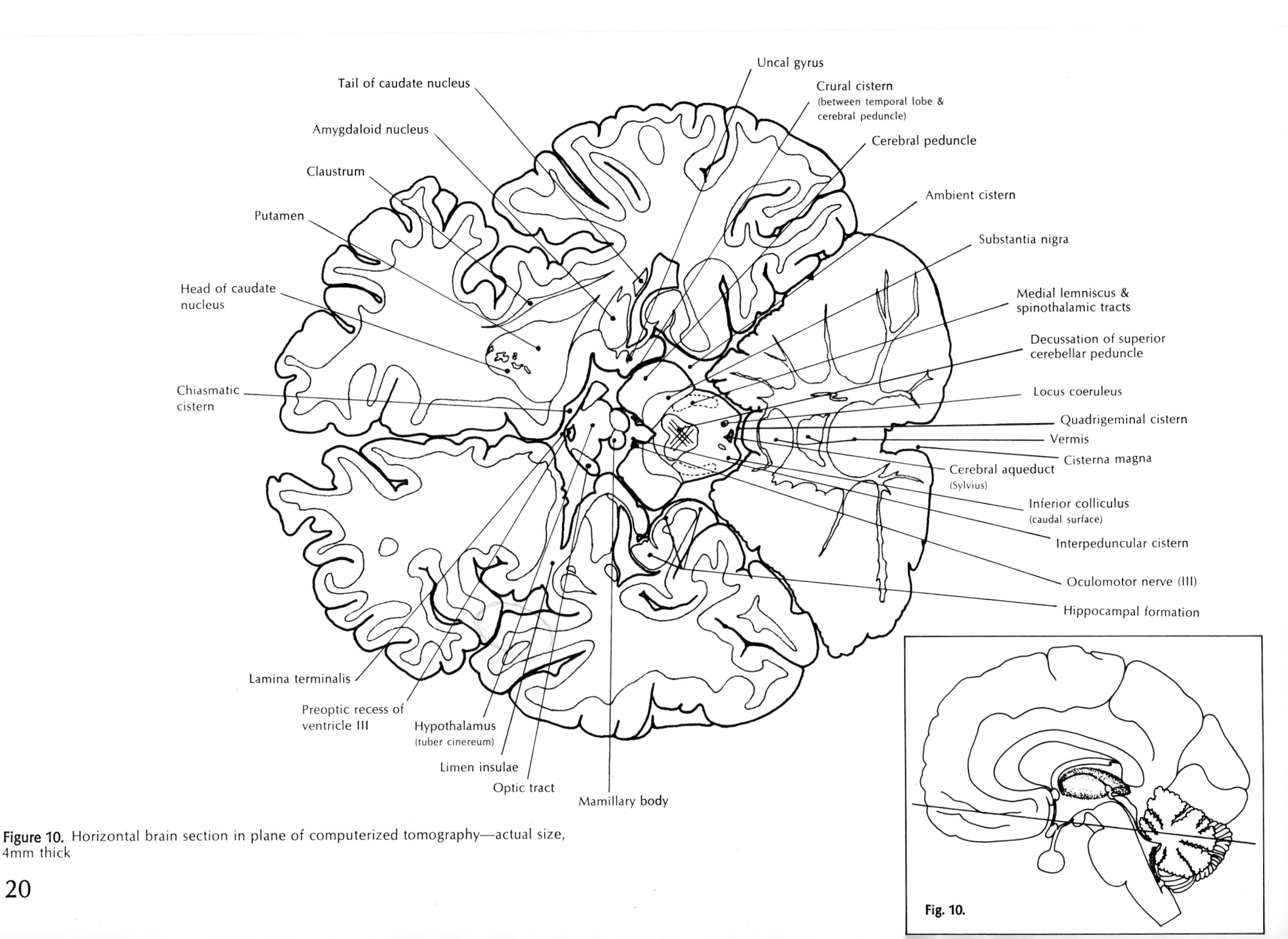

Tail of caudate nucleus

Amygdaloid nucleus

Claustrum

Putamen

Head of caudate nucleus

Chiasmatic cistern

Uncal gyrus

Crural cistern
(between temporal lobe & cerebral peduncle)

Cerebral peduncle

Ambient cistern

Substantia nigra

Medial lemniscus & spinothalamic tracts

Decussation of superior cerebellar peduncle

Locus coeruleus

Quadrigeminal cistern

Vermis

Cisterna magna

Cerebral aqueduct (Sylvius)

Inferior colliculus (caudal surface)

Interpeduncular cistern

Oculomotor nerve (III)

Hippocampal formation

Lamina terminalis

Preoptic recess of ventricle III

Hypothalamus (tuber cinereum)

Limen insulae

Optic tract

Mamillary body

Figure 10. Horizontal brain section in plane of computerized tomography—actual size, 4mm thick

20

Fig. 10.

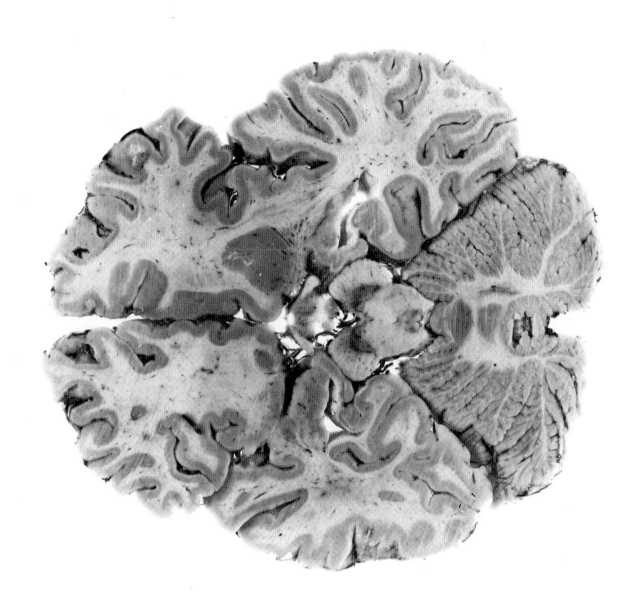

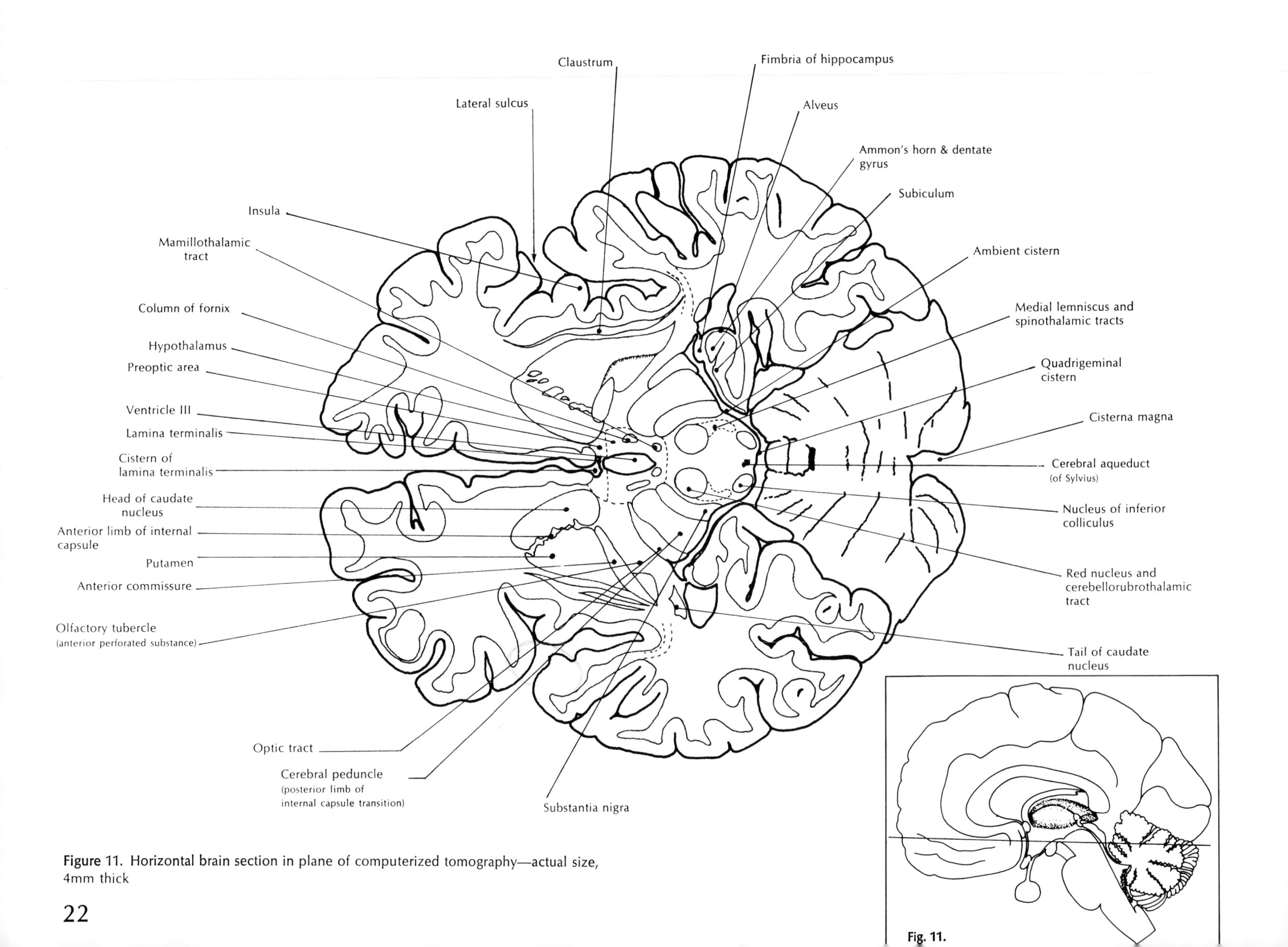

Claustrum

Fimbria of hippocampus

Lateral sulcus

Alveus

Ammon's horn & dentate gyrus

Subiculum

Insula

Mamillothalamic tract

Ambient cistern

Medial lemniscus and spinothalamic tracts

Column of fornix

Quadrigeminal cistern

Hypothalamus

Preoptic area

Cisterna magna

Ventricle III

Lamina terminalis

Cerebral aqueduct (of Sylvius)

Cistern of lamina terminalis

Head of caudate nucleus

Nucleus of inferior colliculus

Anterior limb of internal capsule

Putamen

Red nucleus and cerebellorubrothalamic tract

Anterior commissure

Olfactory tubercle (anterior perforated substance)

Tail of caudate nucleus

Optic tract

Cerebral peduncle (posterior limb of internal capsule transition)

Substantia nigra

Figure 11. Horizontal brain section in plane of computerized tomography—actual size, 4mm thick

22

Fig. 11.

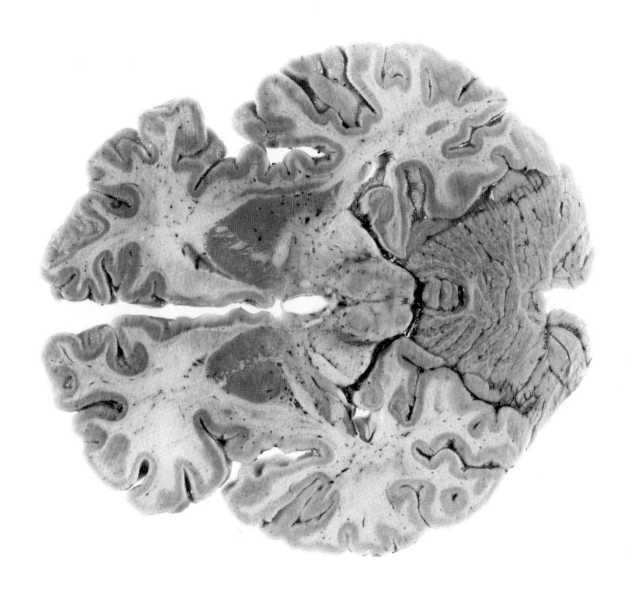

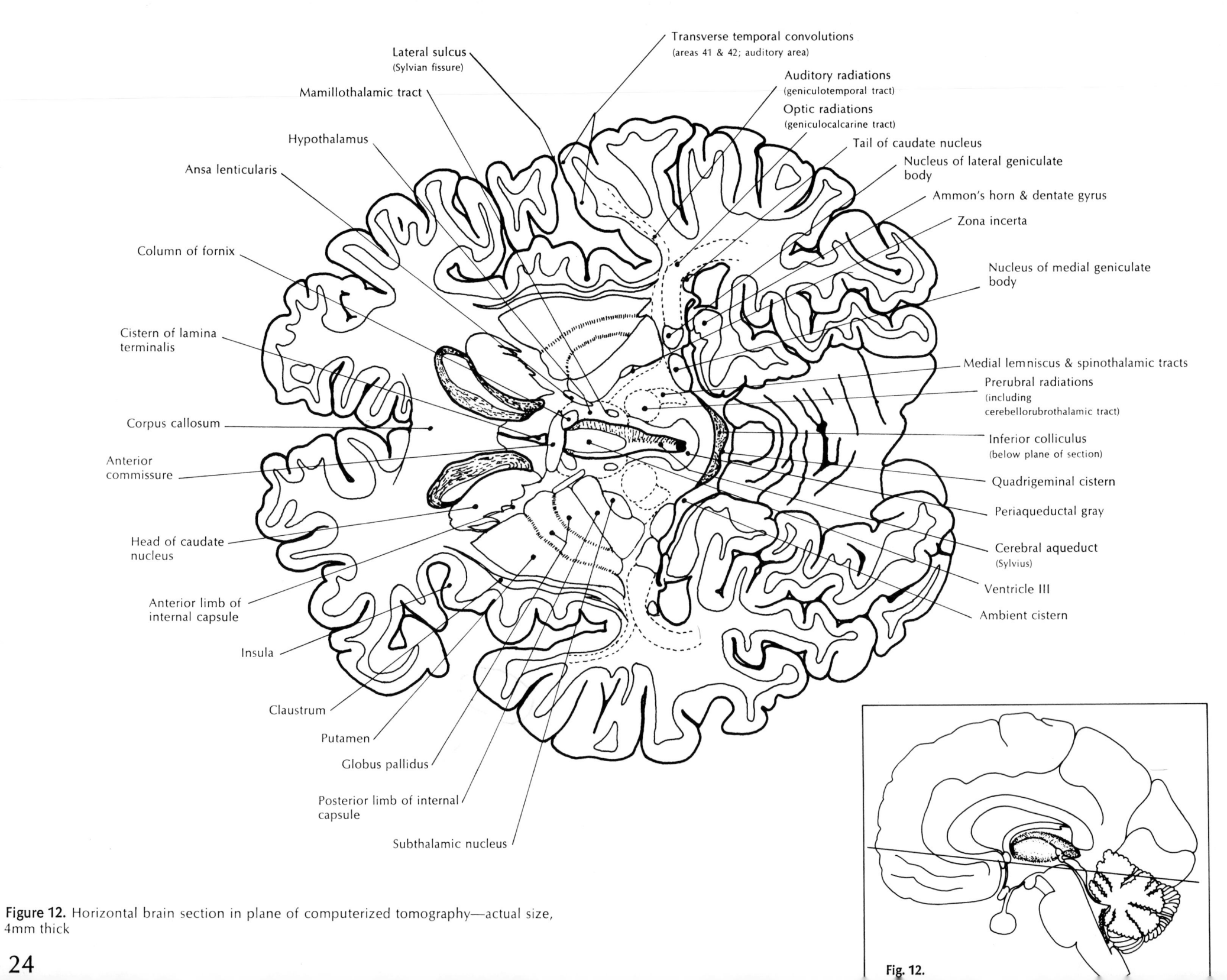

Lateral sulcus
(Sylvian fissure)

Transverse temporal convolutions
(areas 41 & 42; auditory area)

Auditory radiations
(geniculotemporal tract)

Optic radiations
(geniculocalcarine tract)

Mamillothalamic tract

Tail of caudate nucleus

Nucleus of lateral geniculate
body

Hypothalamus

Ammon's horn & dentate gyrus

Ansa lenticularis

Zona incerta

Column of fornix

Nucleus of medial geniculate
body

Cistern of lamina
terminalis

Medial lemniscus & spinothalamic tracts

Prerubral radiations
(including
cerebellorubrothalamic tract)

Corpus callosum

Inferior colliculus
(below plane of section)

Anterior
commissure

Quadrigeminal cistern

Periaqueductal gray

Head of caudate
nucleus

Cerebral aqueduct
(Sylvius)

Anterior limb of
internal capsule

Ventricle III

Insula

Ambient cistern

Claustrum

Putamen

Globus pallidus

Posterior limb of internal
capsule

Subthalamic nucleus

Figure 12. Horizontal brain section in plane of computerized tomography—actual size, 4mm thick

24

Fig. 12.

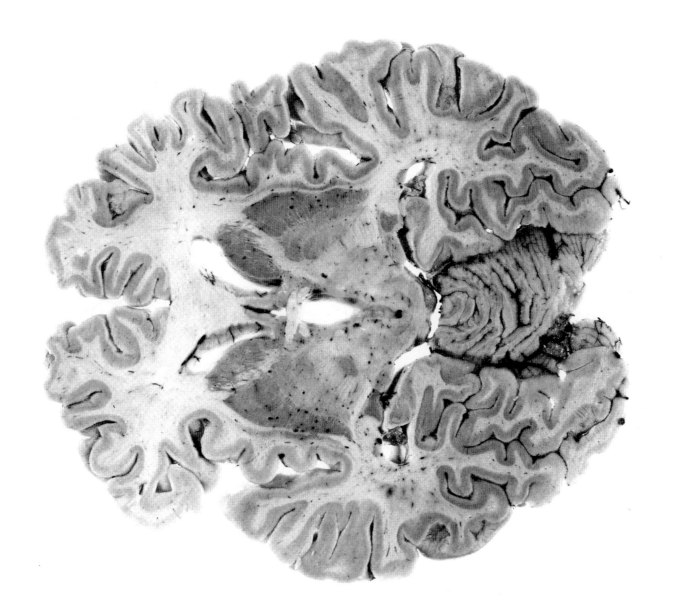

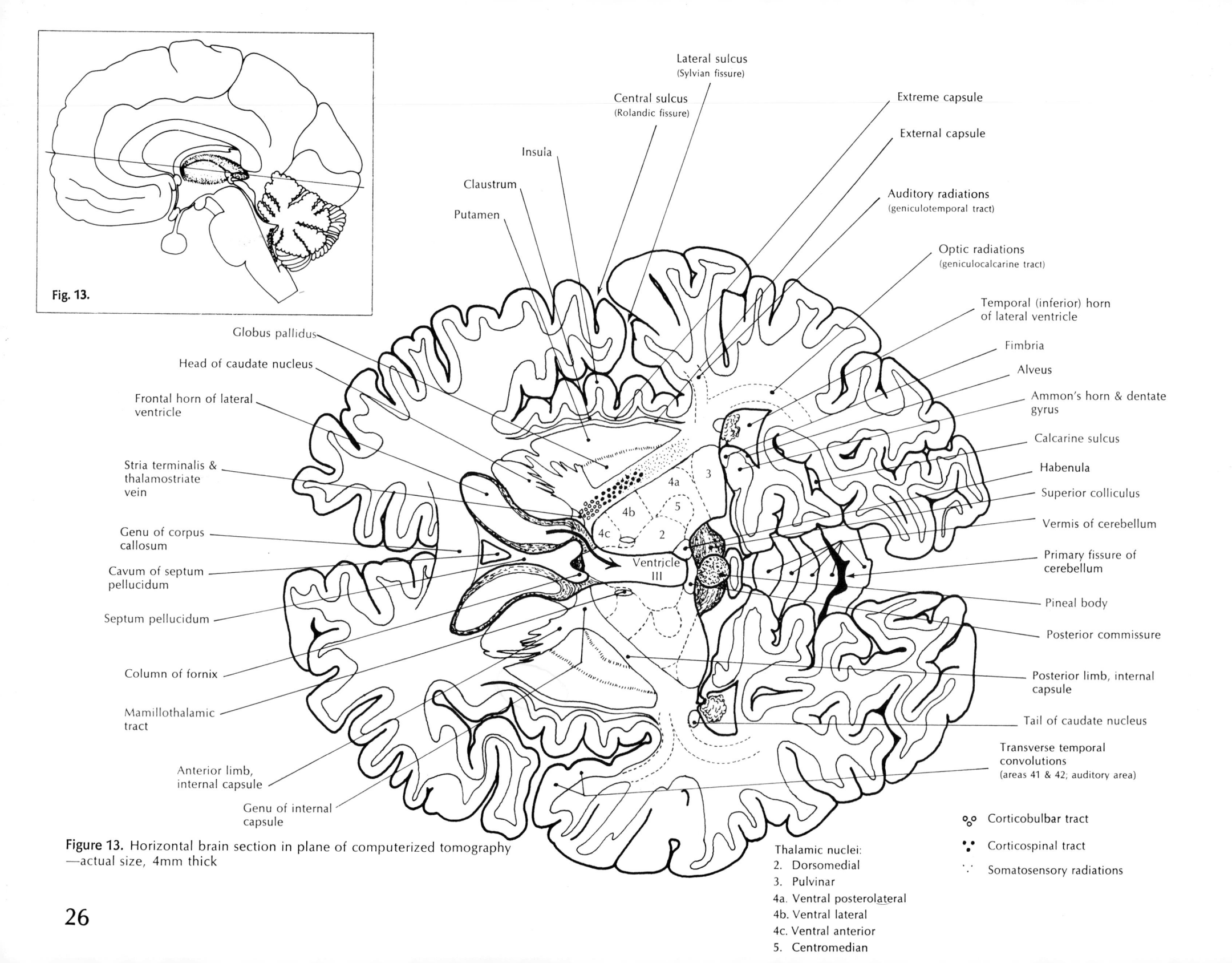

Lateral sulcus
(Sylvian fissure)

Central sulcus
(Rolandic fissure)

Insula

Claustrum

Putamen

Extreme capsule

External capsule

Auditory radiations
(geniculotemporal tract)

Optic radiations
(geniculocalcarine tract)

Temporal (inferior) horn
of lateral ventricle

Fimbria

Alveus

Ammon's horn & dentate
gyrus

Calcarine sulcus

Habenula

Superior colliculus

Vermis of cerebellum

Primary fissure of
cerebellum

Pineal body

Posterior commissure

Posterior limb, internal
capsule

Tail of caudate nucleus

Transverse temporal
convolutions
(areas 41 & 42; auditory area)

Globus pallidus

Head of caudate nucleus

Frontal horn of lateral
ventricle

Stria terminalis &
thalamostriate
vein

Genu of corpus
callosum

Cavum of septum
pellucidum

Septum pellucidum

Column of fornix

Mamillothalamic
tract

Anterior limb,
internal capsule

Genu of internal
capsule

Ventricle
III

4a

4b

4c

5

2

3

Fig. 13.

Figure 13. Horizontal brain section in plane of computerized tomography
—actual size, 4mm thick

Thalamic nuclei:
2. Dorsomedial
3. Pulvinar
4a. Ventral posterolateral
4b. Ventral lateral
4c. Ventral anterior
5. Centromedian

Corticobulbar tract

Corticospinal tract

Somatosensory radiations

26

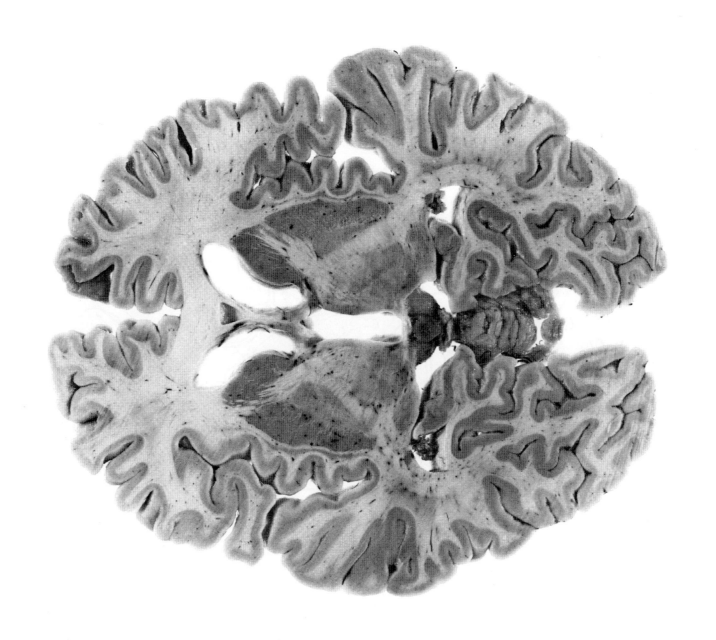

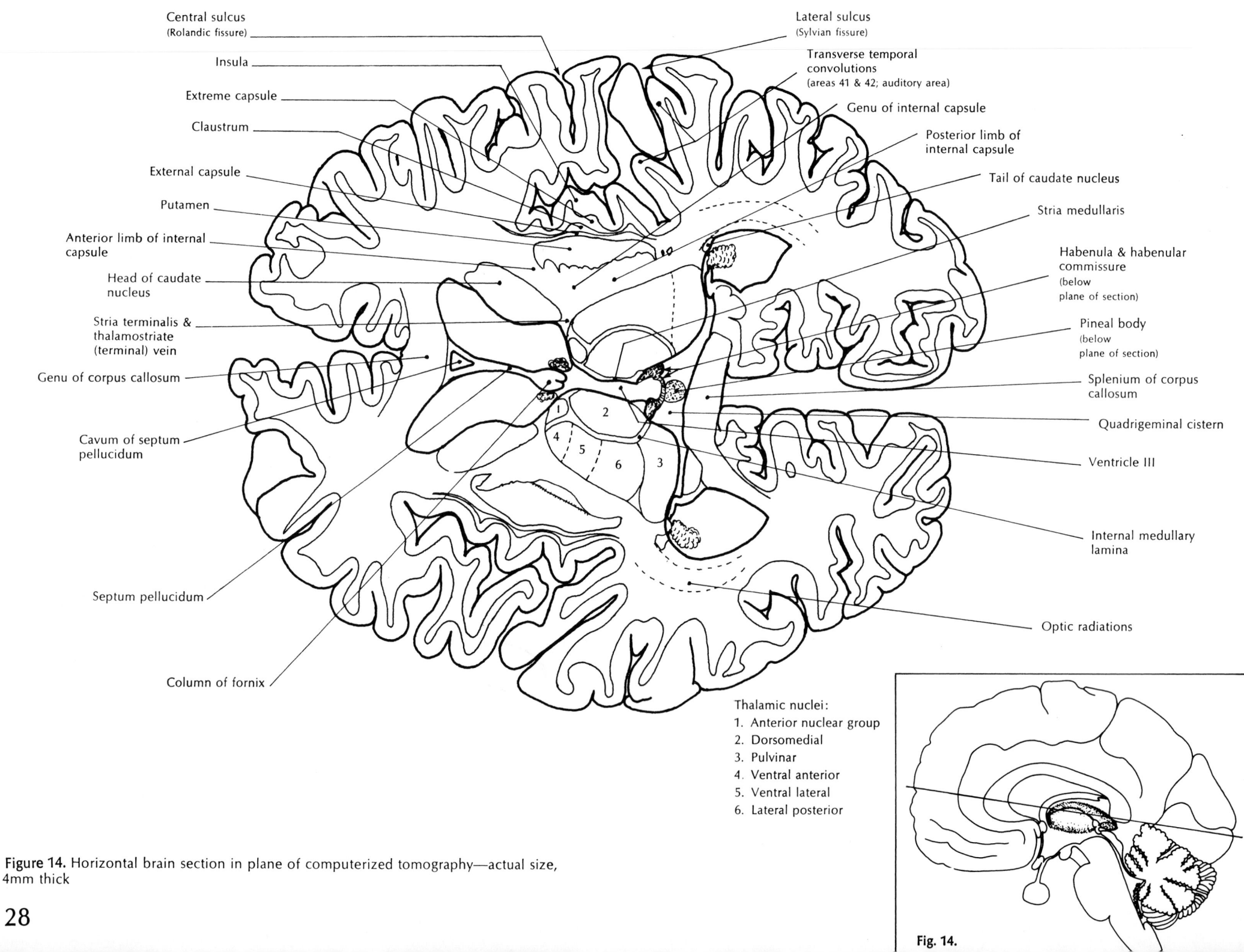

Central sulcus
(Rolandic fissure)

Insula

Extreme capsule

Claustrum

External capsule

Putamen

Anterior limb of internal
capsule

Head of caudate
nucleus

Stria terminalis &
thalamostriate
(terminal) vein

Genu of corpus callosum

Cavum of septum
pellucidum

Septum pellucidum

Column of fornix

Lateral sulcus
(Sylvian fissure)

Transverse temporal
convolutions
(areas 41 & 42; auditory area)

Genu of internal capsule

Posterior limb of
internal capsule

Tail of caudate nucleus

Stria medullaris

Habenula & habenular
commissure
(below
plane of section)

Pineal body
(below
plane of section)

Splenium of corpus
callosum

Quadrigeminal cistern

Ventricle III

Internal medullary
lamina

Optic radiations

Thalamic nuclei:
1. Anterior nuclear group
2. Dorsomedial
3. Pulvinar
4. Ventral anterior
5. Ventral lateral
6. Lateral posterior

Figure 14. Horizontal brain section in plane of computerized tomography—actual size,
4mm thick

28

Fig. 14.

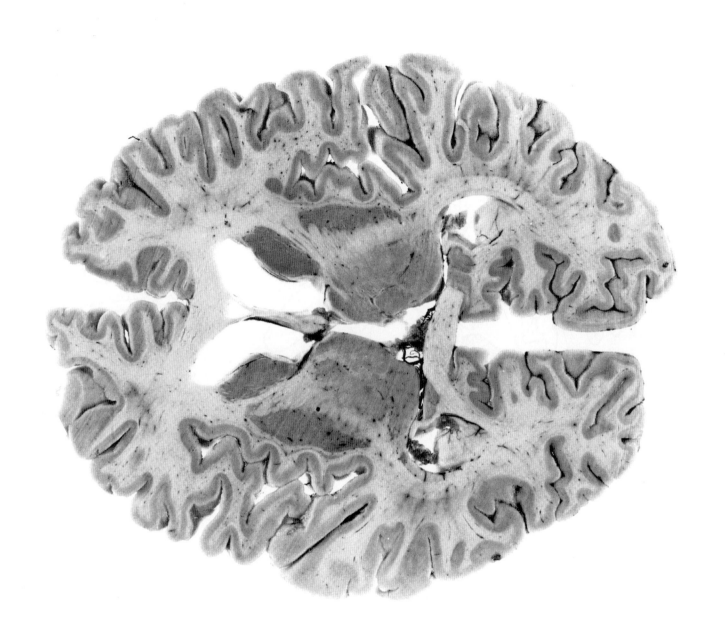

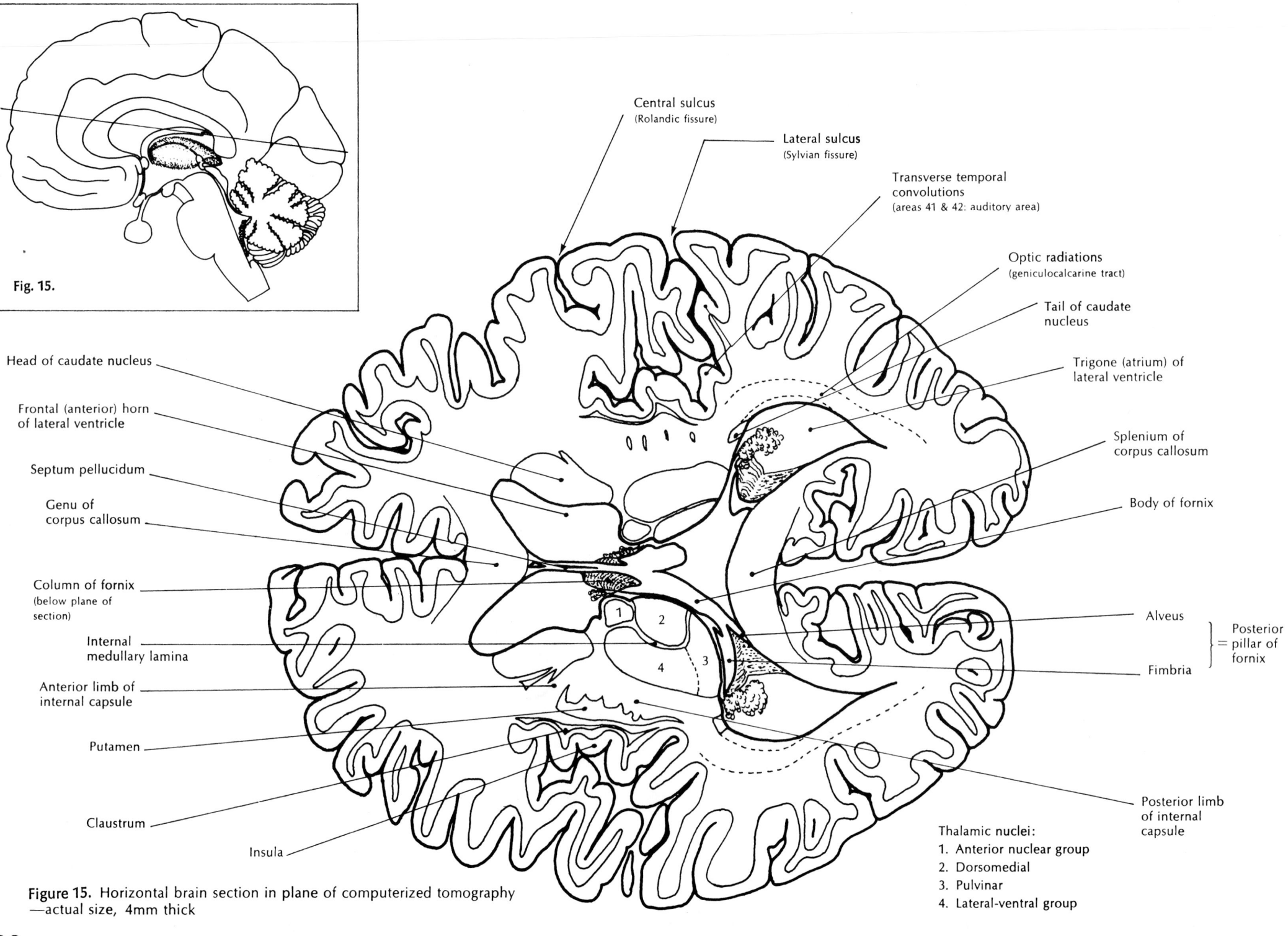

Central sulcus
(Rolandic fissure)

Lateral sulcus
(Sylvian fissure)

Transverse temporal
convolutions
(areas 41 & 42: auditory area)

Optic radiations
(geniculocalcarine tract)

Tail of caudate
nucleus

Trigone (atrium) of
lateral ventricle

Splenium of
corpus callosum

Body of fornix

Alveus

Posterior
= pillar of
fornix

Fimbria

Posterior limb
of internal
capsule

Head of caudate nucleus

Frontal (anterior) horn
of lateral ventricle

Septum pellucidum

Genu of
corpus callosum

Column of fornix
(below plane of
section)

Internal
medullary lamina

Anterior limb of
internal capsule

Putamen

Claustrum

Insula

Fig. 15.

Thalamic nuclei:
1. Anterior nuclear group
2. Dorsomedial
3. Pulvinar
4. Lateral-ventral group

Figure 15. Horizontal brain section in plane of computerized tomography
—actual size, 4mm thick

30

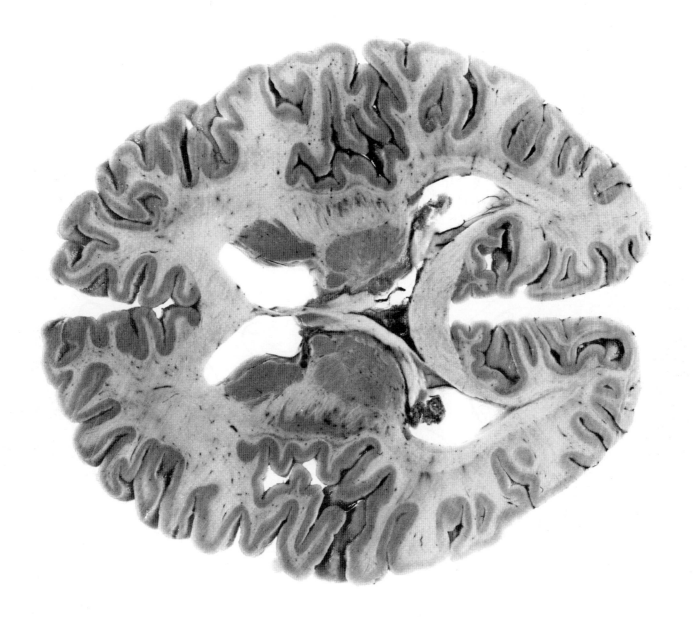

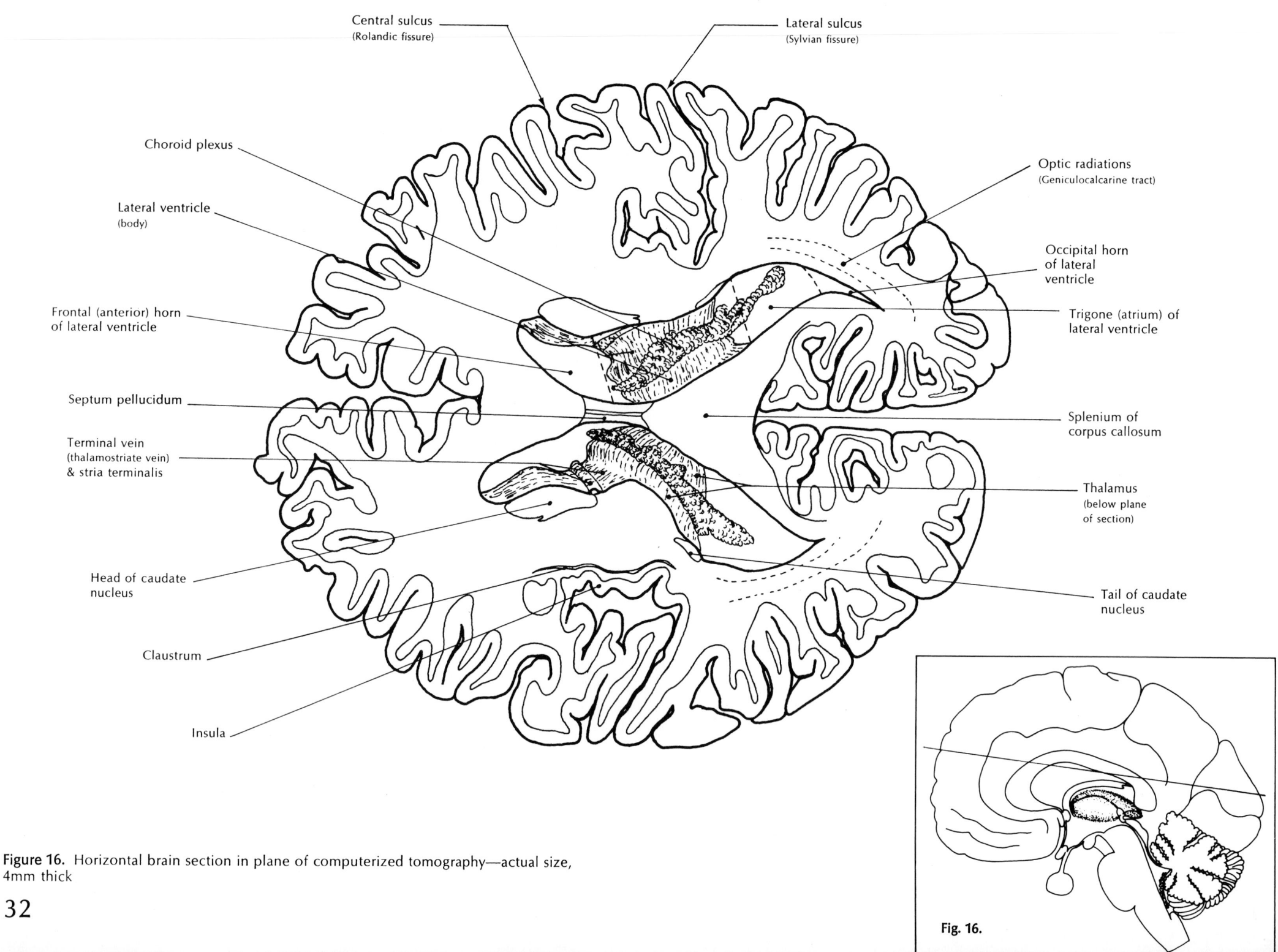

Central sulcus (Rolandic fissure)

Lateral sulcus (Sylvian fissure)

Choroid plexus

Optic radiations (Geniculocalcarine tract)

Lateral ventricle (body)

Occipital horn of lateral ventricle

Frontal (anterior) horn of lateral ventricle

Trigone (atrium) of lateral ventricle

Septum pellucidum

Splenium of corpus callosum

Terminal vein (thalamostriate vein) & stria terminalis

Thalamus (below plane of section)

Head of caudate nucleus

Tail of caudate nucleus

Claustrum

Insula

Figure 16. Horizontal brain section in plane of computerized tomography—actual size, 4mm thick

32

Fig. 16.

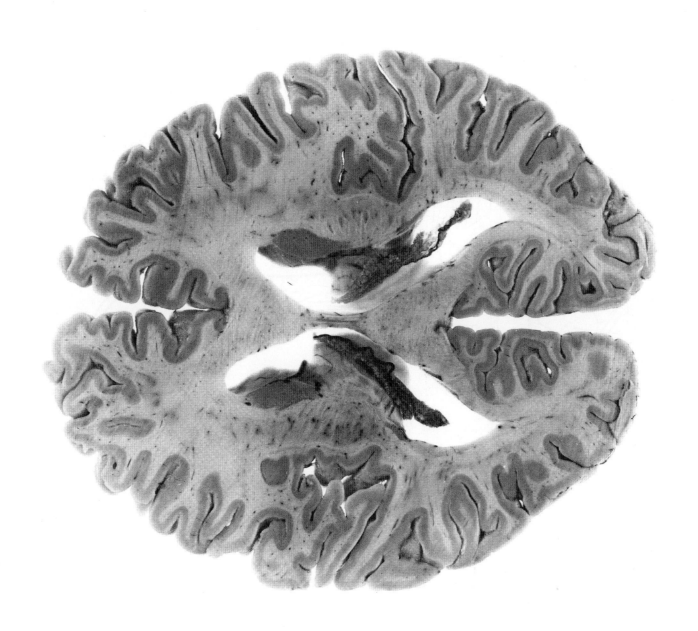

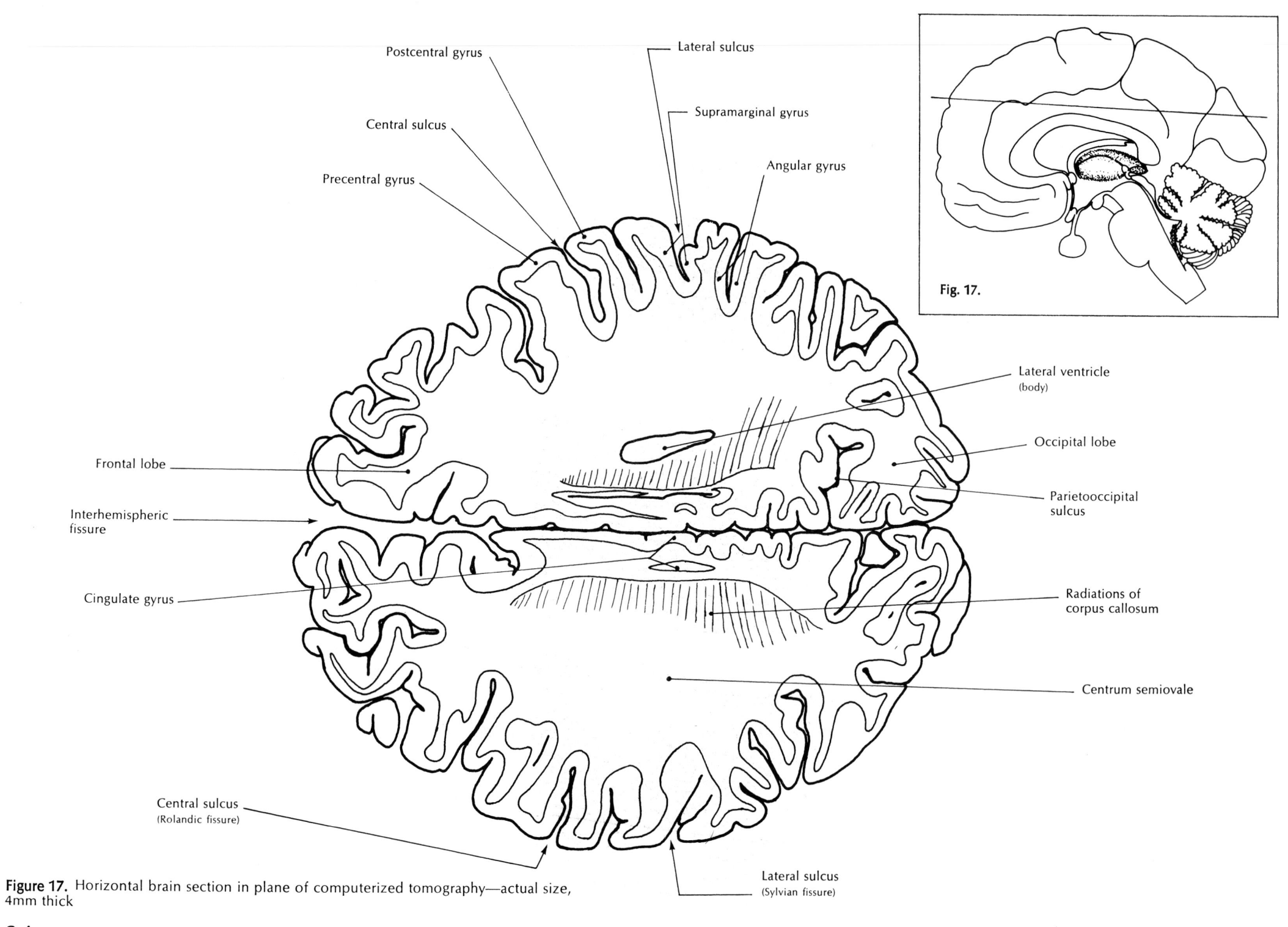

Postcentral gyrus

Central sulcus

Precentral gyrus

Lateral sulcus

Supramarginal gyrus

Angular gyrus

Fig. 17.

Frontal lobe

Interhemispheric
fissure

Cingulate gyrus

Lateral ventricle
(body)

Occipital lobe

Parietooccipital
sulcus

Radiations of
corpus callosum

Centrum semiovale

Central sulcus
(Rolandic fissure)

Lateral sulcus
(Sylvian fissure)

Figure 17. Horizontal brain section in plane of computerized tomography—actual size,
4mm thick

34

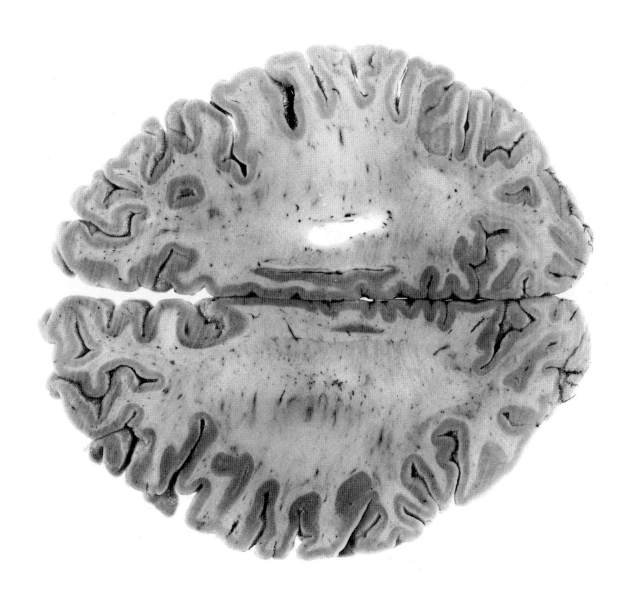

CORONAL SECTIONS OF THE GROSS BRAIN AND BRAIN STEM

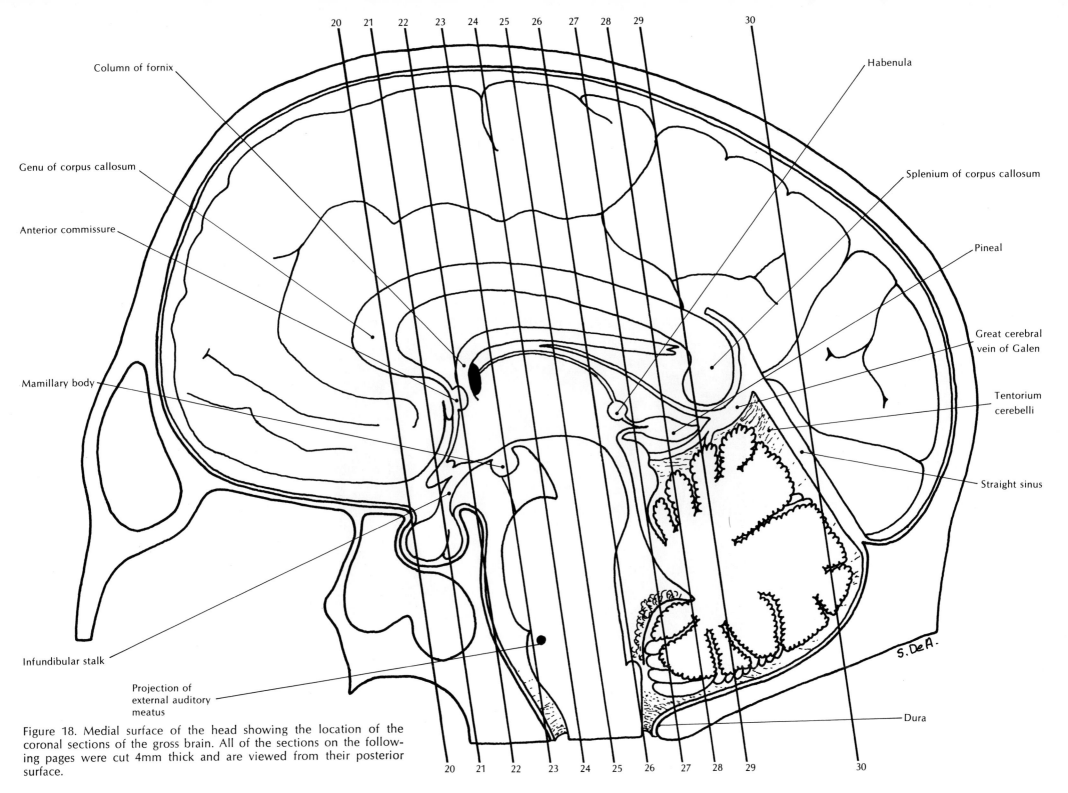

Figure 18. Medial surface of the head showing the location of the coronal sections of the gross brain. All of the sections on the following pages were cut 4mm thick and are viewed from their posterior surface.

37

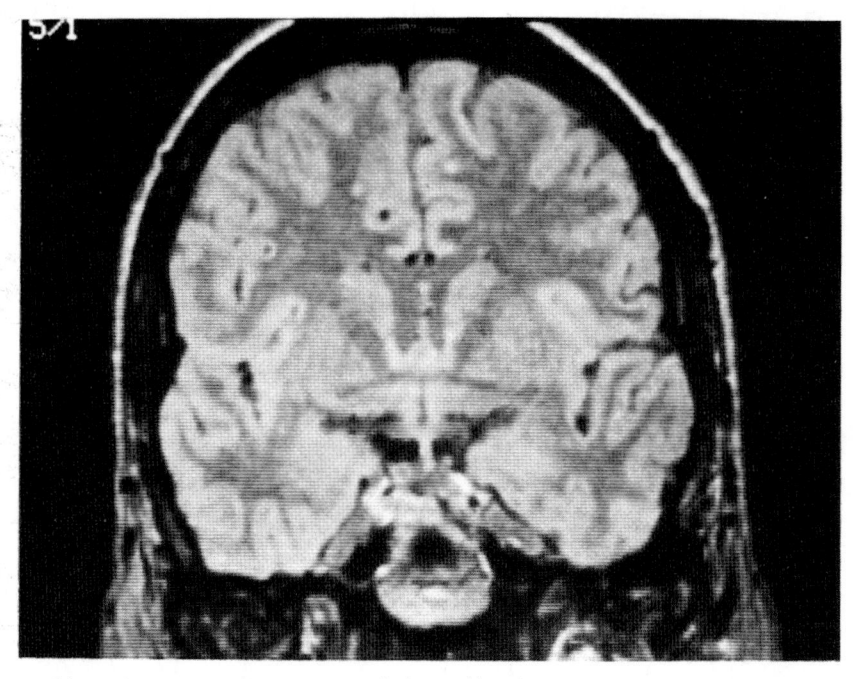

a. Magnetic resonance image, coronal plane of head

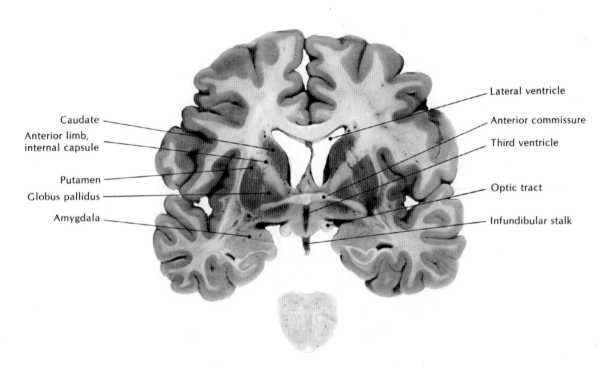

Caudate

Anterior limb,
internal capsule

Putamen

Globus pallidus

Amygdala

Lateral ventricle

Anterior commissure

Third ventricle

Optic tract

Infundibular stalk

b. Coronal section of gross brain (see Fig. 22)

Figure 19. Comparison of the magnetic resonance image of the head in
the coronal plane with a section of gross brain cut in the same plane

39

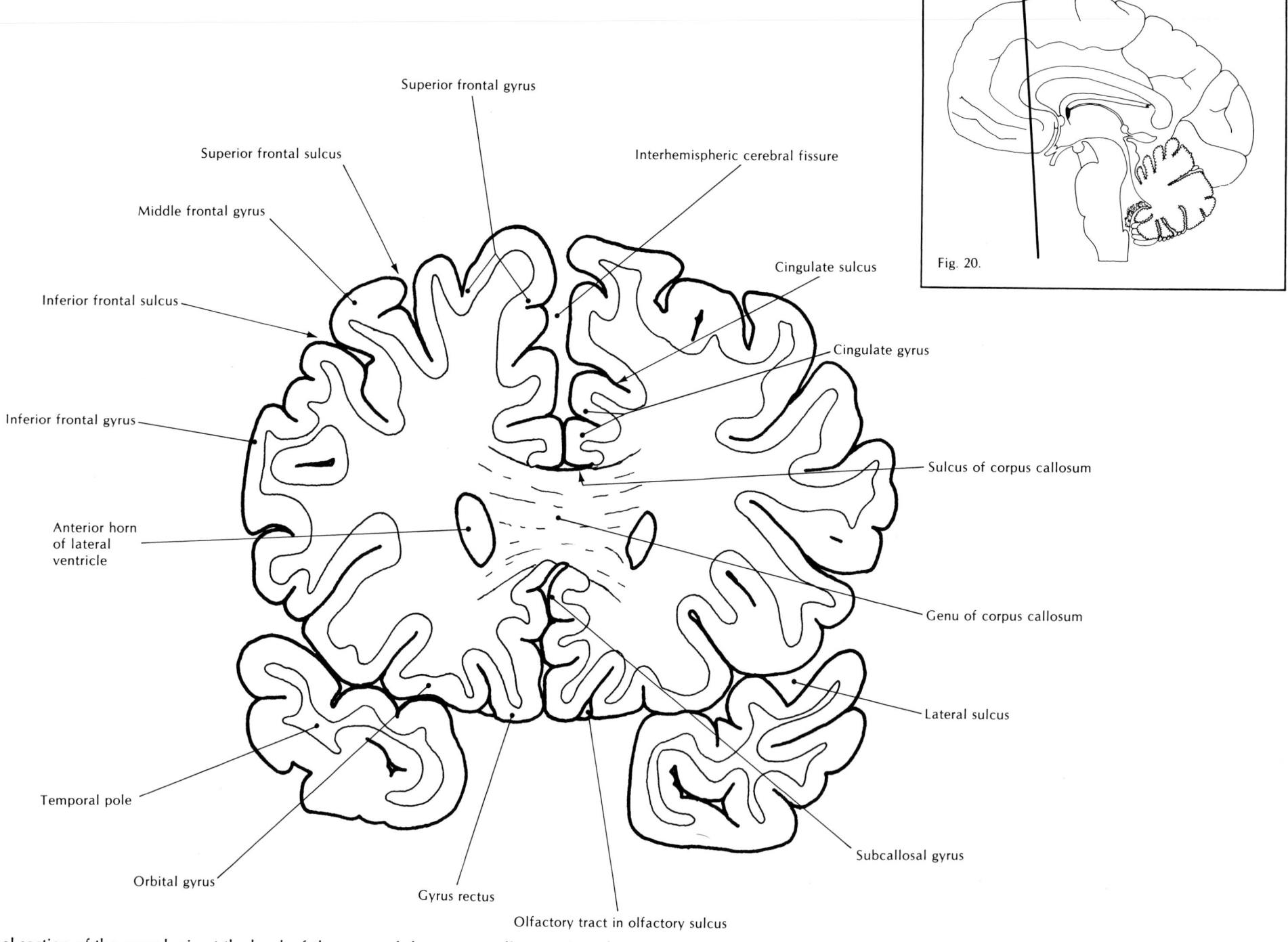

Superior frontal gyrus

Superior frontal sulcus

Middle frontal gyrus

Interhemispheric cerebral fissure

Inferior frontal sulcus

Cingulate sulcus

Inferior frontal gyrus

Cingulate gyrus

Sulcus of corpus callosum

Anterior horn of lateral ventricle

Genu of corpus callosum

Temporal pole

Lateral sulcus

Subcallosal gyrus

Orbital gyrus

Gyrus rectus

Olfactory tract in olfactory sulcus

Fig. 20.

Figure 20. Coronal section of the gross brain at the level of the genu of the corpus callosum viewed from its posterior surface—1.3×

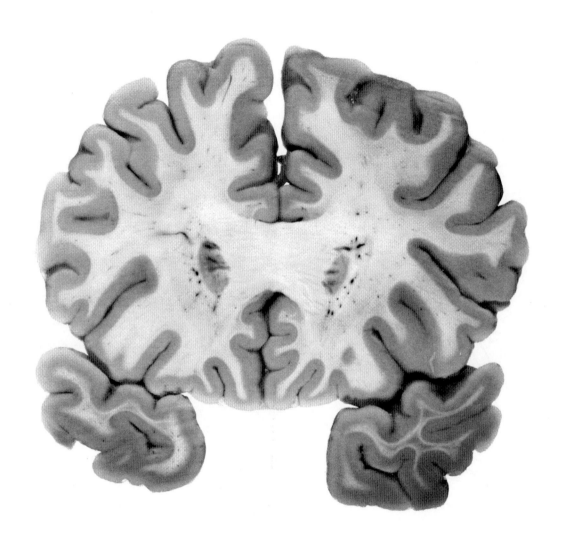

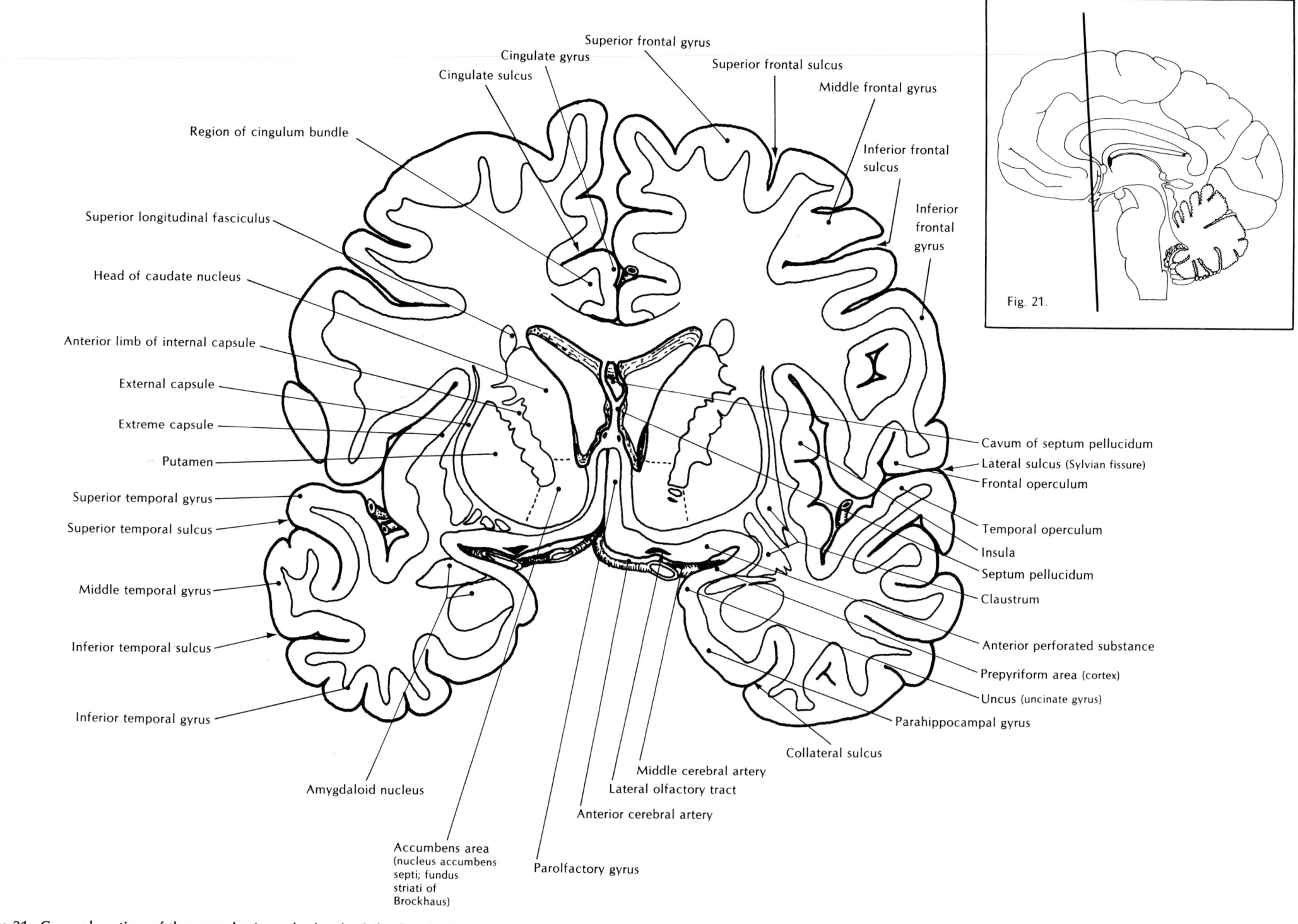

Cingulate gyrus

Cingulate sulcus

Superior frontal gyrus

Superior frontal sulcus

Middle frontal gyrus

Inferior frontal sulcus

Inferior frontal gyrus

Region of cingulum bundle

Superior longitudinal fasciculus

Head of caudate nucleus

Anterior limb of internal capsule

External capsule

Extreme capsule

Putamen

Superior temporal gyrus

Superior temporal sulcus

Middle temporal gyrus

Inferior temporal sulcus

Inferior temporal gyrus

Cavum of septum pellucidum

Lateral sulcus (Sylvian fissure)

Frontal operculum

Temporal operculum

Insula

Septum pellucidum

Claustrum

Anterior perforated substance

Prepyriform area (cortex)

Uncus (uncinate gyrus)

Parahippocampal gyrus

Collateral sulcus

Middle cerebral artery

Lateral olfactory tract

Anterior cerebral artery

Amygdaloid nucleus

Accumbens area (nucleus accumbens septi; fundus striati of Brockhaus)

Parolfactory gyrus

Fig. 21.

Figure 21. Coronal section of the gross brain at the level of the head of the caudate nucleus viewed from its posterior surface—1.3×

42

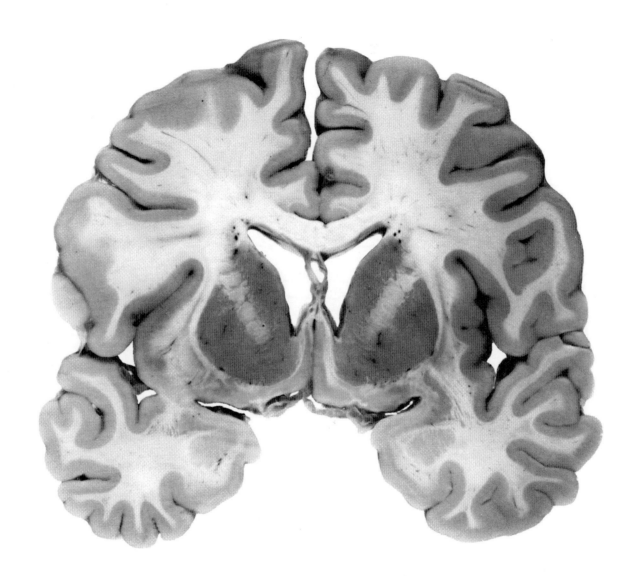

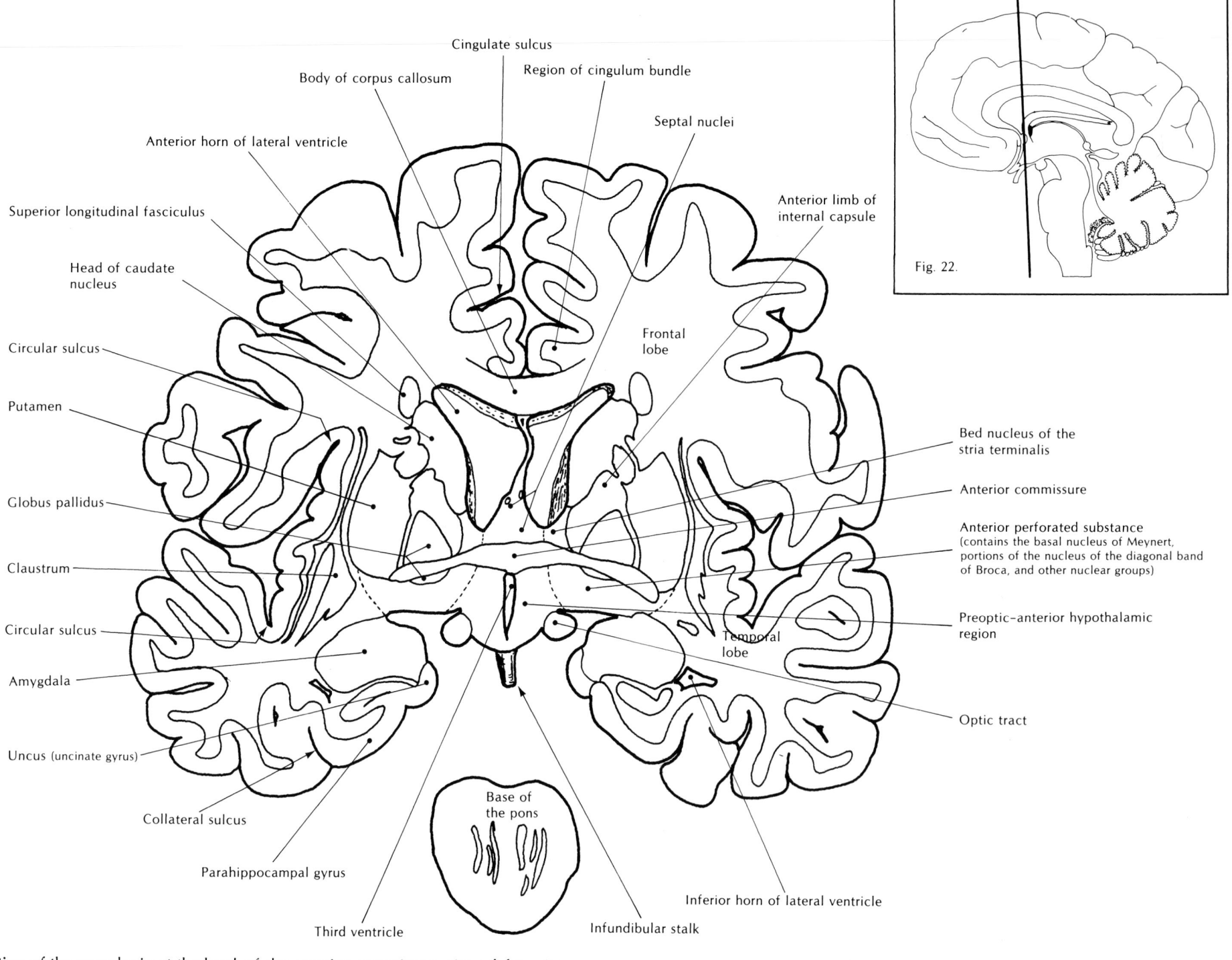

Cingulate sulcus

Region of cingulum bundle

Body of corpus callosum

Septal nuclei

Anterior horn of lateral ventricle

Superior longitudinal fasciculus

Anterior limb of internal capsule

Head of caudate nucleus

Frontal lobe

Circular sulcus

Putamen

Bed nucleus of the stria terminalis

Anterior commissure

Globus pallidus

Anterior perforated substance (contains the basal nucleus of Meynert, portions of the nucleus of the diagonal band of Broca, and other nuclear groups)

Claustrum

Preoptic–anterior hypothalamic region

Circular sulcus

Amygdala

Temporal lobe

Optic tract

Uncus (uncinate gyrus)

Collateral sulcus

Base of the pons

Parahippocampal gyrus

Inferior horn of lateral ventricle

Third ventricle

Infundibular stalk

Fig. 22.

Figure 22. Coronal section of the gross brain at the level of the anterior commissure viewed from its posterior surface—1.3×

44

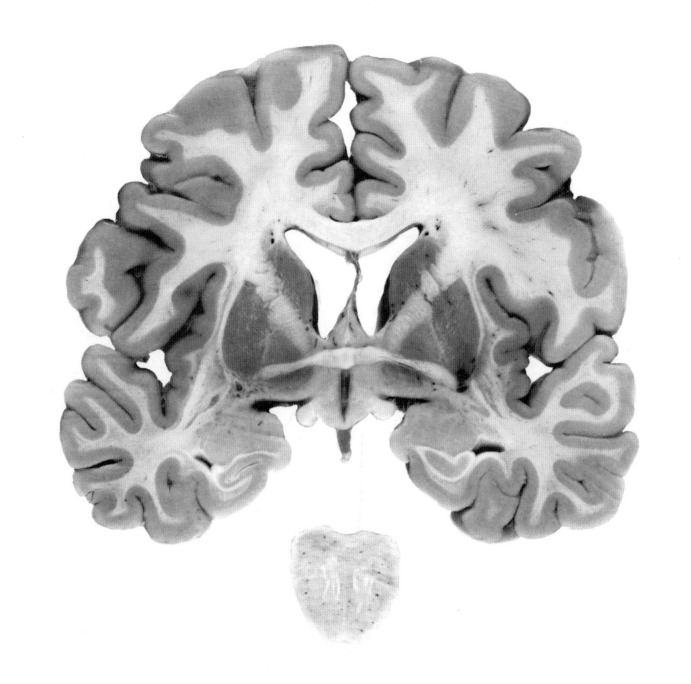

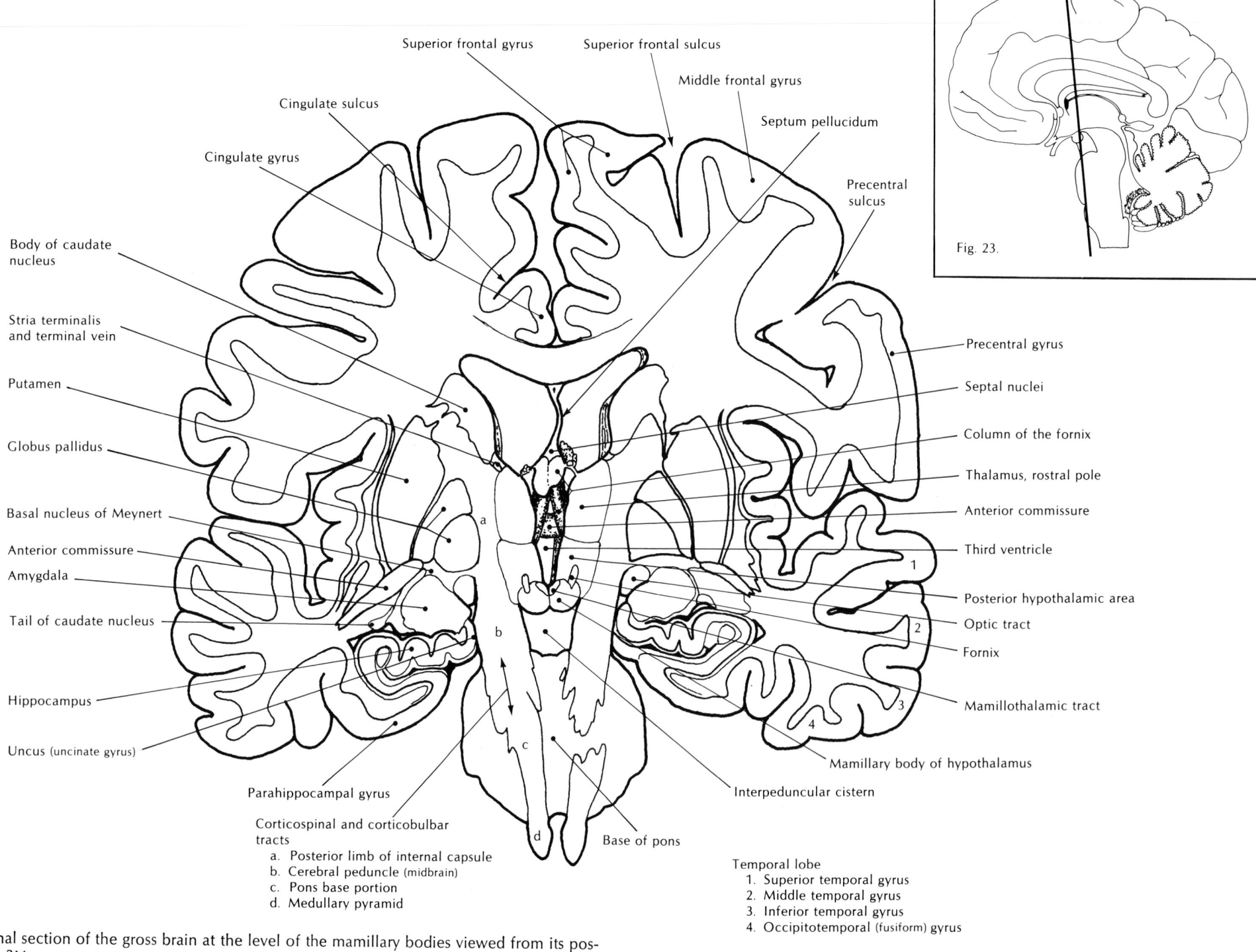

Superior frontal gyrus
Superior frontal sulcus
Middle frontal gyrus
Cingulate sulcus
Septum pellucidum
Cingulate gyrus
Precentral sulcus
Body of caudate nucleus
Precentral gyrus
Stria terminalis and terminal vein
Septal nuclei
Putamen
Column of the fornix
Globus pallidus
Thalamus, rostral pole
Anterior commissure
Basal nucleus of Meynert
Third ventricle
Anterior commissure
Posterior hypothalamic area
Amygdala
Optic tract
Tail of caudate nucleus
Fornix
Hippocampus
Mamillothalamic tract
Uncus (uncinate gyrus)
Mamillary body of hypothalamus
Parahippocampal gyrus
Interpeduncular cistern
Corticospinal and corticobulbar tracts
Base of pons

a. Posterior limb of internal capsule
b. Cerebral peduncle (midbrain)
c. Pons base portion
d. Medullary pyramid

Temporal lobe
1. Superior temporal gyrus
2. Middle temporal gyrus
3. Inferior temporal gyrus
4. Occipitotemporal (fusiform) gyrus

Fig. 23.

Figure 23. Coronal section of the gross brain at the level of the mamillary bodies viewed from its posterior surface—1.3×

46

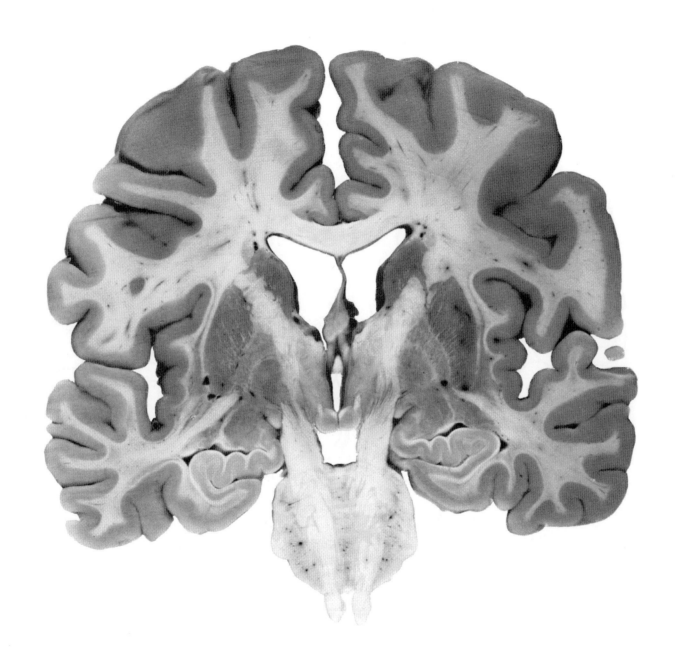

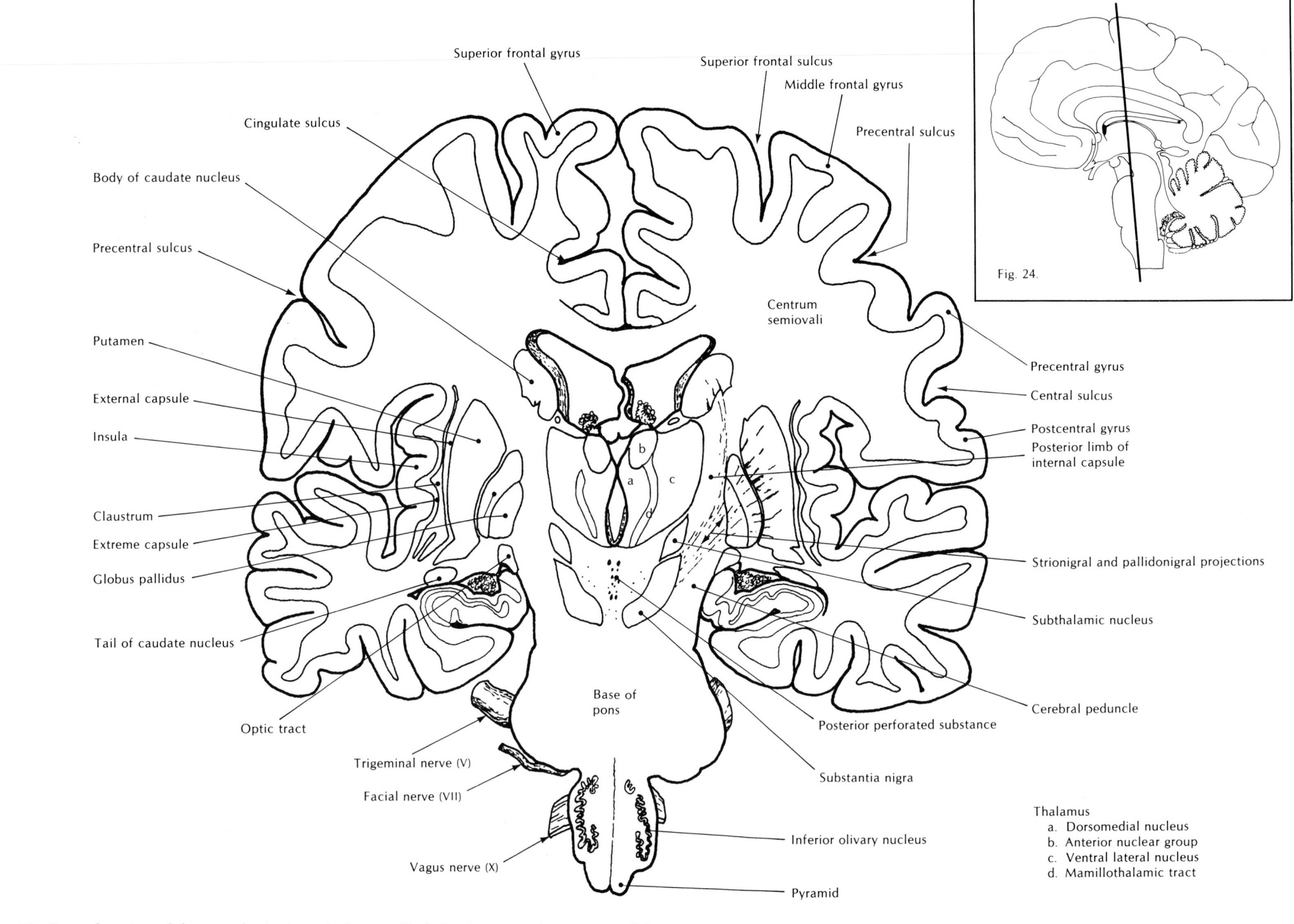

Superior frontal gyrus

Superior frontal sulcus

Middle frontal gyrus

Precentral sulcus

Cingulate sulcus

Body of caudate nucleus

Precentral sulcus

Putamen

External capsule

Insula

Claustrum

Extreme capsule

Globus pallidus

Tail of caudate nucleus

Optic tract

Trigeminal nerve (V)

Facial nerve (VII)

Vagus nerve (X)

Centrum
semiovali

Precentral gyrus

Central sulcus

Postcentral gyrus

Posterior limb of
internal capsule

Strionigral and pallidonigral projections

Subthalamic nucleus

Cerebral peduncle

Base of
pons

Posterior perforated substance

Substantia nigra

Inferior olivary nucleus

Pyramid

Fig. 24.

Thalamus
  a. Dorsomedial nucleus
  b. Anterior nuclear group
  c. Ventral lateral nucleus
  d. Mamillothalamic tract

Figure 24. Coronal section of the gross brain through the mamillothalamic tract and main mass of the substantia nigra viewed from its posterior surface—1.3✕

48

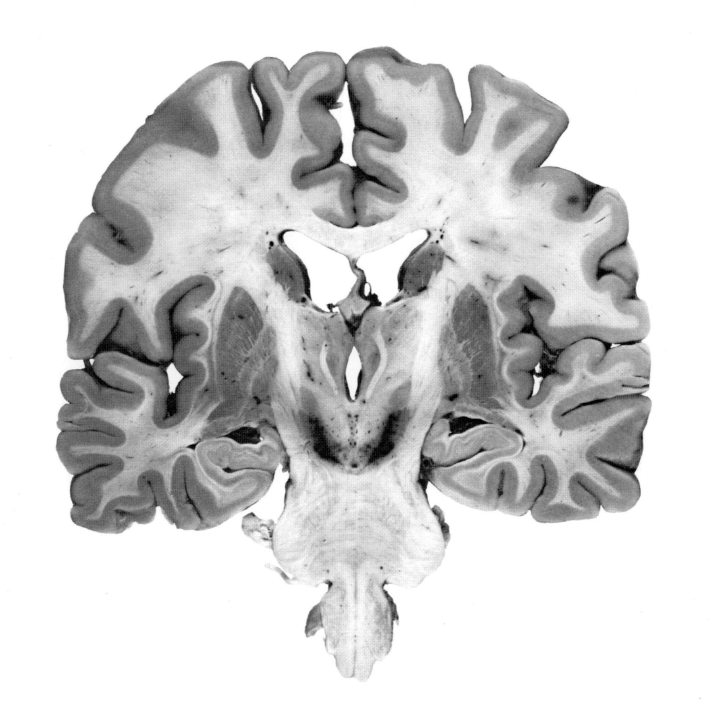

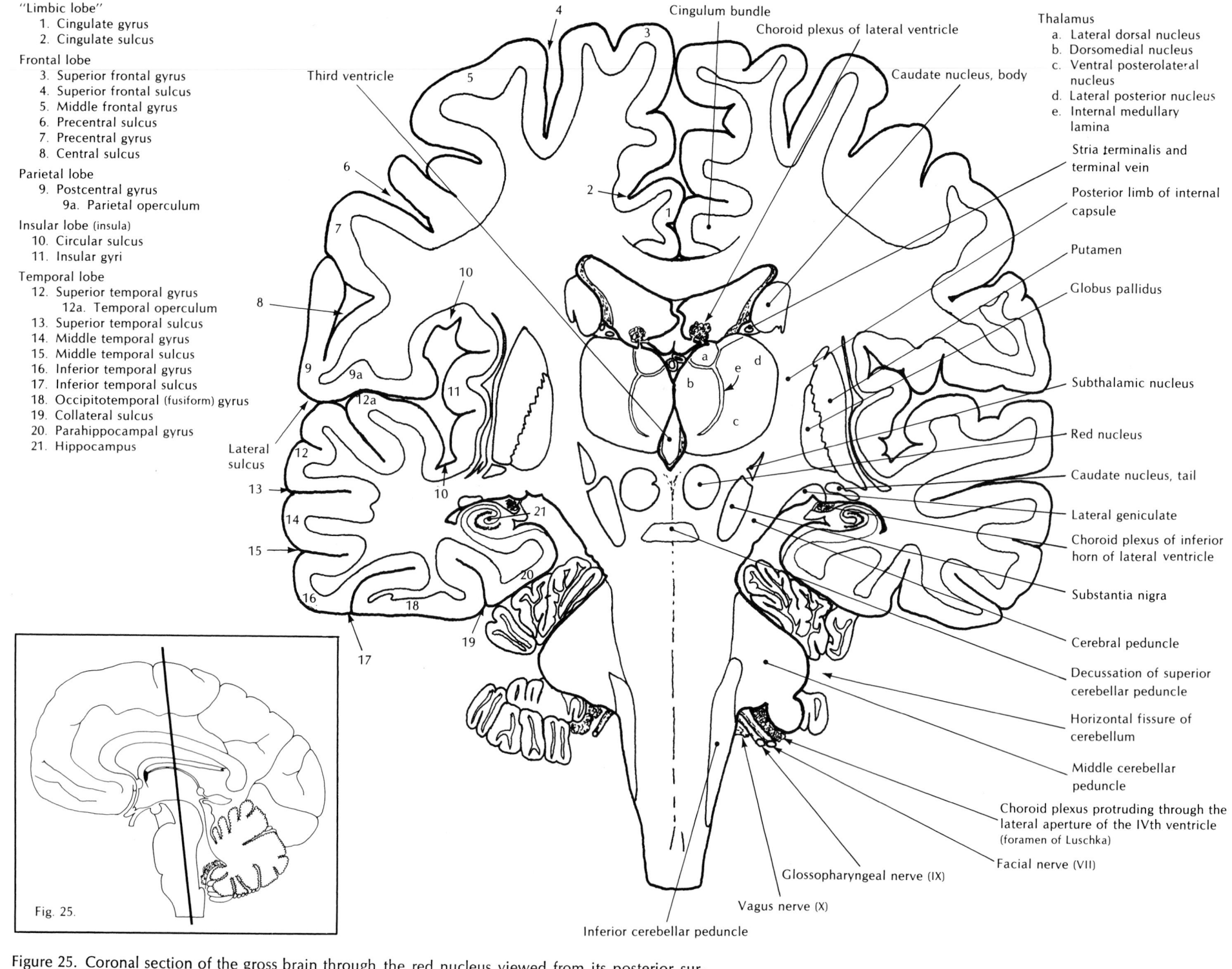

"Limbic lobe"
  1. Cingulate gyrus
  2. Cingulate sulcus
Frontal lobe
  3. Superior frontal gyrus
  4. Superior frontal sulcus
  5. Middle frontal gyrus
  6. Precentral sulcus
  7. Precentral gyrus
  8. Central sulcus
Parietal lobe
  9. Postcentral gyrus
    9a. Parietal operculum
Insular lobe (insula)
  10. Circular sulcus
  11. Insular gyri
Temporal lobe
  12. Superior temporal gyrus
    12a. Temporal operculum
  13. Superior temporal sulcus
  14. Middle temporal gyrus
  15. Middle temporal sulcus
  16. Inferior temporal gyrus
  17. Inferior temporal sulcus
  18. Occipitotemporal (fusiform) gyrus
  19. Collateral sulcus
  20. Parahippocampal gyrus
  21. Hippocampus

Cingulum bundle
Choroid plexus of lateral ventricle
Caudate nucleus, body

Third ventricle

Thalamus
  a. Lateral dorsal nucleus
  b. Dorsomedial nucleus
  c. Ventral posterolateral nucleus
  d. Lateral posterior nucleus
  e. Internal medullary lamina

Stria terminalis and terminal vein
Posterior limb of internal capsule
Putamen
Globus pallidus
Subthalamic nucleus
Red nucleus
Caudate nucleus, tail
Lateral geniculate
Choroid plexus of inferior horn of lateral ventricle
Substantia nigra
Cerebral peduncle
Decussation of superior cerebellar peduncle
Horizontal fissure of cerebellum
Middle cerebellar peduncle
Choroid plexus protruding through the lateral aperture of the IVth ventricle (foramen of Luschka)
Facial nerve (VII)

Lateral sulcus

Glossopharyngeal nerve (IX)
Vagus nerve (X)
Inferior cerebellar peduncle

Fig. 25.

Figure 25. Coronal section of the gross brain through the red nucleus viewed from its posterior surface—1.3×

50

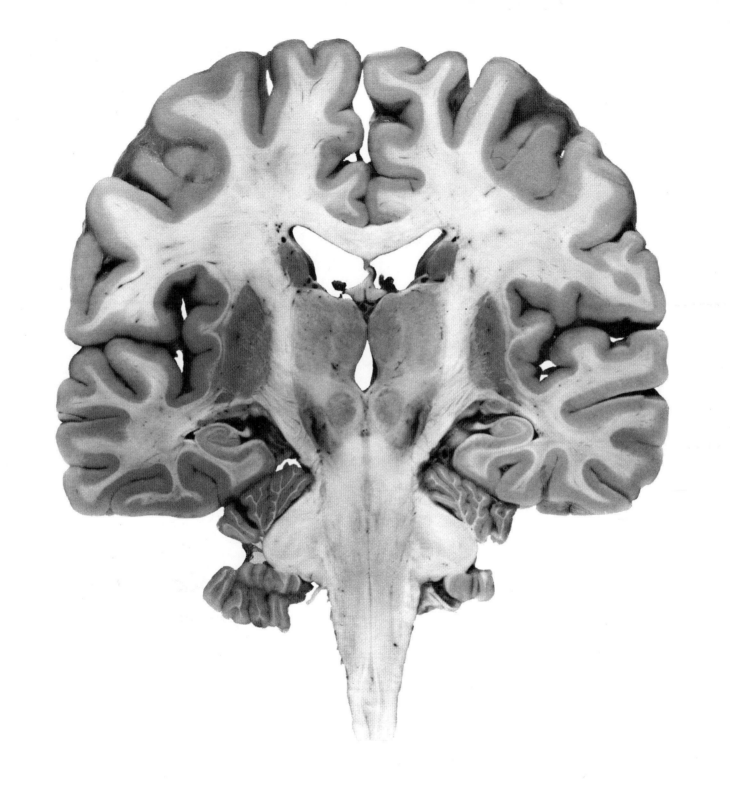

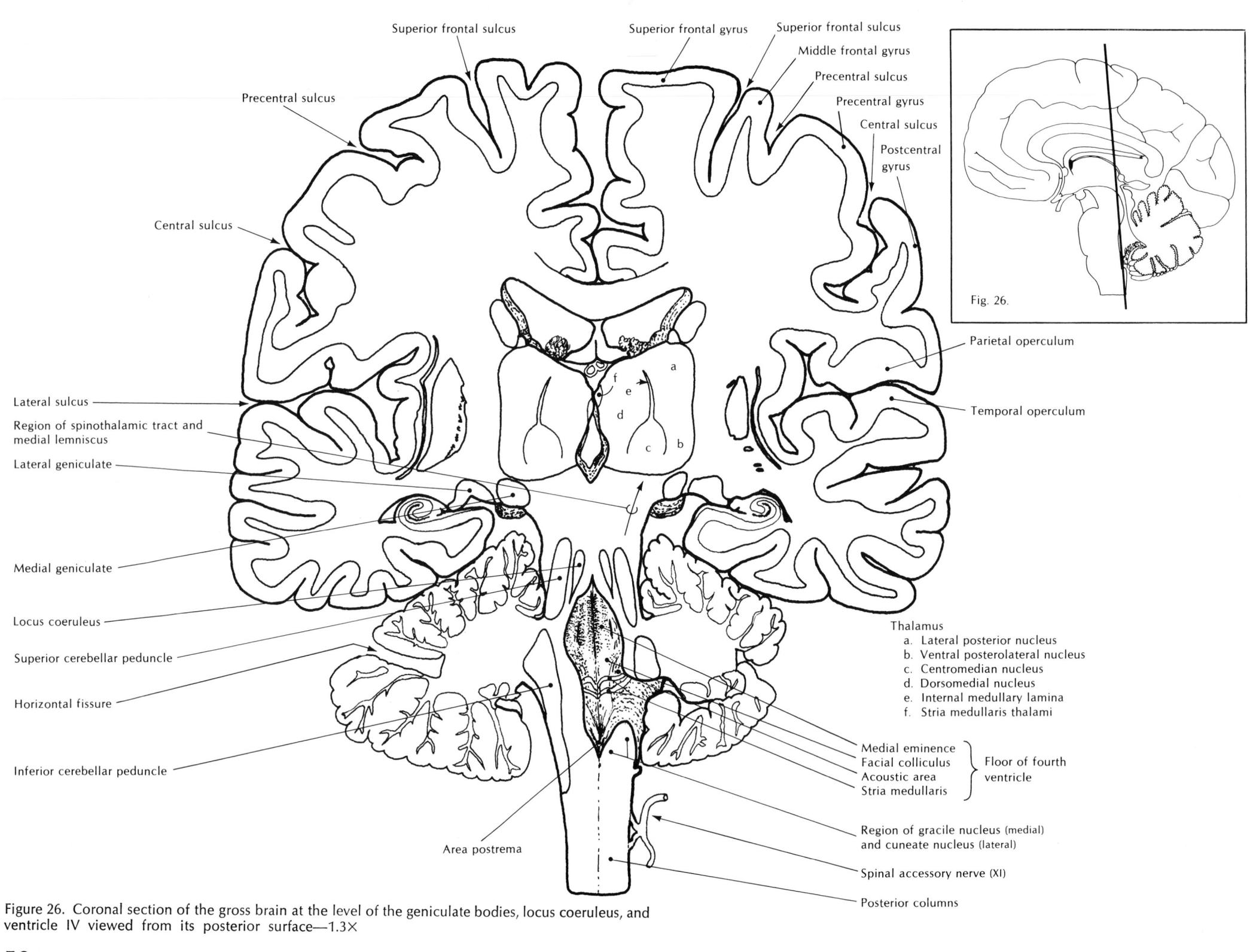

Superior frontal sulcus

Superior frontal gyrus

Superior frontal sulcus

Middle frontal gyrus

Precentral sulcus

Precentral gyrus

Central sulcus

Postcentral gyrus

Precentral sulcus

Central sulcus

Lateral sulcus

Region of spinothalamic tract and medial lemniscus

Lateral geniculate

Medial geniculate

Locus coeruleus

Superior cerebellar peduncle

Horizontal fissure

Inferior cerebellar peduncle

Area postrema

Fig. 26.

Parietal operculum

Temporal operculum

Thalamus
a. Lateral posterior nucleus
b. Ventral posterolateral nucleus
c. Centromedian nucleus
d. Dorsomedial nucleus
e. Internal medullary lamina
f. Stria medullaris thalami

Medial eminence
Facial colliculus   } Floor of fourth
Acoustic area   } ventricle
Stria medullaris

Region of gracile nucleus (medial)
and cuneate nucleus (lateral)

Spinal accessory nerve (XI)

Posterior columns

Figure 26. Coronal section of the gross brain at the level of the geniculate bodies, locus coeruleus, and ventricle IV viewed from its posterior surface—1.3×

52

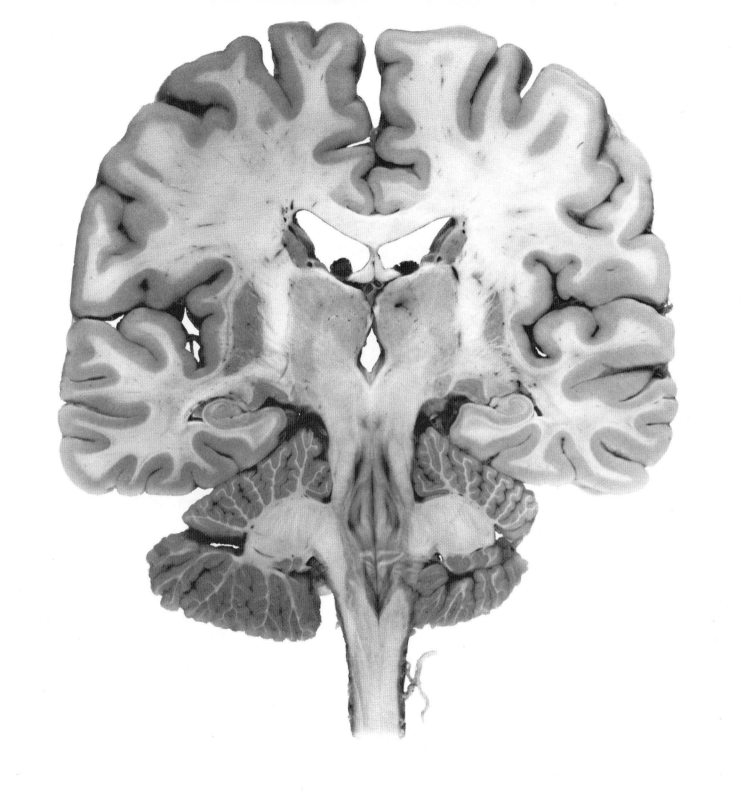

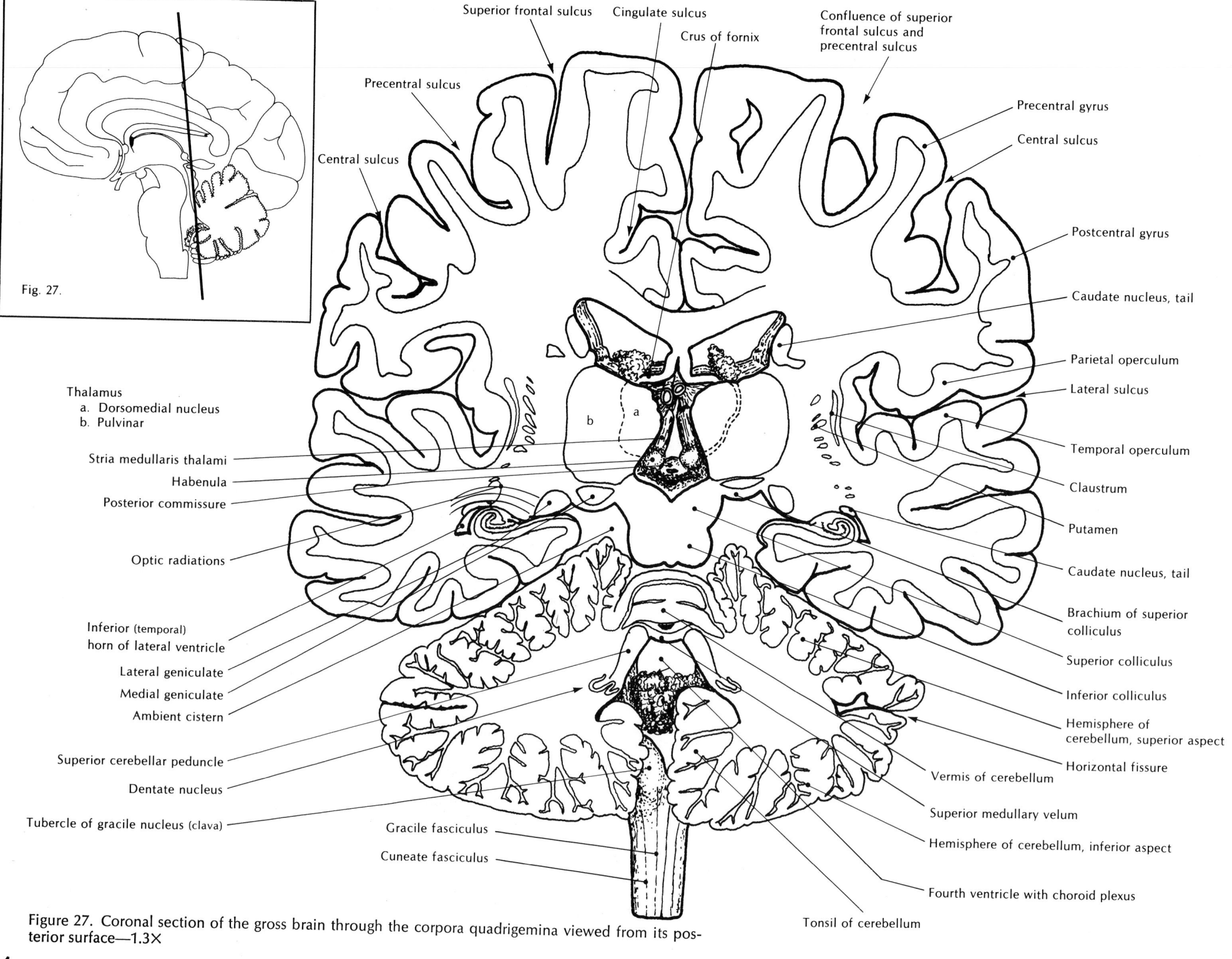

Fig. 27.

Superior frontal sulcus

Cingulate sulcus

Crus of fornix

Confluence of superior frontal sulcus and precentral sulcus

Precentral sulcus

Precentral gyrus

Central sulcus

Central sulcus

Postcentral gyrus

Caudate nucleus, tail

Parietal operculum

Lateral sulcus

Temporal operculum

Claustrum

Putamen

Caudate nucleus, tail

Brachium of superior colliculus

Superior colliculus

Inferior colliculus

Hemisphere of cerebellum, superior aspect

Horizontal fissure

Vermis of cerebellum

Superior medullary velum

Hemisphere of cerebellum, inferior aspect

Fourth ventricle with choroid plexus

Tonsil of cerebellum

Thalamus
a. Dorsomedial nucleus
b. Pulvinar

Stria medullaris thalami

Habenula

Posterior commissure

Optic radiations

Inferior (temporal) horn of lateral ventricle

Lateral geniculate

Medial geniculate

Ambient cistern

Superior cerebellar peduncle

Dentate nucleus

Tubercle of gracile nucleus (clava)

Gracile fasciculus

Cuneate fasciculus

Figure 27. Coronal section of the gross brain through the corpora quadrigemina viewed from its posterior surface—1.3×

54

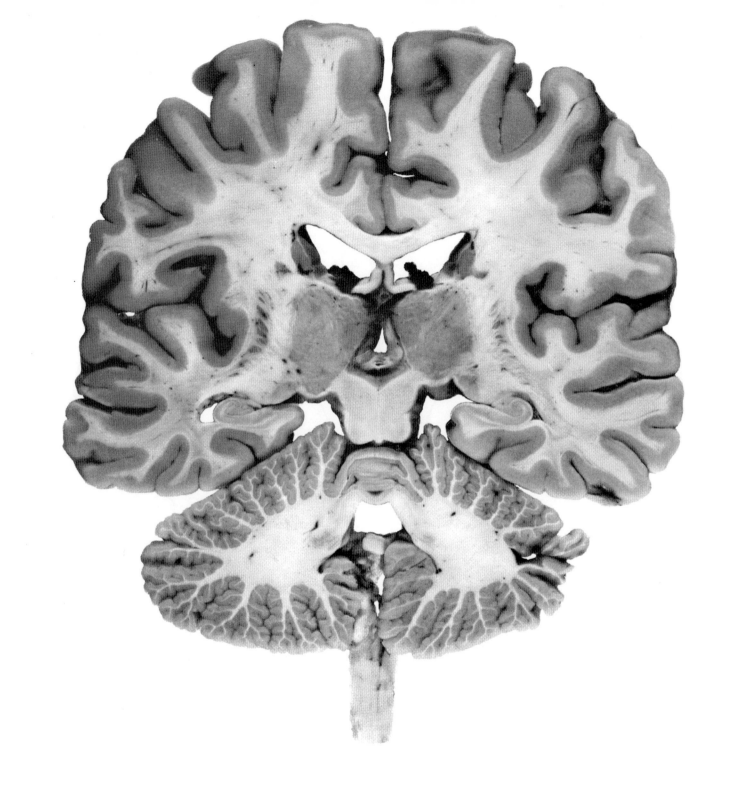

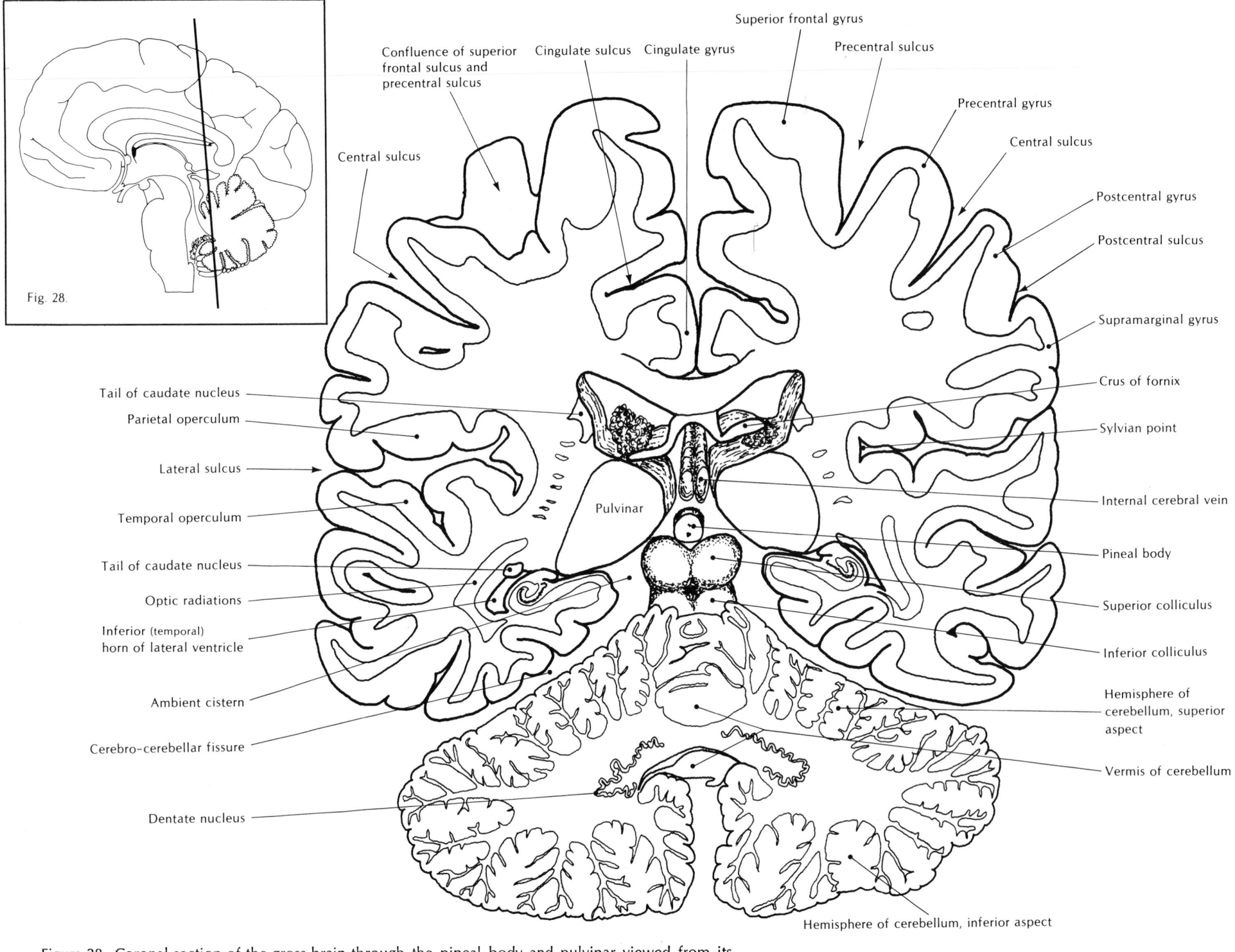

Figure 28. Coronal section of the gross brain through the pineal body and pulvinar viewed from its posterior surface—1.3×

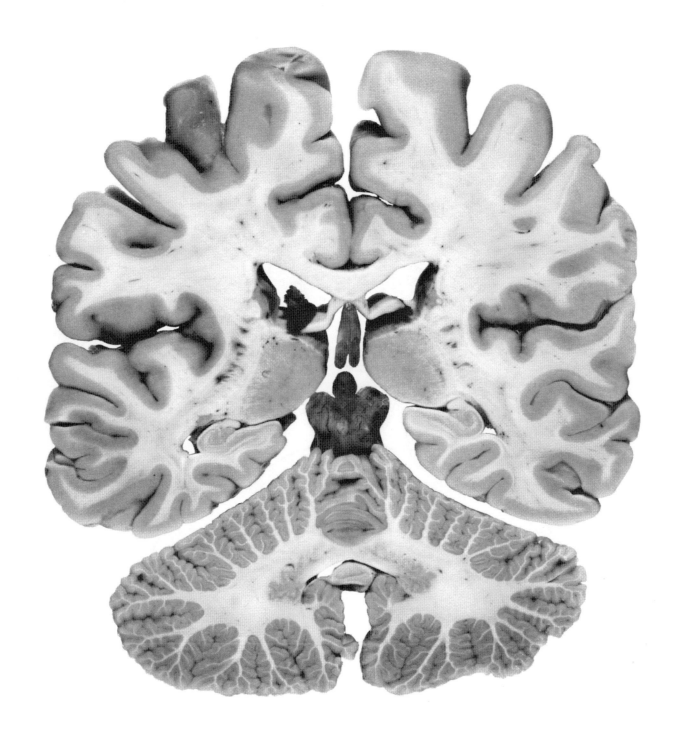

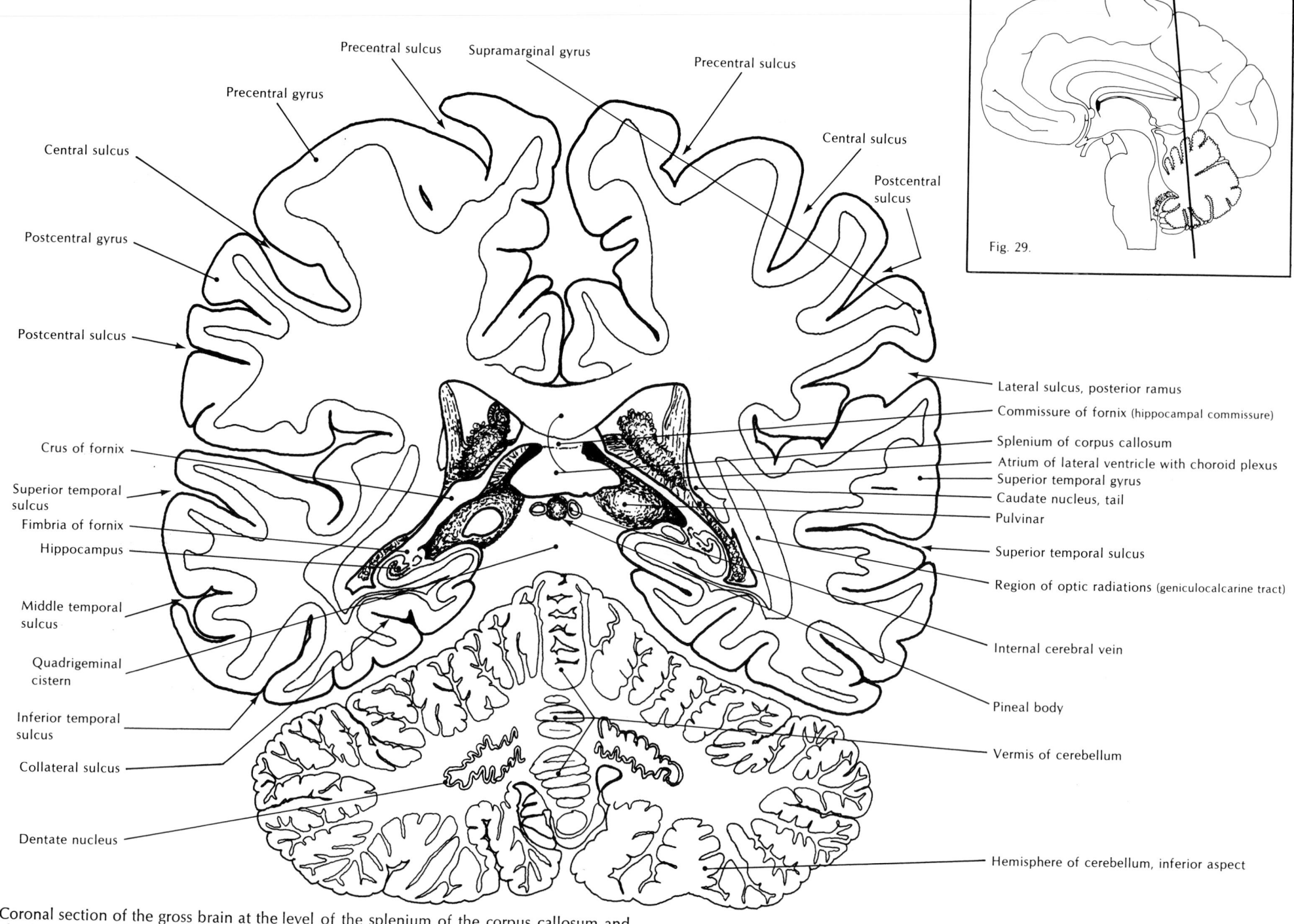

Precentral sulcus

Supramarginal gyrus

Precentral gyrus

Precentral sulcus

Central sulcus

Central sulcus

Postcentral sulcus

Postcentral gyrus

Postcentral sulcus

Fig. 29.

Lateral sulcus, posterior ramus

Commissure of fornix (hippocampal commissure)

Crus of fornix

Splenium of corpus callosum

Atrium of lateral ventricle with choroid plexus

Superior temporal sulcus

Superior temporal gyrus

Fimbria of fornix

Caudate nucleus, tail

Hippocampus

Pulvinar

Middle temporal sulcus

Superior temporal sulcus

Quadrigeminal cistern

Region of optic radiations (geniculocalcarine tract)

Inferior temporal sulcus

Internal cerebral vein

Collateral sulcus

Pineal body

Vermis of cerebellum

Dentate nucleus

Hemisphere of cerebellum, inferior aspect

Figure 29. Coronal section of the gross brain at the level of the splenium of the corpus callosum and the crus of the fornix viewed from its posterior surface—1.3×

58

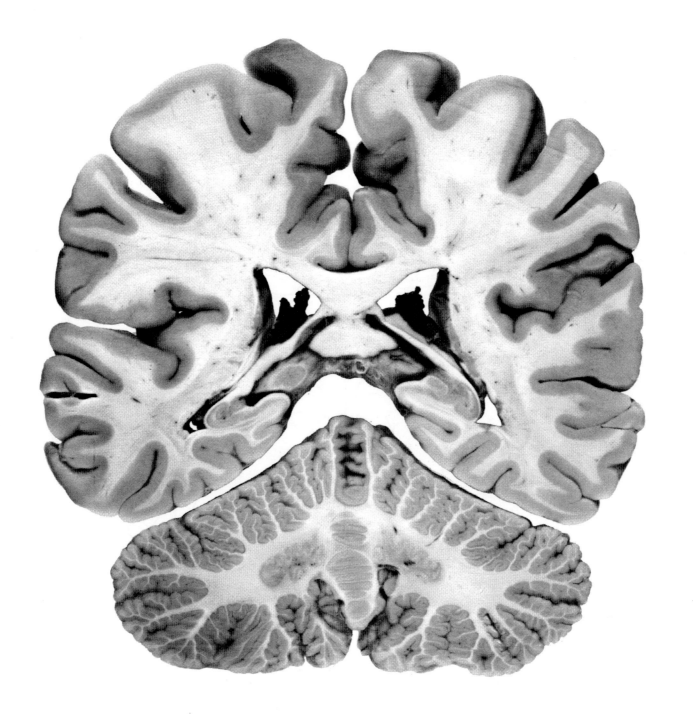

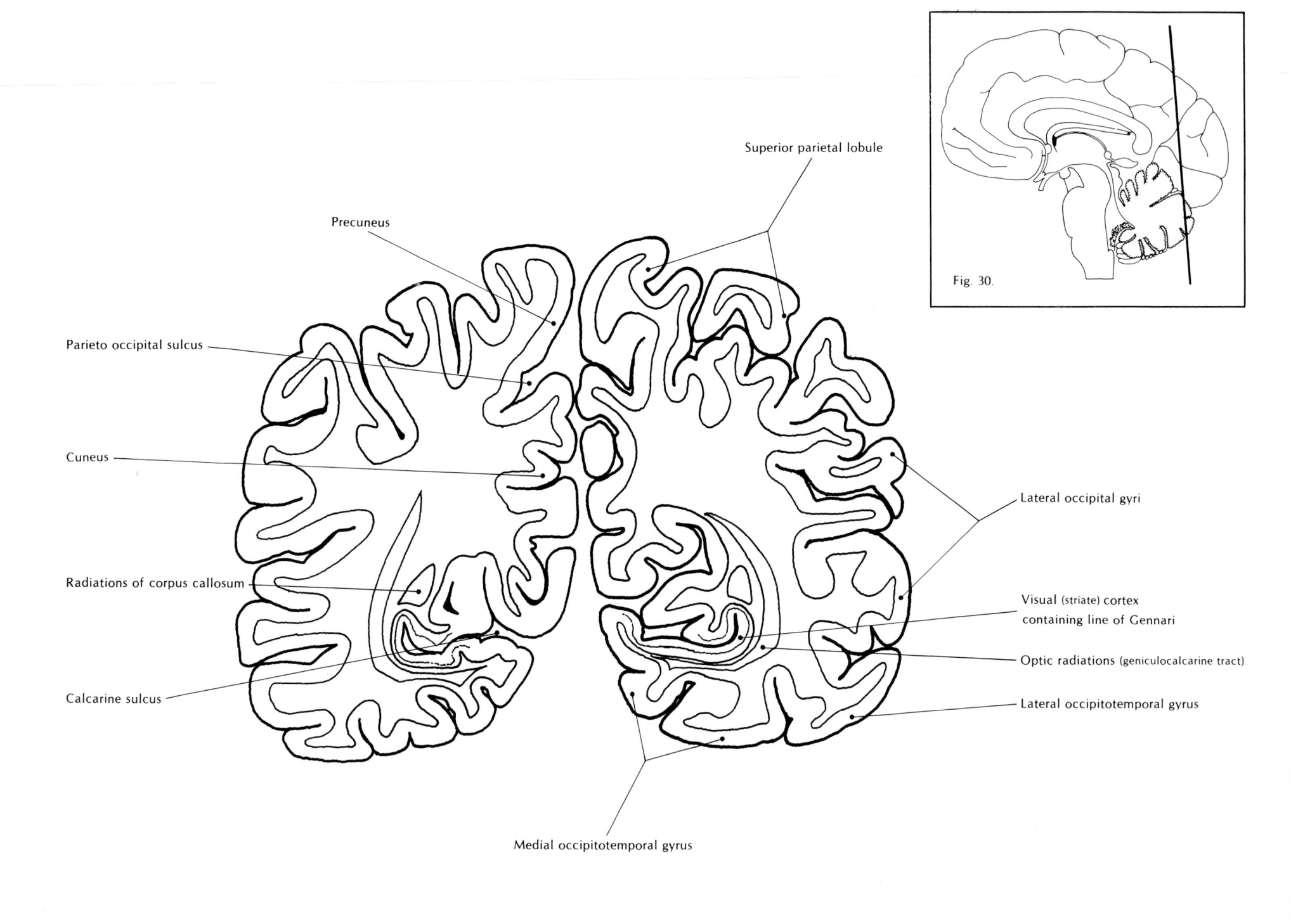

Precuneus

Superior parietal lobule

Parieto occipital sulcus

Cuneus

Lateral occipital gyri

Radiations of corpus callosum

Visual (striate) cortex containing line of Gennari

Optic radiations (geniculocalcarine tract)

Lateral occipitotemporal gyrus

Calcarine sulcus

Fig. 30.

Medial occipitotemporal gyrus

Figure 30. Coronal section of the gross brain through the optic radiations and calcarine fissure viewed from its posterior surface—1.3×

60

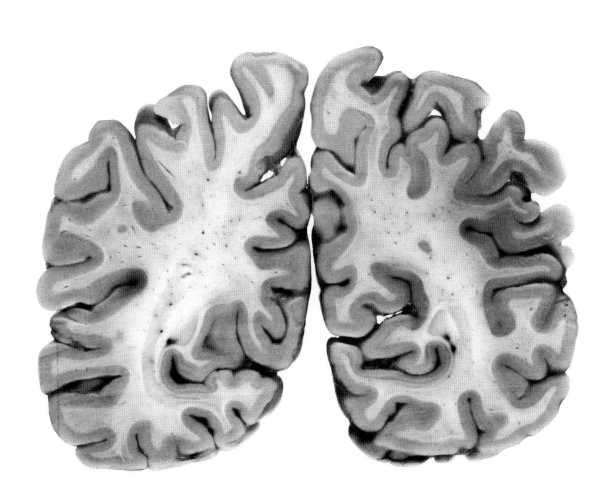

TRANSVERSE MICROSCOPIC SECTIONS OF THE SPINAL CORD

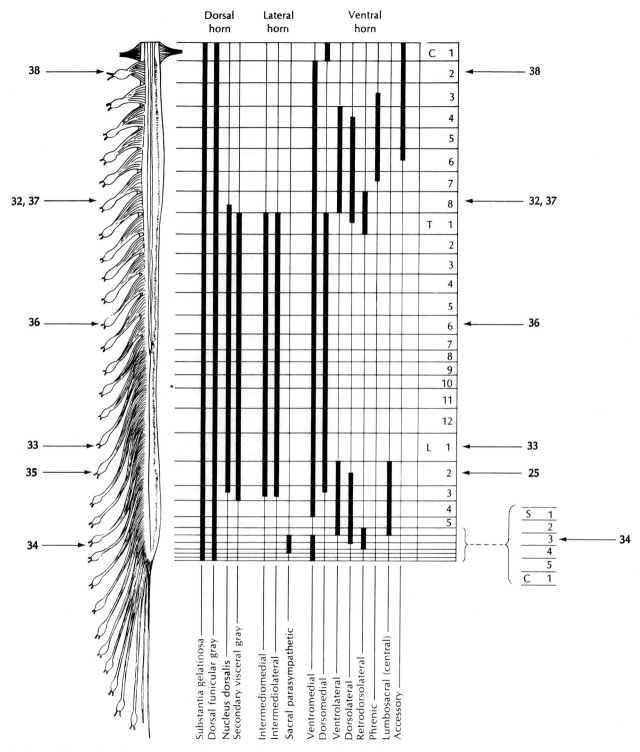

Figure 31. Nuclear columns of the spinal cord, adapted from Crosby, E. C., Humphrey, T., and Lauer, E. W. *Correlative Anatomy of the Nervous System*. Macmillan, New York, 1962. The pages on which figures are located are noted

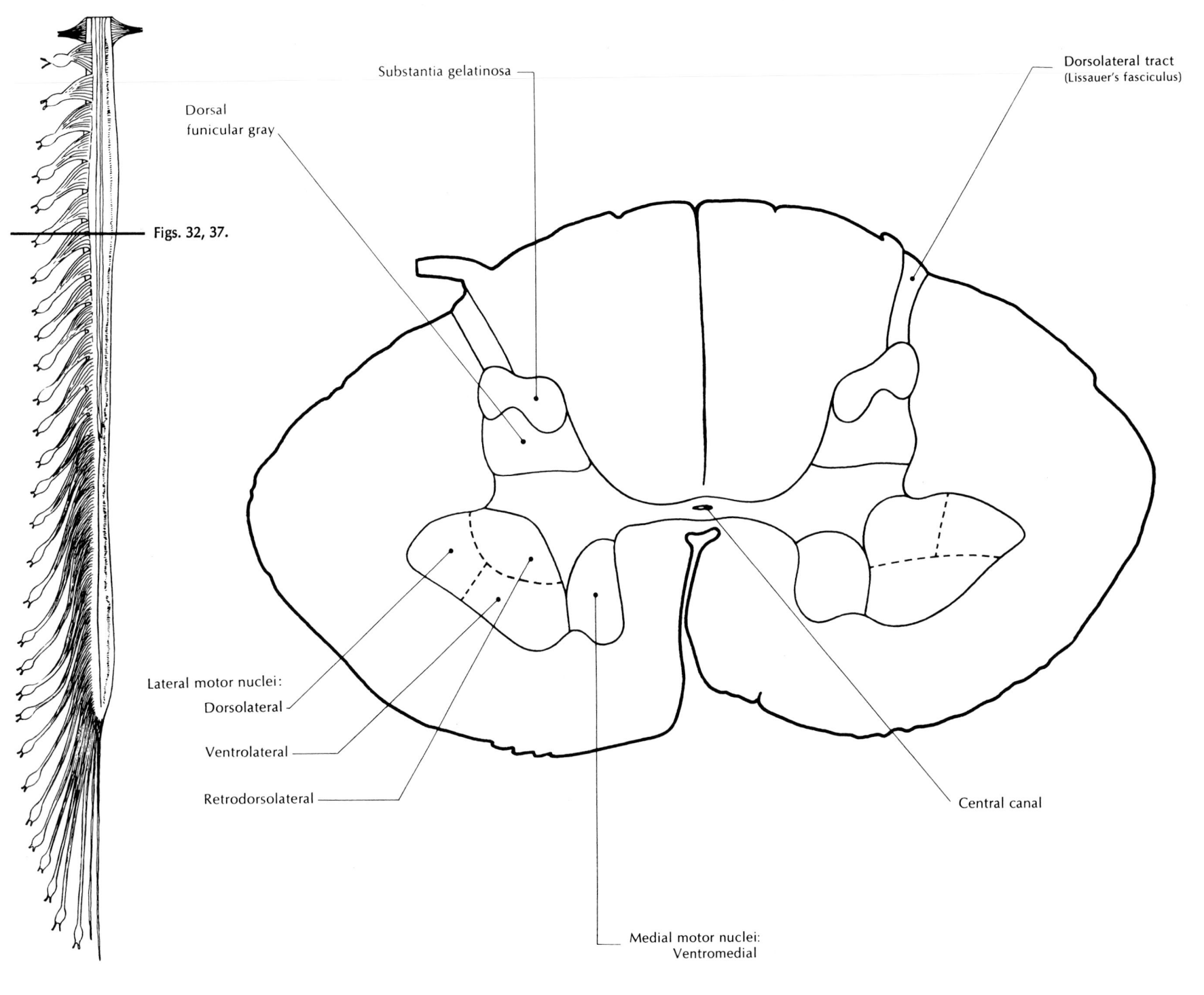

Dorsal
funicular gray

Substantia gelatinosa

Dorsolateral tract
(Lissauer's fasciculus)

Figs. 32, 37.

Lateral motor nuclei:

Dorsolateral

Ventrolateral

Retrodorsolateral

Central canal

Medial motor nuclei:
Ventromedial

Figure 32. Nuclear organization of the spinal cord in the cervical enlargement
(C8)—Nissl, 18X

64

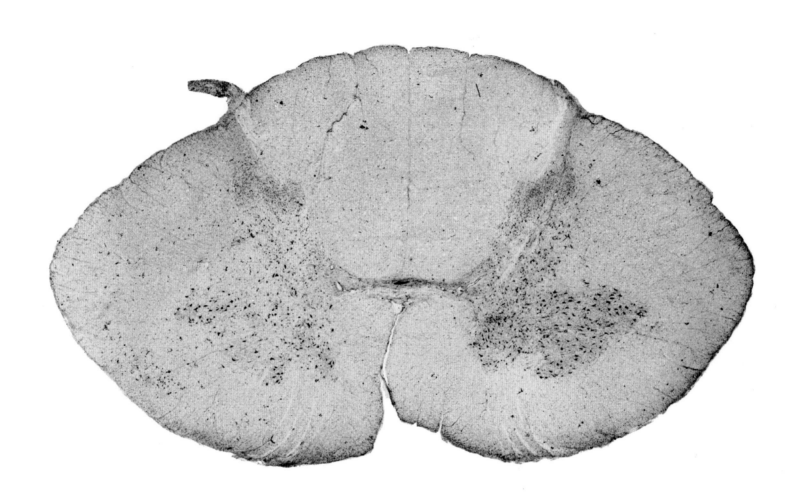

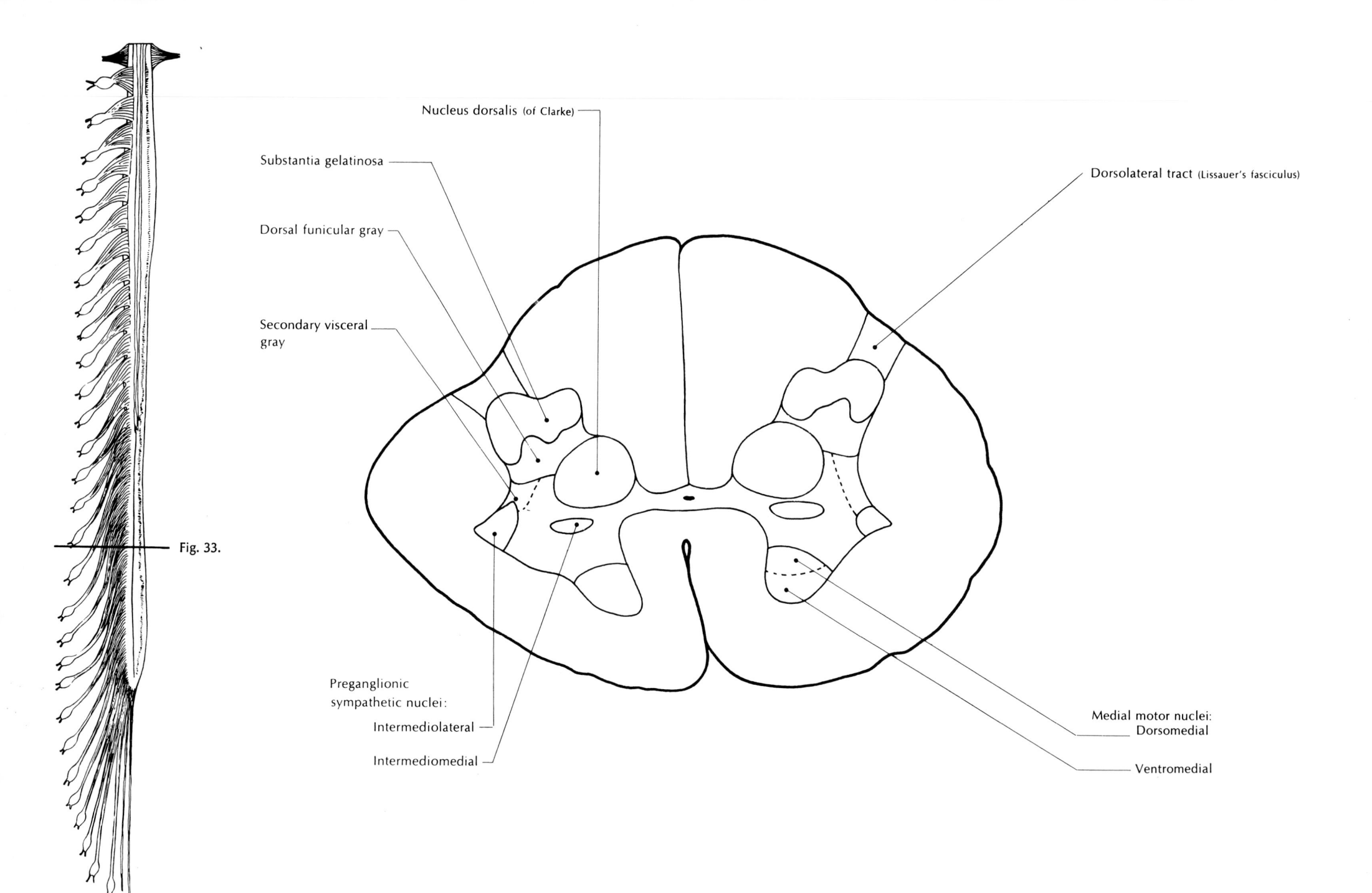

Nucleus dorsalis (of Clarke)

Substantia gelatinosa

Dorsolateral tract (Lissauer's fasciculus)

Dorsal funicular gray

Secondary visceral gray

Preganglionic sympathetic nuclei:

Intermediolateral

Intermediomedial

Medial motor nuclei:
Dorsomedial

Ventromedial

Fig. 33.

Figure 33. Nuclear organization of the upper lumbar cord (L1)—Nissl, 18×

66

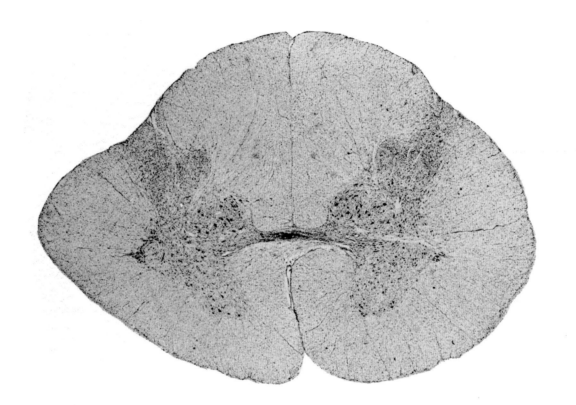

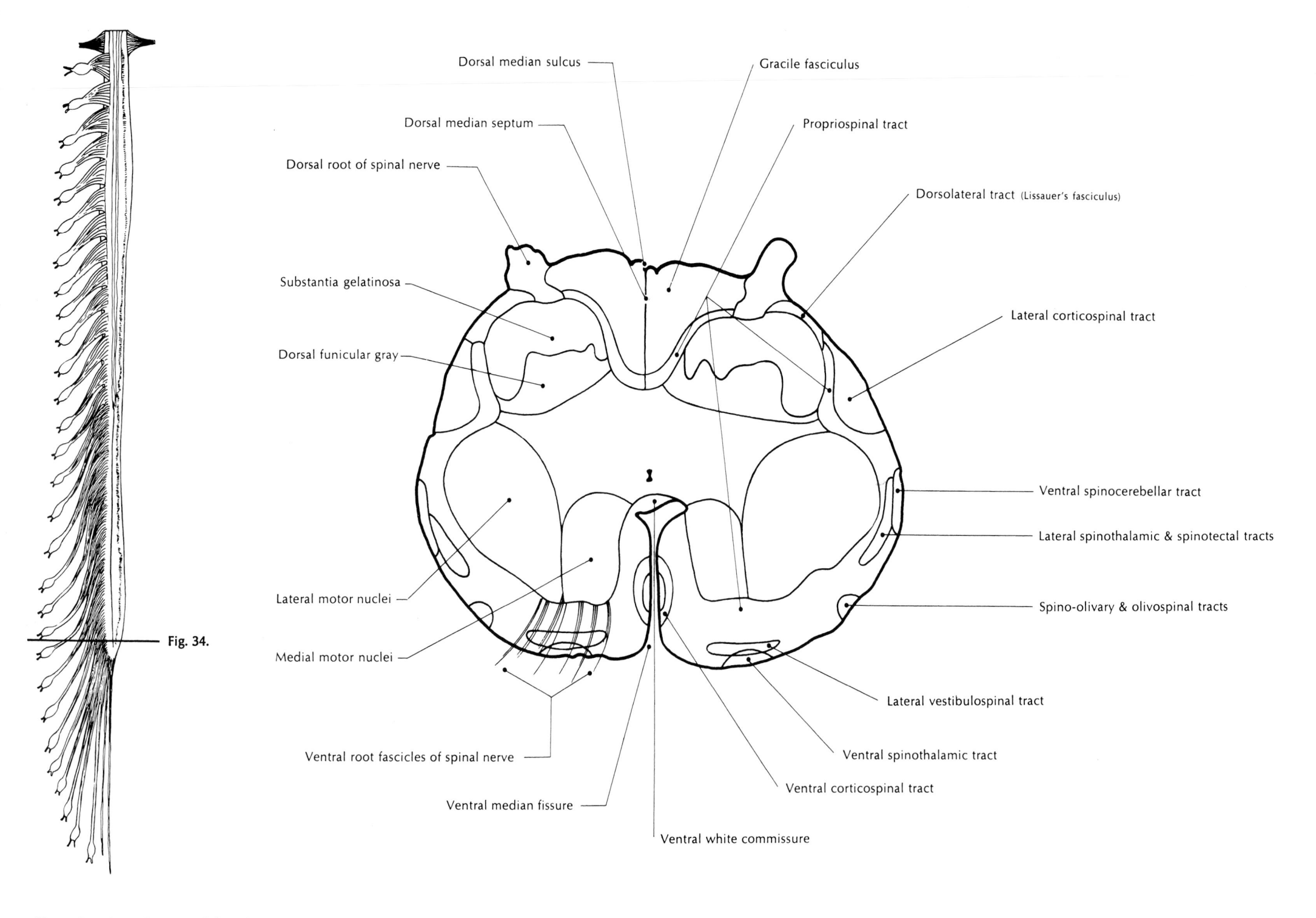

Dorsal median sulcus

Gracile fasciculus

Dorsal median septum

Propriospinal tract

Dorsal root of spinal nerve

Dorsolateral tract (Lissauer's fasciculus)

Substantia gelatinosa

Lateral corticospinal tract

Dorsal funicular gray

Ventral spinocerebellar tract

Lateral spinothalamic & spinotectal tracts

Spino-olivary & olivospinal tracts

Lateral motor nuclei

Medial motor nuclei

Lateral vestibulospinal tract

Ventral root fascicles of spinal nerve

Ventral spinothalamic tract

Ventral corticospinal tract

Ventral median fissure

Ventral white commissure

Fig. 34.

Figure 34. Organization of the white matter: Sacral cord (S3)—Weil, 18✕

68

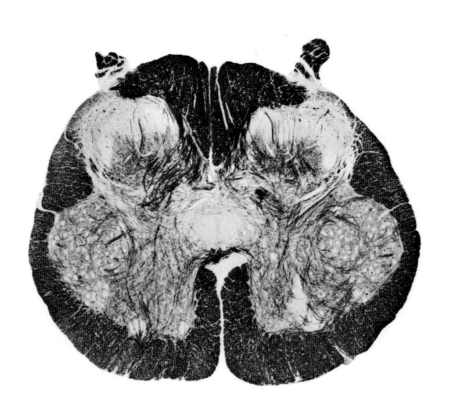

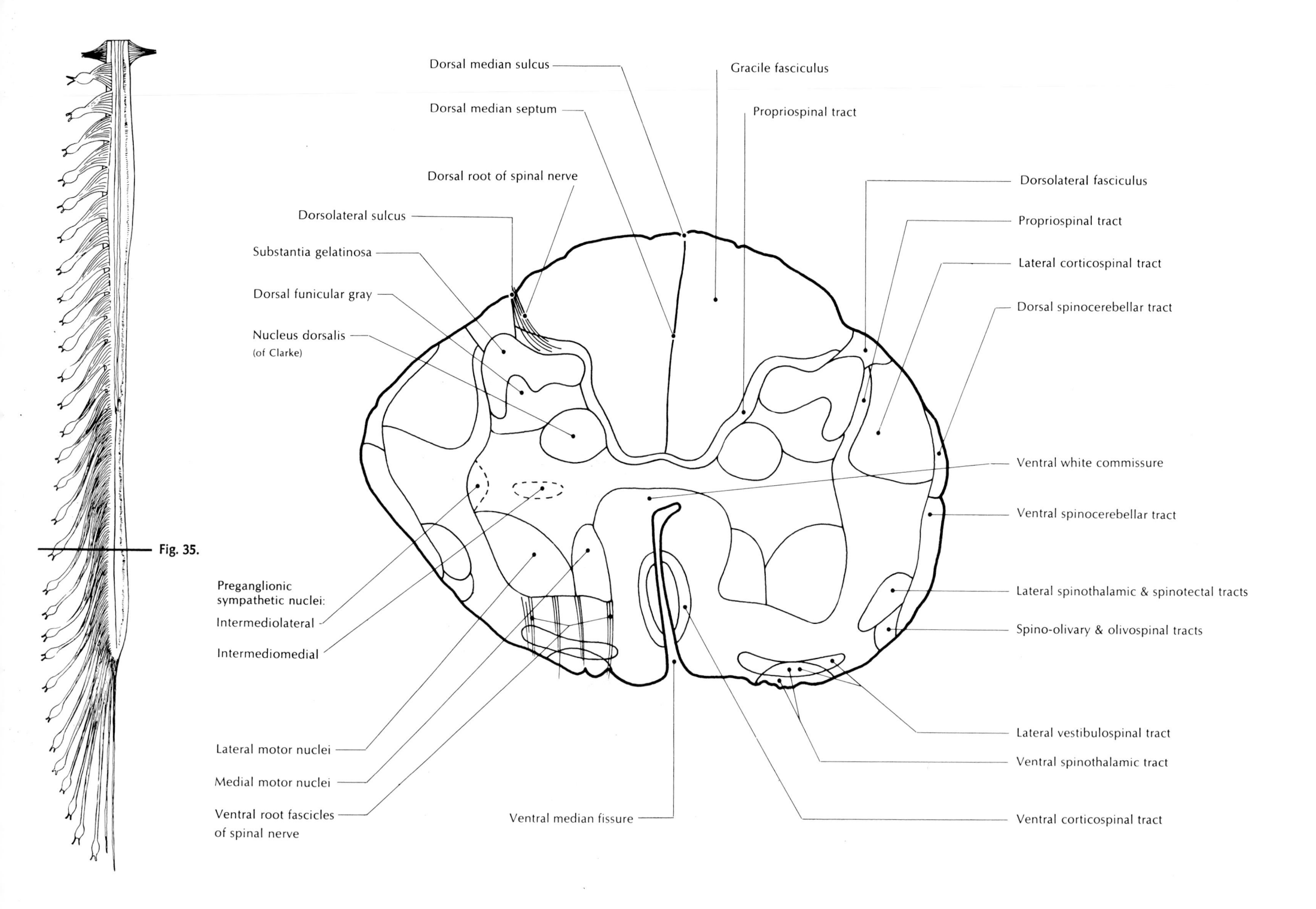

Dorsal median sulcus

Dorsal median septum

Dorsal root of spinal nerve

Dorsolateral sulcus

Substantia gelatinosa

Dorsal funicular gray

Nucleus dorsalis
(of Clarke)

Gracile fasciculus

Propriospinal tract

Dorsolateral fasciculus

Propriospinal tract

Lateral corticospinal tract

Dorsal spinocerebellar tract

Ventral white commissure

Ventral spinocerebellar tract

Fig. 35.

Preganglionic
sympathetic nuclei:

Intermediolateral

Intermediomedial

Lateral spinothalamic & spinotectal tracts

Spino-olivary & olivospinal tracts

Lateral vestibulospinal tract

Ventral spinothalamic tract

Lateral motor nuclei

Medial motor nuclei

Ventral root fascicles
of spinal nerve

Ventral median fissure

Ventral corticospinal tract

Figure 35. Organization of the white matter: Lumbar cord (L2)—Weil, 18×

70

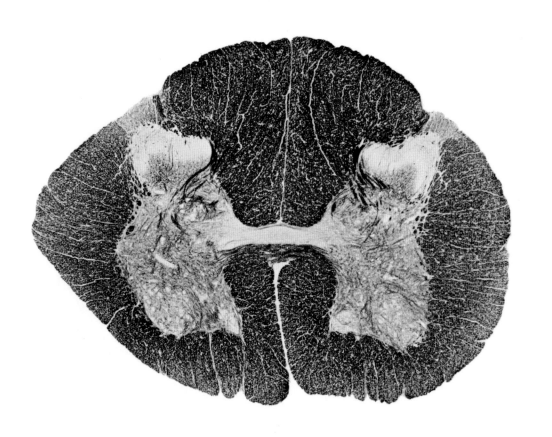

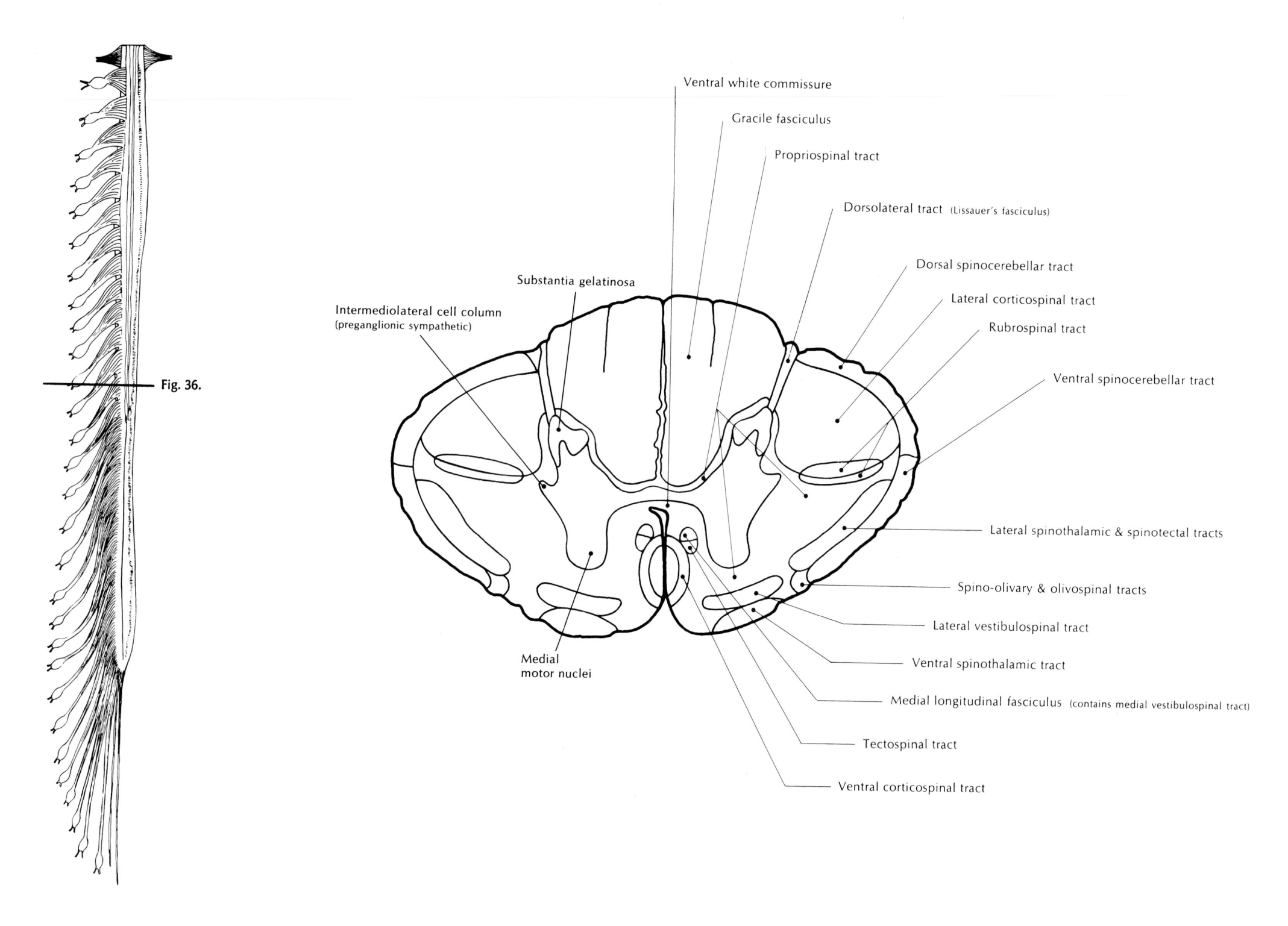

Figure 36. Organization of the white matter: Thoracic cord (T6)—Weil, 18×

Fig. 36.

Ventral white commissure

Gracile fasciculus

Propriospinal tract

Dorsolateral tract (Lissauer's fasciculus)

Dorsal spinocerebellar tract

Lateral corticospinal tract

Rubrospinal tract

Ventral spinocerebellar tract

Substantia gelatinosa

Intermediolateral cell column
(preganglionic sympathetic)

Lateral spinothalamic & spinotectal tracts

Spino-olivary & olivospinal tracts

Lateral vestibulospinal tract

Ventral spinothalamic tract

Medial longitudinal fasciculus (contains medial vestibulospinal tract)

Medial
motor nuclei

Tectospinal tract

Ventral corticospinal tract

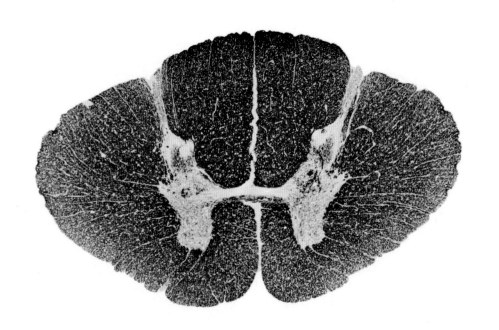

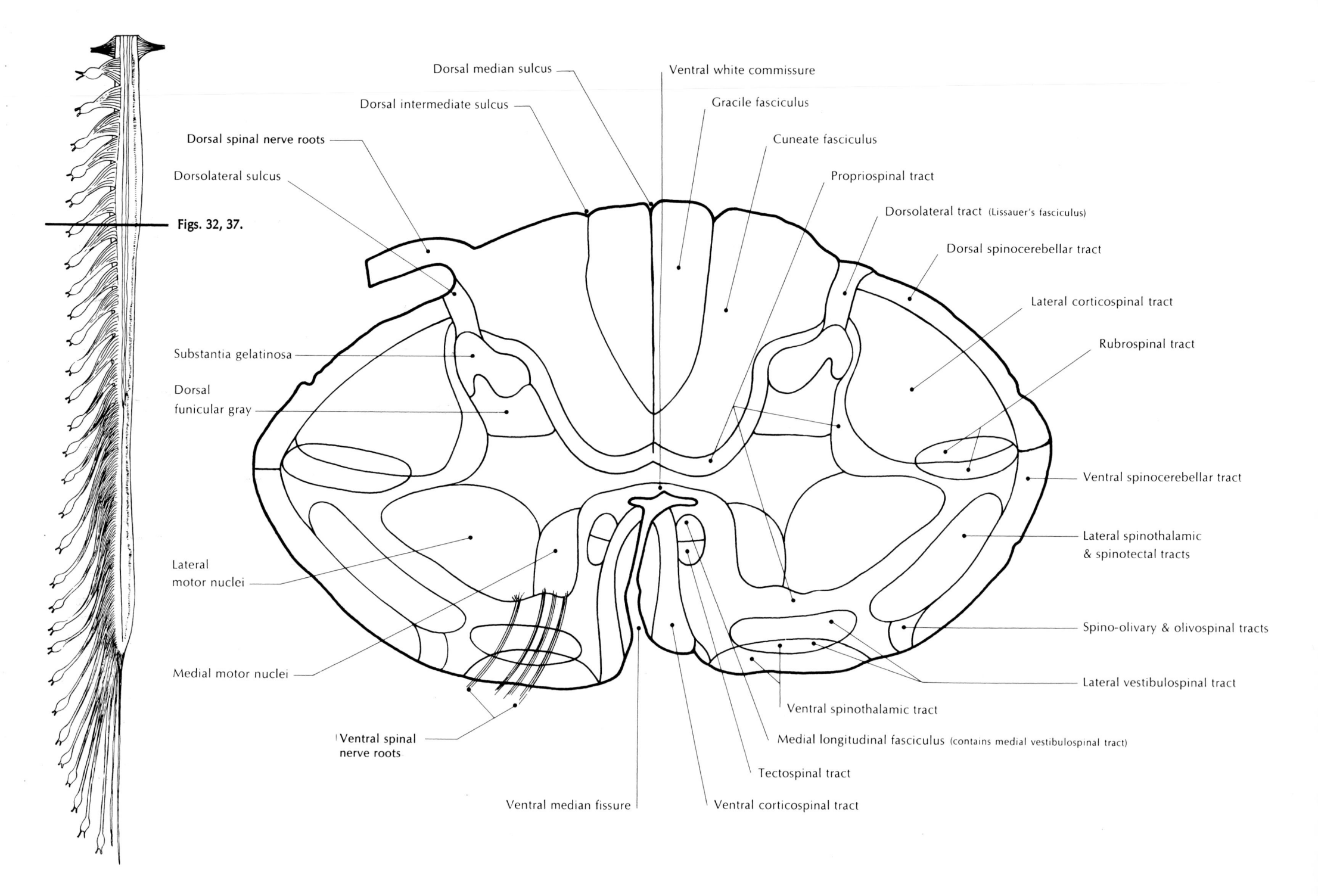

Dorsal median sulcus
Ventral white commissure
Dorsal intermediate sulcus
Gracile fasciculus
Dorsal spinal nerve roots
Cuneate fasciculus
Dorsolateral sulcus
Propriospinal tract
Dorsolateral tract (Lissauer's fasciculus)
Dorsal spinocerebellar tract
Figs. 32, 37.
Lateral corticospinal tract
Substantia gelatinosa
Rubrospinal tract
Dorsal funicular gray
Ventral spinocerebellar tract
Lateral spinothalamic & spinotectal tracts
Lateral motor nuclei
Spino-olivary & olivospinal tracts
Medial motor nuclei
Lateral vestibulospinal tract
Ventral spinothalamic tract
Ventral spinal nerve roots
Medial longitudinal fasciculus (contains medial vestibulospinal tract)
Tectospinal tract
Ventral median fissure
Ventral corticospinal tract

Figure 37. Organization of the white matter: Cervical cord enlargement (C8)—Weil, 18×

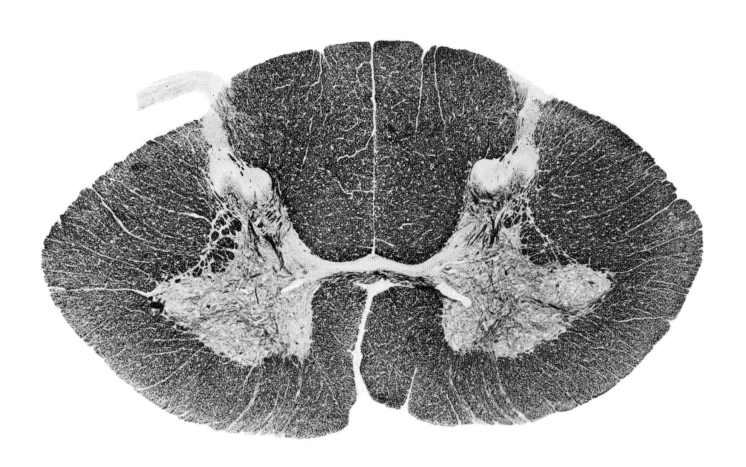

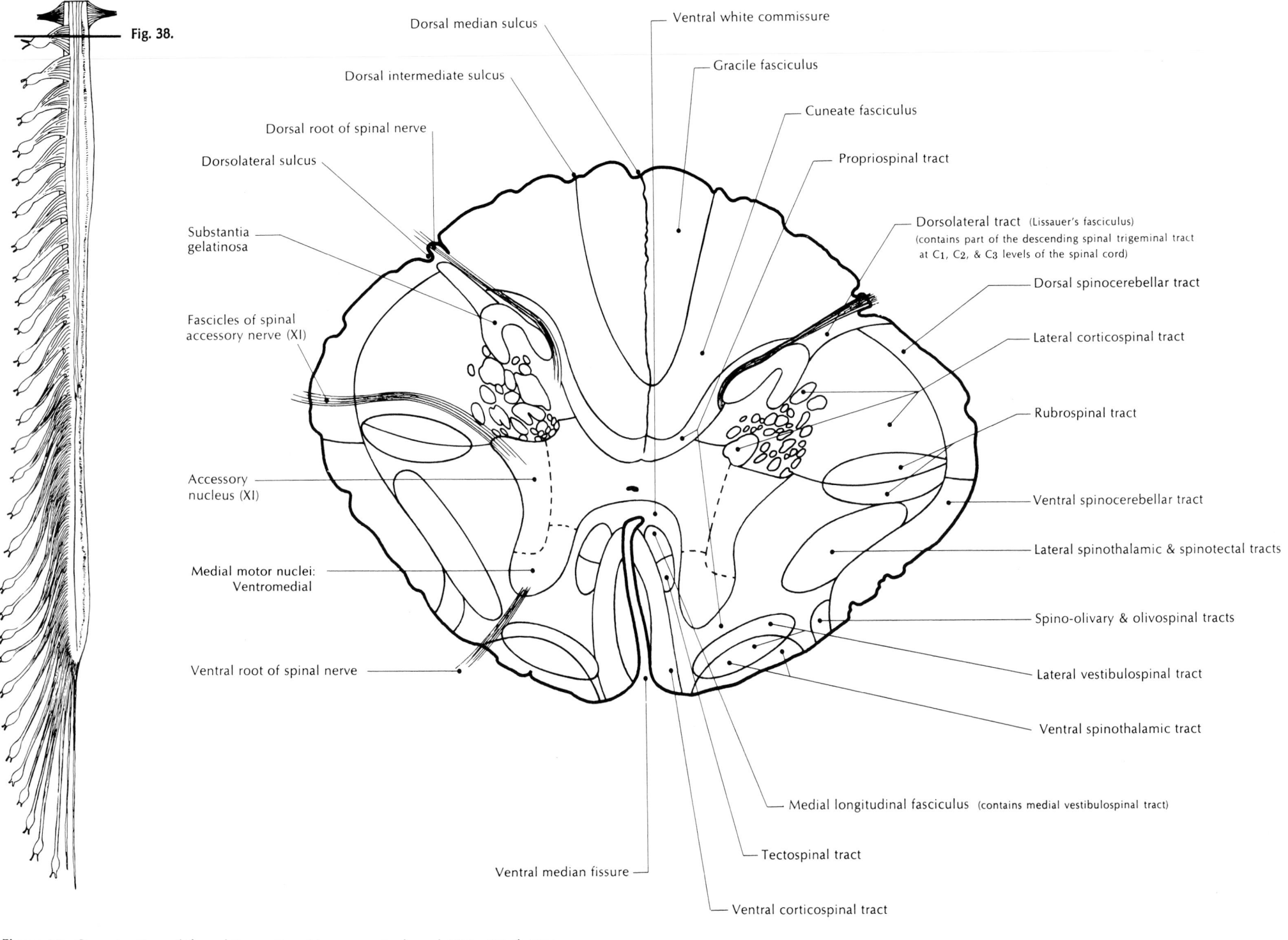

Fig. 38.

Dorsal median sulcus

Dorsal intermediate sulcus

Dorsal root of spinal nerve

Dorsolateral sulcus

Substantia gelatinosa

Fascicles of spinal accessory nerve (XI)

Accessory nucleus (XI)

Medial motor nuclei: Ventromedial

Ventral root of spinal nerve

Ventral white commissure

Gracile fasciculus

Cuneate fasciculus

Propriospinal tract

Dorsolateral tract (Lissauer's fasciculus) (contains part of the descending spinal trigeminal tract at C₁, C₂, & C₃ levels of the spinal cord)

Dorsal spinocerebellar tract

Lateral corticospinal tract

Rubrospinal tract

Ventral spinocerebellar tract

Lateral spinothalamic & spinotectal tracts

Spino-olivary & olivospinal tracts

Lateral vestibulospinal tract

Ventral spinothalamic tract

Medial longitudinal fasciculus (contains medial vestibulospinal tract)

Tectospinal tract

Ventral median fissure

Ventral corticospinal tract

Figure 38. Organization of the white matter: Upper cervical cord (C2)—Weil, 18×

76

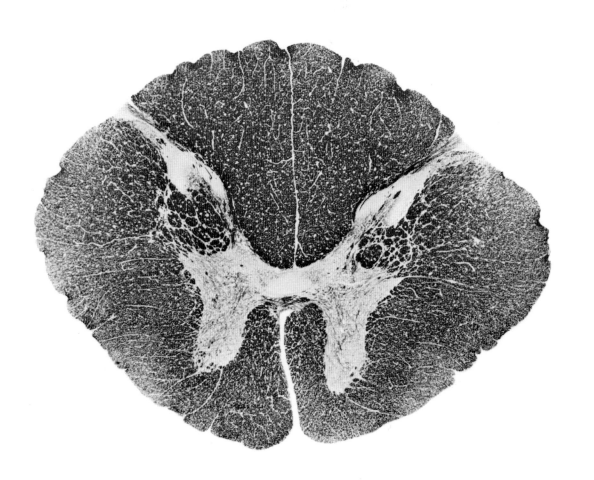

TRANSVERSE MICROSCOPIC SECTIONS OF THE BRAIN STEM

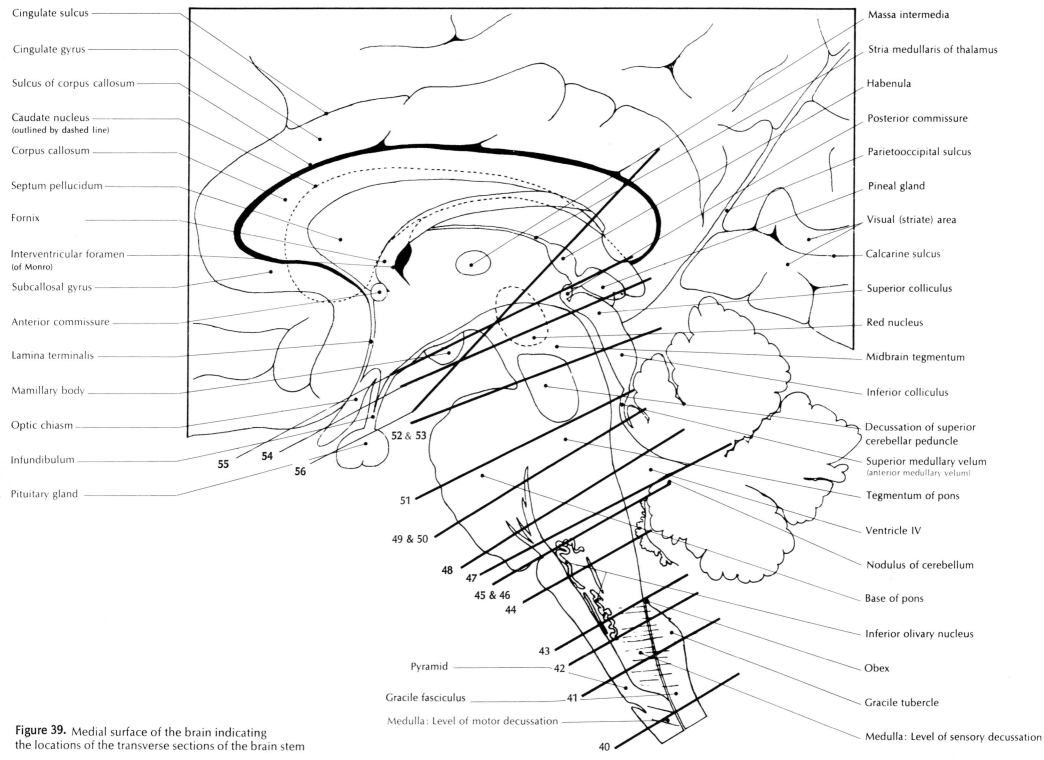

Figure 39. Medial surface of the brain indicating the locations of the transverse sections of the brain stem

Cingulate sulcus

Cingulate gyrus

Sulcus of corpus callosum

Caudate nucleus
(outlined by dashed line)

Corpus callosum

Septum pellucidum

Fornix

Interventricular foramen
(of Monro)

Subcallosal gyrus

Anterior commissure

Lamina terminalis

Mamillary body

Optic chiasm

Infundibulum

Pituitary gland

Massa intermedia

Stria medullaris of thalamus

Habenula

Posterior commissure

Parietooccipital sulcus

Pineal gland

Visual (striate) area

Calcarine sulcus

Superior colliculus

Red nucleus

Midbrain tegmentum

Inferior colliculus

Decussation of superior
cerebellar peduncle

Superior medullary velum
(anterior medullary velum)

Tegmentum of pons

Ventricle IV

Nodulus of cerebellum

Base of pons

Inferior olivary nucleus

Obex

Gracile tubercle

Medulla: Level of sensory decussation

Pyramid

Gracile fasciculus

Medulla: Level of motor decussation

52 & 53

55   54

56

51

49 & 50

48   47

45 & 46

44

43

42

41

40

79

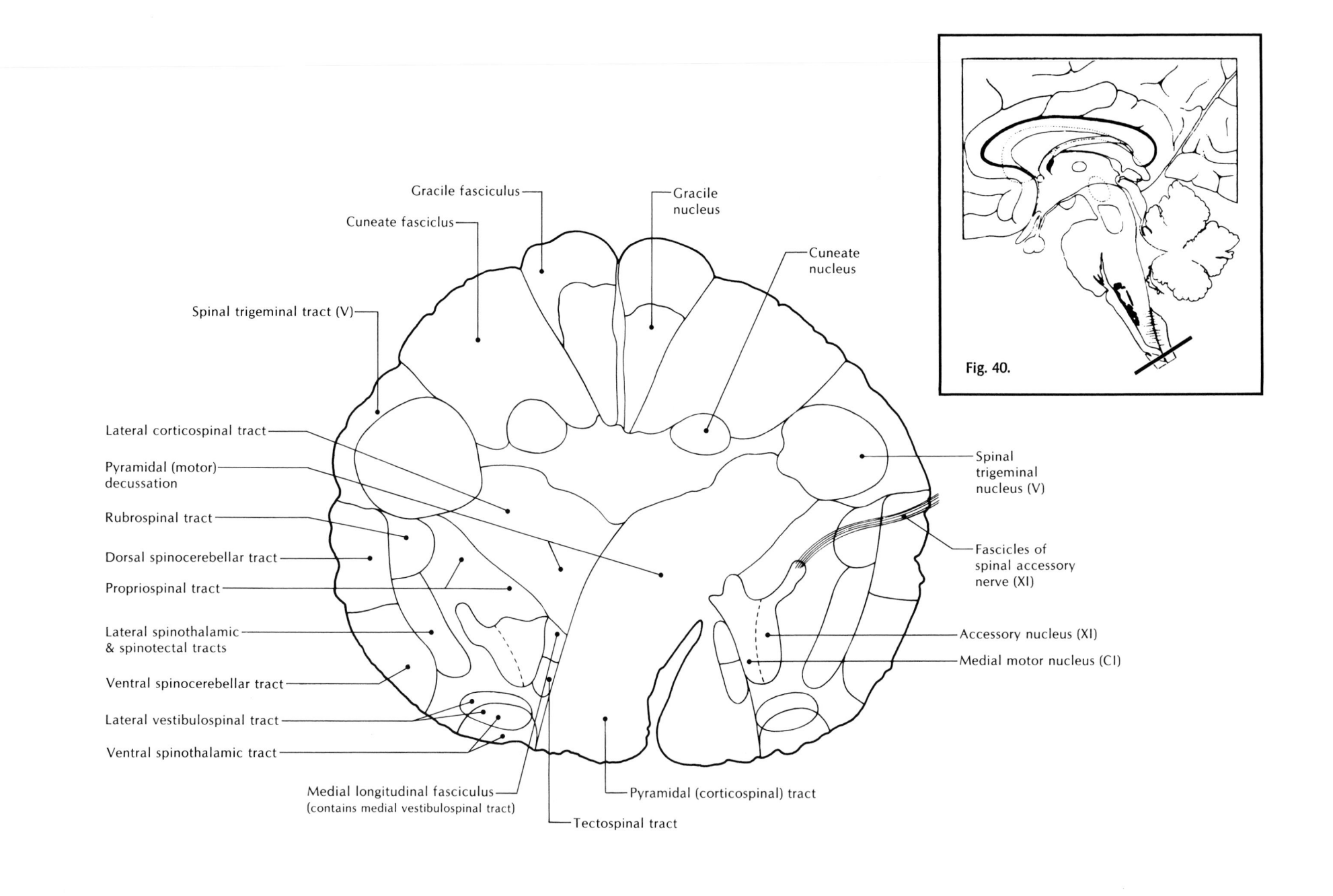

Gracile fasciculus

Gracile nucleus

Cuneate fasciclus

Cuneate nucleus

Spinal trigeminal tract (V)

Lateral corticospinal tract

Pyramidal (motor) decussation

Rubrospinal tract

Dorsal spinocerebellar tract

Propriospinal tract

Lateral spinothalamic & spinotectal tracts

Ventral spinocerebellar tract

Lateral vestibulospinal tract

Ventral spinothalamic tract

Spinal trigeminal nucleus (V)

Fascicles of spinal accessory nerve (XI)

Accessory nucleus (XI)

Medial motor nucleus (CI)

Medial longitudinal fasciculus (contains medial vestibulospinal tract)

Pyramidal (corticospinal) tract

Tectospinal tract

Fig. 40.

Figure 40. Medulla: Motor decussation—Weil, 10×

80

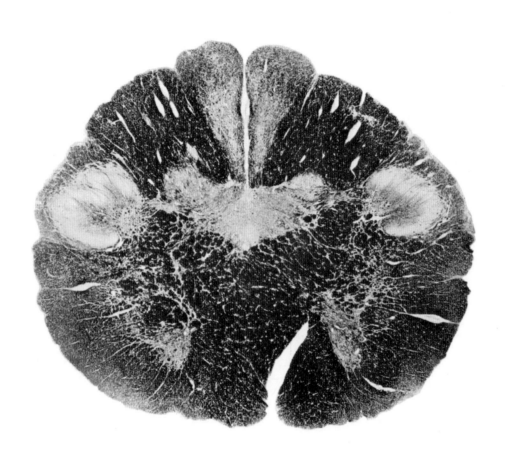

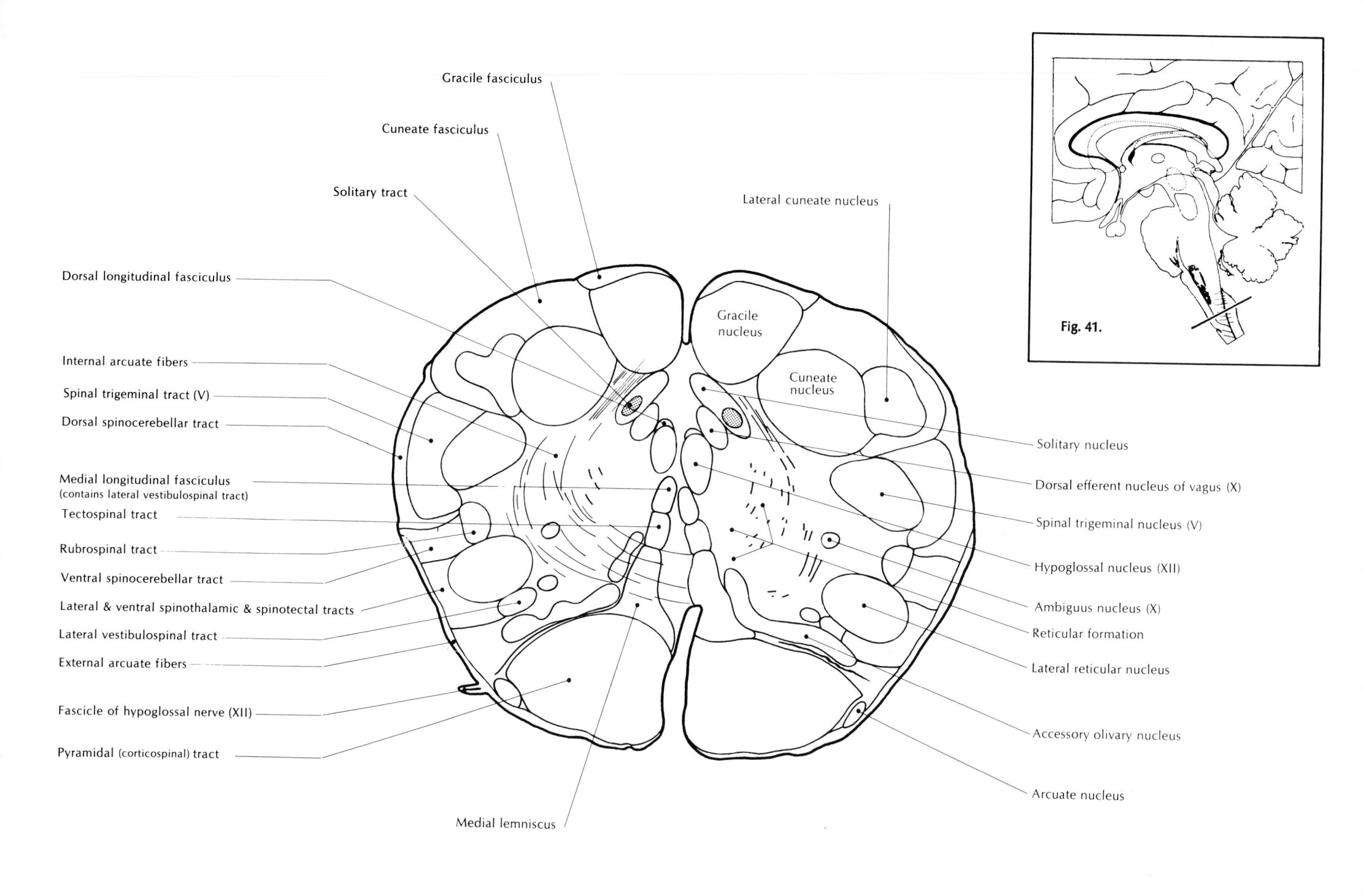

Gracile fasciculus

Cuneate fasciculus

Solitary tract

Lateral cuneate nucleus

Dorsal longitudinal fasciculus

Internal arcuate fibers

Spinal trigeminal tract (V)

Dorsal spinocerebellar tract

Medial longitudinal fasciculus
(contains lateral vestibulospinal tract)

Tectospinal tract

Rubrospinal tract

Ventral spinocerebellar tract

Lateral & ventral spinothalamic & spinotectal tracts

Lateral vestibulospinal tract

External arcuate fibers

Fascicle of hypoglossal nerve (XII)

Pyramidal (corticospinal) tract

Gracile
nucleus

Cuneate
nucleus

Solitary nucleus

Dorsal efferent nucleus of vagus (X)

Spinal trigeminal nucleus (V)

Hypoglossal nucleus (XII)

Ambiguus nucleus (X)

Reticular formation

Lateral reticular nucleus

Accessory olivary nucleus

Arcuate nucleus

Medial lemniscus

Fig. 41.

Figure 41. Medulla: Sensory decussation—Weil, 10×

82

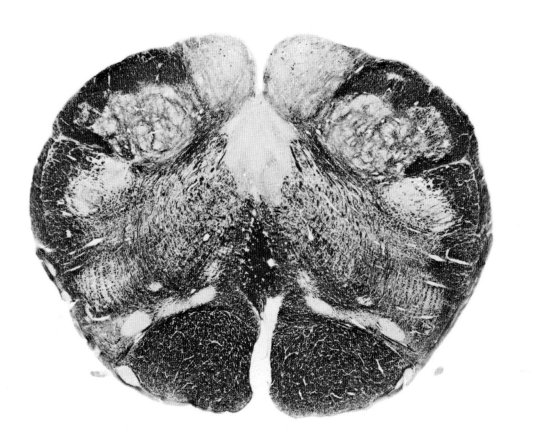

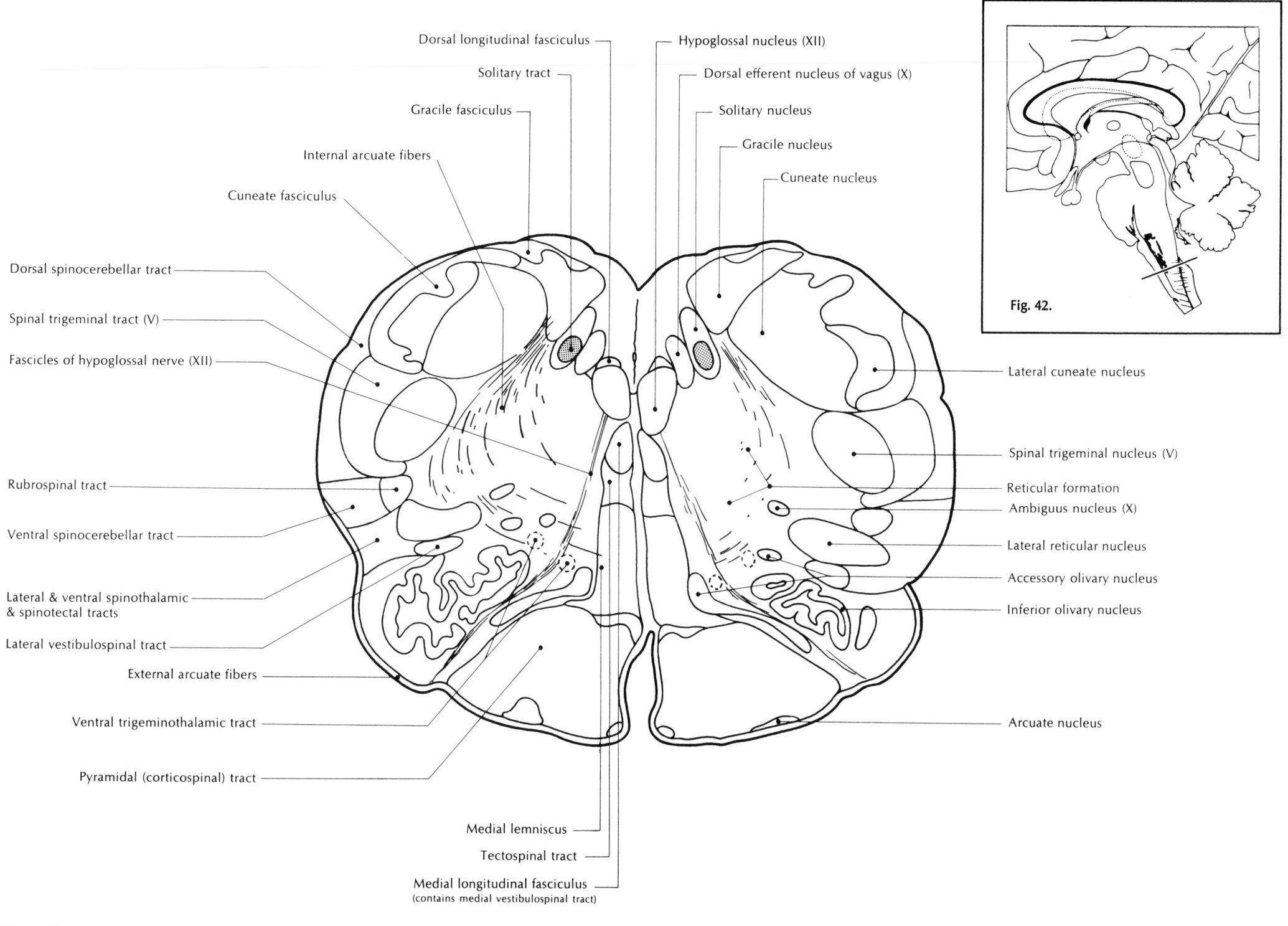

Dorsal longitudinal fasciculus

Solitary tract

Gracile fasciculus

Internal arcuate fibers

Cuneate fasciculus

Hypoglossal nucleus (XII)

Dorsal efferent nucleus of vagus (X)

Solitary nucleus

Gracile nucleus

Cuneate nucleus

Dorsal spinocerebellar tract

Spinal trigeminal tract (V)

Fascicles of hypoglossal nerve (XII)

Rubrospinal tract

Ventral spinocerebellar tract

Lateral & ventral spinothalamic & spinotectal tracts

Lateral vestibulospinal tract

External arcuate fibers

Ventral trigeminothalamic tract

Pyramidal (corticospinal) tract

Fig. 42.

Lateral cuneate nucleus

Spinal trigeminal nucleus (V)

Reticular formation

Ambiguus nucleus (X)

Lateral reticular nucleus

Accessory olivary nucleus

Inferior olivary nucleus

Arcuate nucleus

Medial lemniscus

Tectospinal tract

Medial longitudinal fasciculus
(contains medial vestibulospinal tract)

Figure 42. Medulla: Rostral sensory decussation—Weil, 10X

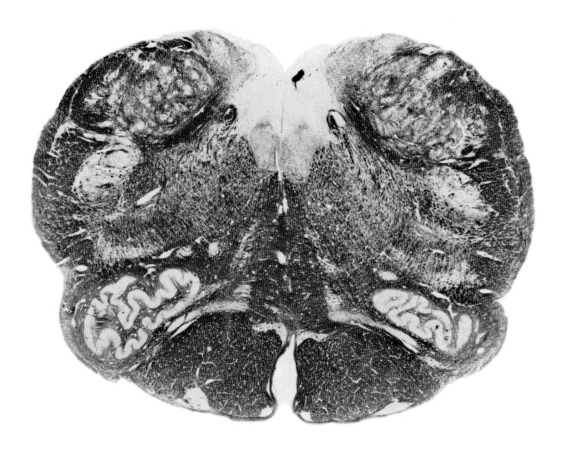

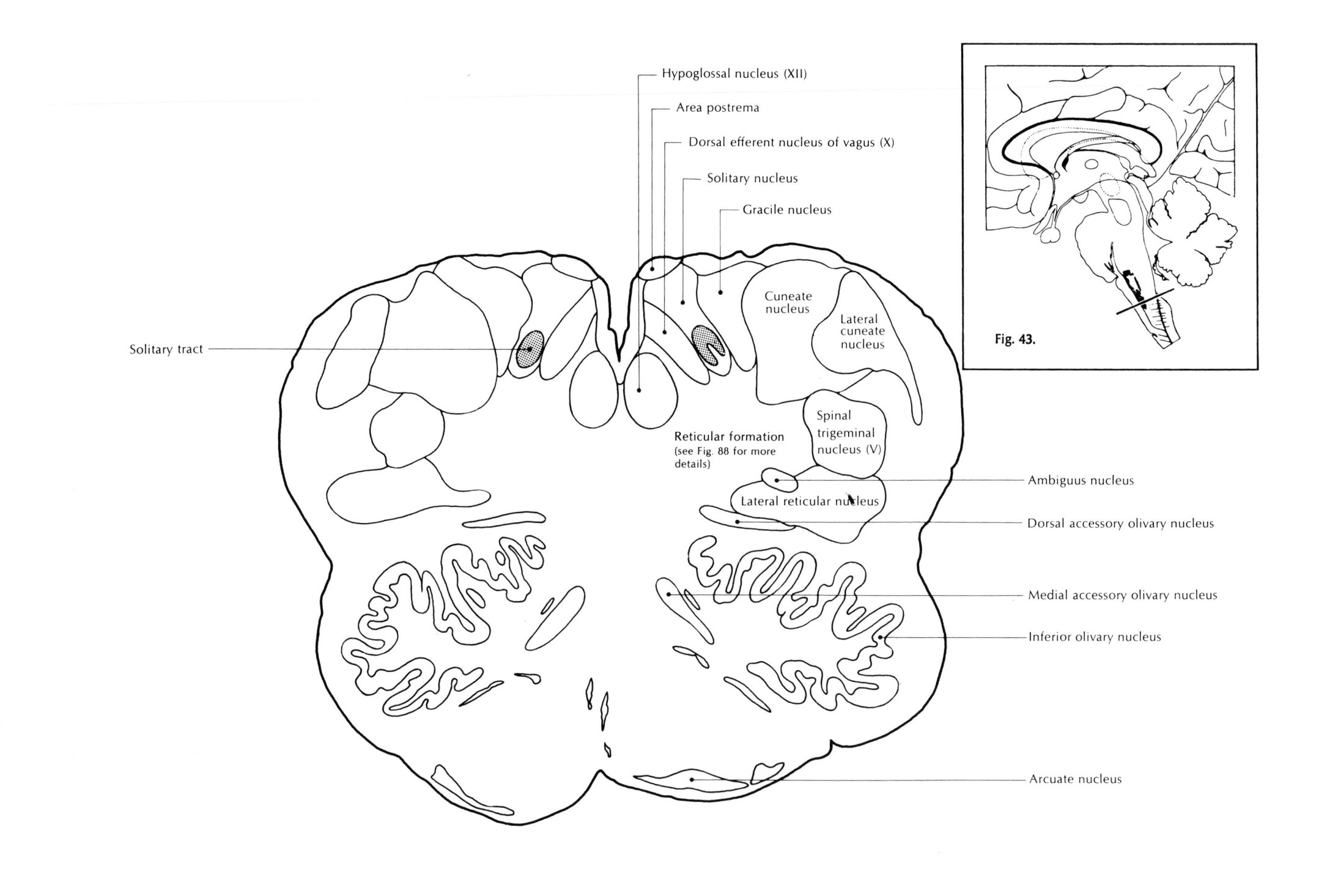

Hypoglossal nucleus (XII)

Area postrema

Dorsal efferent nucleus of vagus (X)

Solitary nucleus

Gracile nucleus

Cuneate nucleus

Lateral cuneate nucleus

Solitary tract

Spinal trigeminal nucleus (V)

Reticular formation (see Fig. 88 for more details)

Lateral reticular nucleus

Ambiguus nucleus

Dorsal accessory olivary nucleus

Medial accessory olivary nucleus

Inferior olivary nucleus

Arcuate nucleus

Fig. 43.

Figure 43. Medulla (obex; transition from closed to open medulla): Level of cranial nerve nuclei X and XII—Nissl, 10×

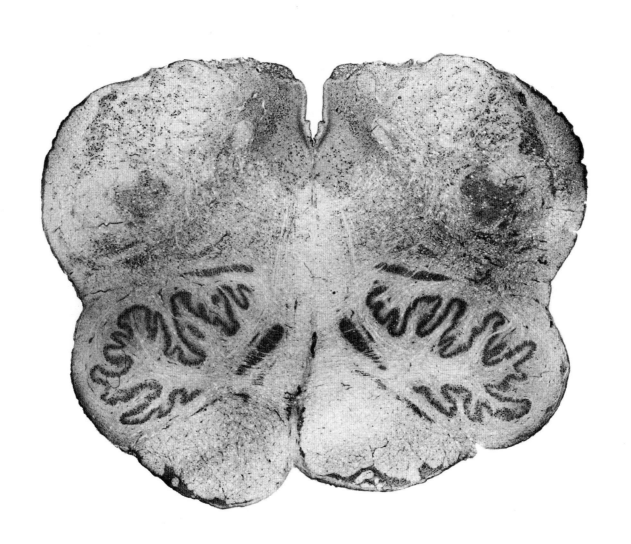

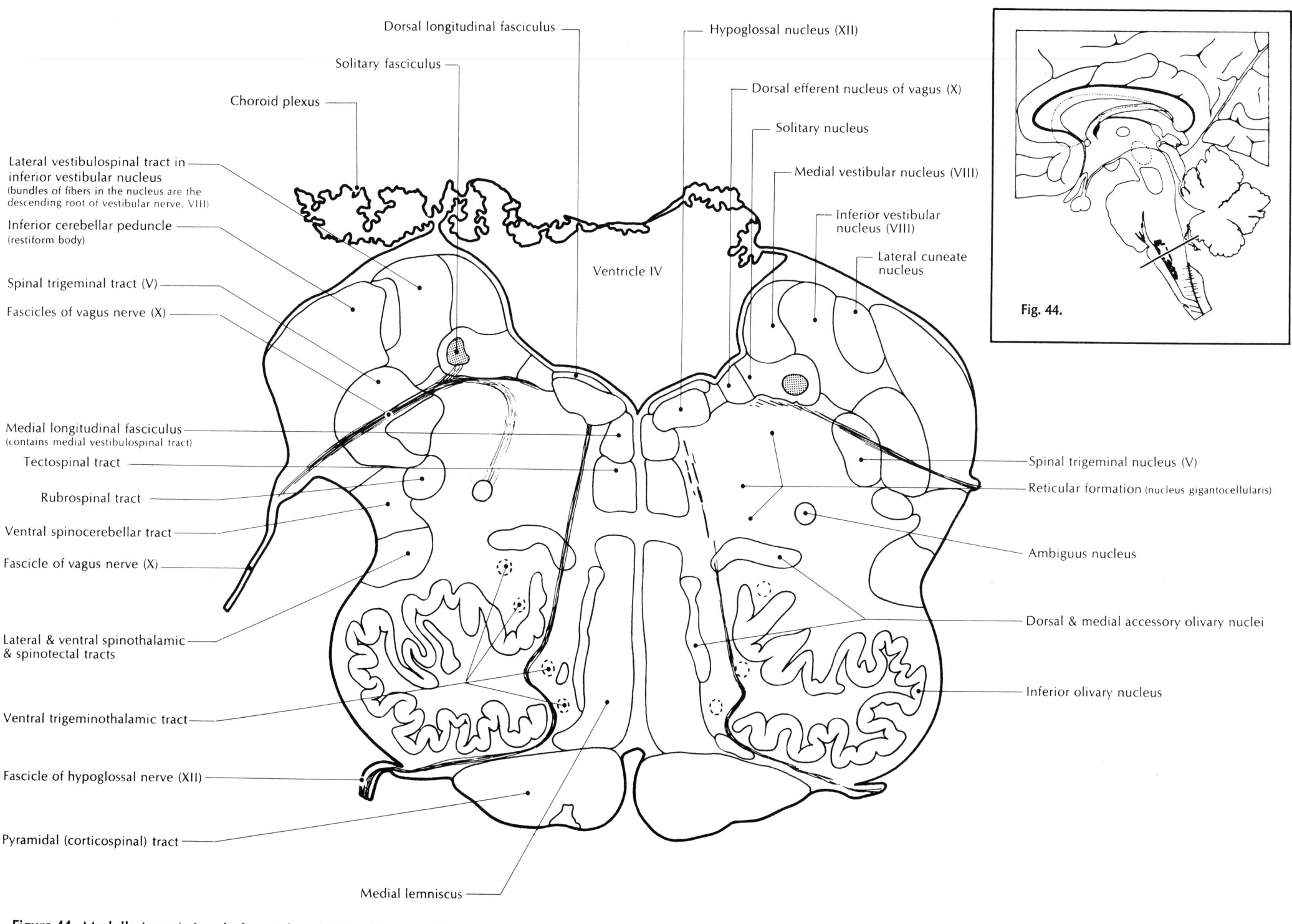

Dorsal longitudinal fasciculus

Solitary fasciculus

Choroid plexus

Hypoglossal nucleus (XII)

Dorsal efferent nucleus of vagus (X)

Solitary nucleus

Medial vestibular nucleus (VIII)

Inferior vestibular nucleus (VIII)

Lateral cuneate nucleus

Lateral vestibulospinal tract in inferior vestibular nucleus
(bundles of fibers in the nucleus are the descending root of vestibular nerve, VIII)

Inferior cerebellar peduncle
(restiform body)

Spinal trigeminal tract (V)

Fascicles of vagus nerve (X)

Ventricle IV

Medial longitudinal fasciculus
(contains medial vestibulospinal tract)

Tectospinal tract

Rubrospinal tract

Ventral spinocerebellar tract

Fascicle of vagus nerve (X)

Lateral & ventral spinothalamic & spinotectal tracts

Ventral trigeminothalamic tract

Fascicle of hypoglossal nerve (XII)

Pyramidal (corticospinal) tract

Medial lemniscus

Spinal trigeminal nucleus (V)

Reticular formation (nucleus gigantocellularis)

Ambiguus nucleus

Dorsal & medial accessory olivary nuclei

Inferior olivary nucleus

Fig. 44.

Figure 44. Medulla (open): Level of cranial nuclei X and XII—Weil, 10X

88

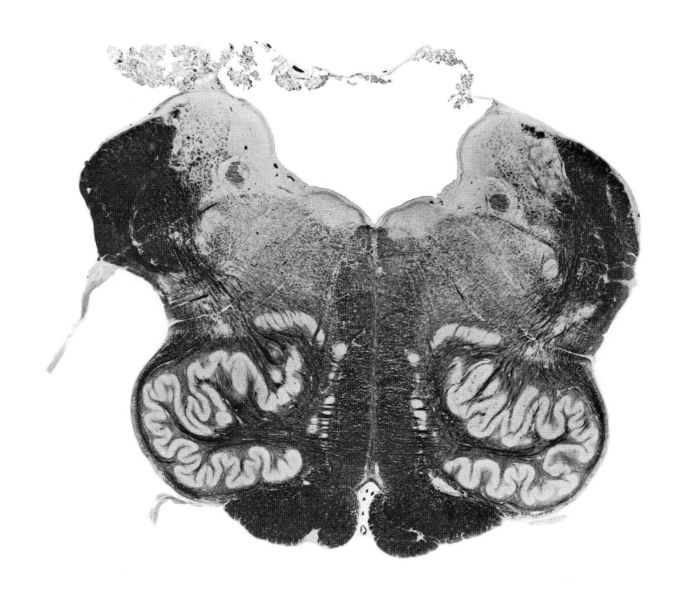

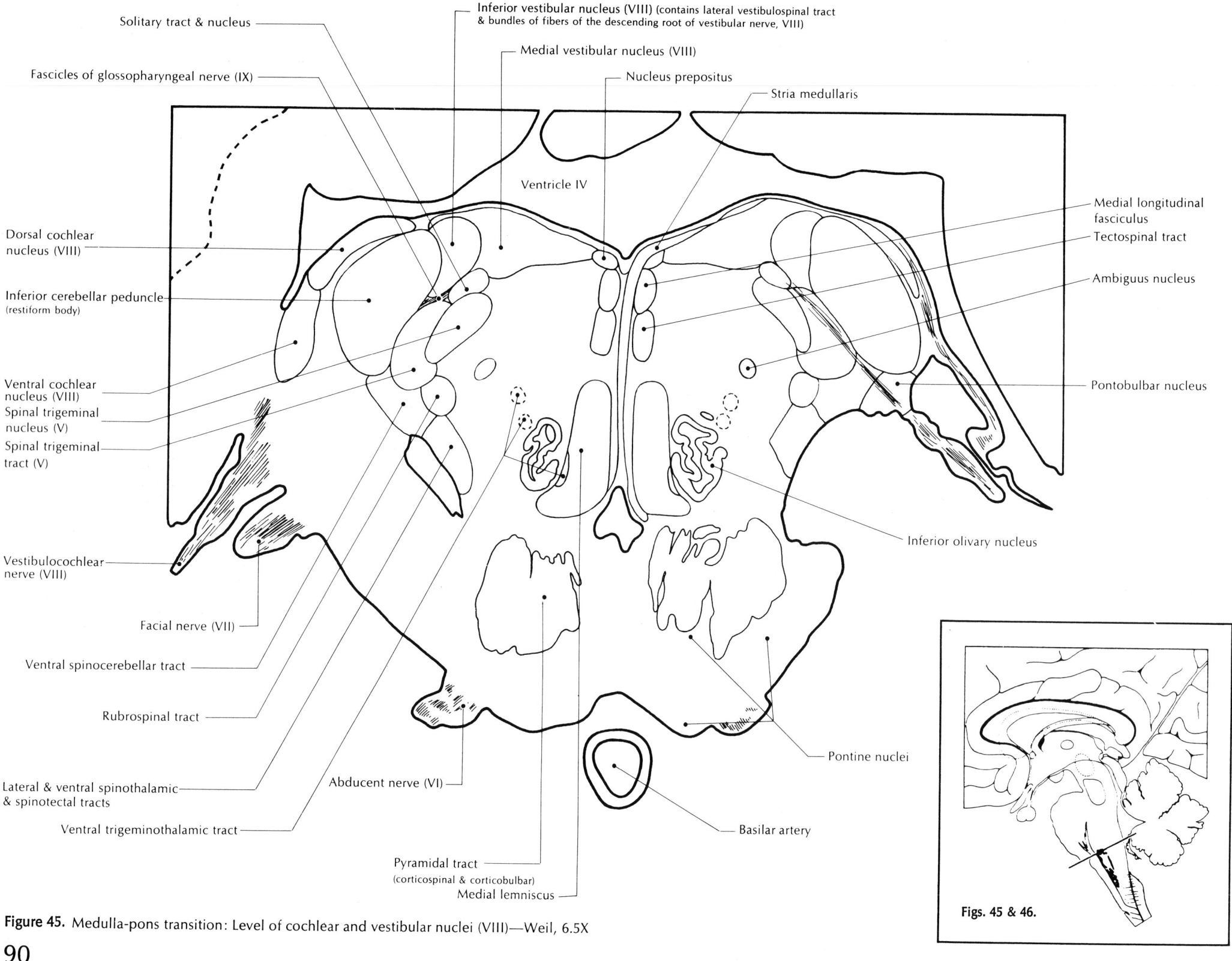

Solitary tract & nucleus

Inferior vestibular nucleus (VIII) (contains lateral vestibulospinal tract & bundles of fibers of the descending root of vestibular nerve, VIII)

Medial vestibular nucleus (VIII)

Nucleus prepositus

Stria medullaris

Fascicles of glossopharyngeal nerve (IX)

Ventricle IV

Medial longitudinal fasciculus

Dorsal cochlear nucleus (VIII)

Tectospinal tract

Inferior cerebellar peduncle (restiform body)

Ambiguus nucleus

Ventral cochlear nucleus (VIII)

Pontobulbar nucleus

Spinal trigeminal nucleus (V)

Spinal trigeminal tract (V)

Inferior olivary nucleus

Vestibulocochlear nerve (VIII)

Facial nerve (VII)

Ventral spinocerebellar tract

Rubrospinal tract

Pontine nuclei

Lateral & ventral spinothalamic & spinotectal tracts

Abducent nerve (VI)

Ventral trigeminothalamic tract

Basilar artery

Pyramidal tract (corticospinal & corticobulbar)

Medial lemniscus

Figs. 45 & 46.

Figure 45. Medulla-pons transition: Level of cochlear and vestibular nuclei (VIII)—Weil, 6.5X

90

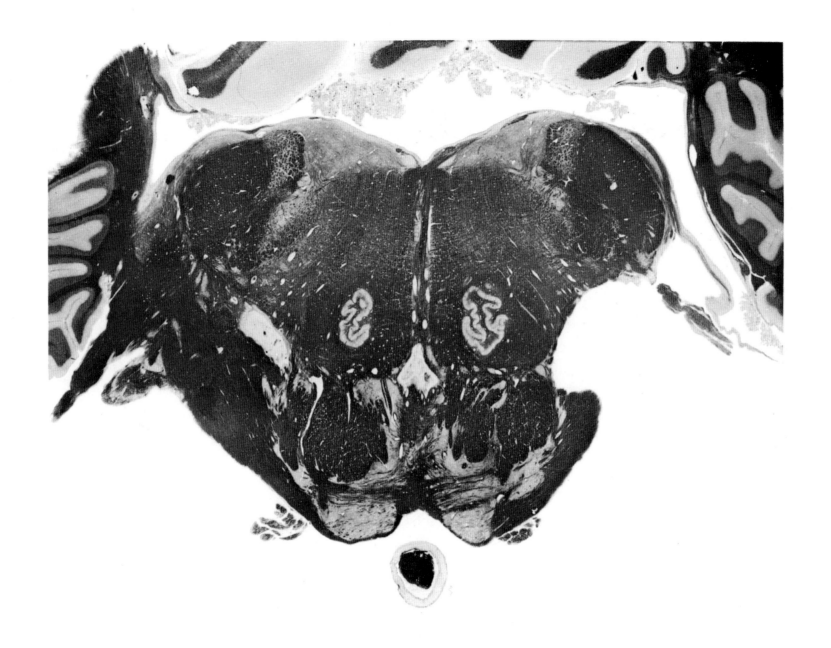

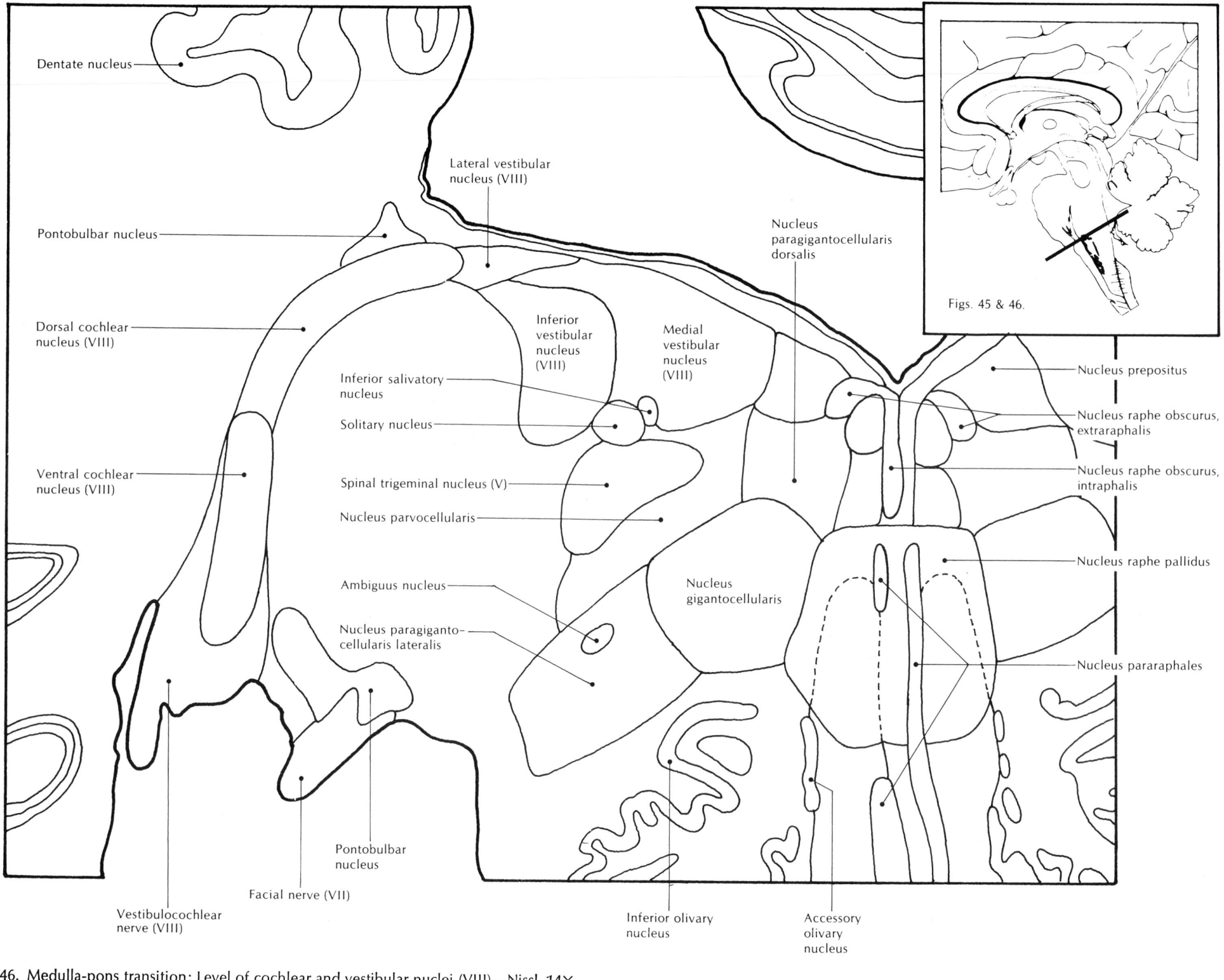

Figure 46. Medulla-pons transition: Level of cochlear and vestibular nuclei (VIII)—Nissl, 14×

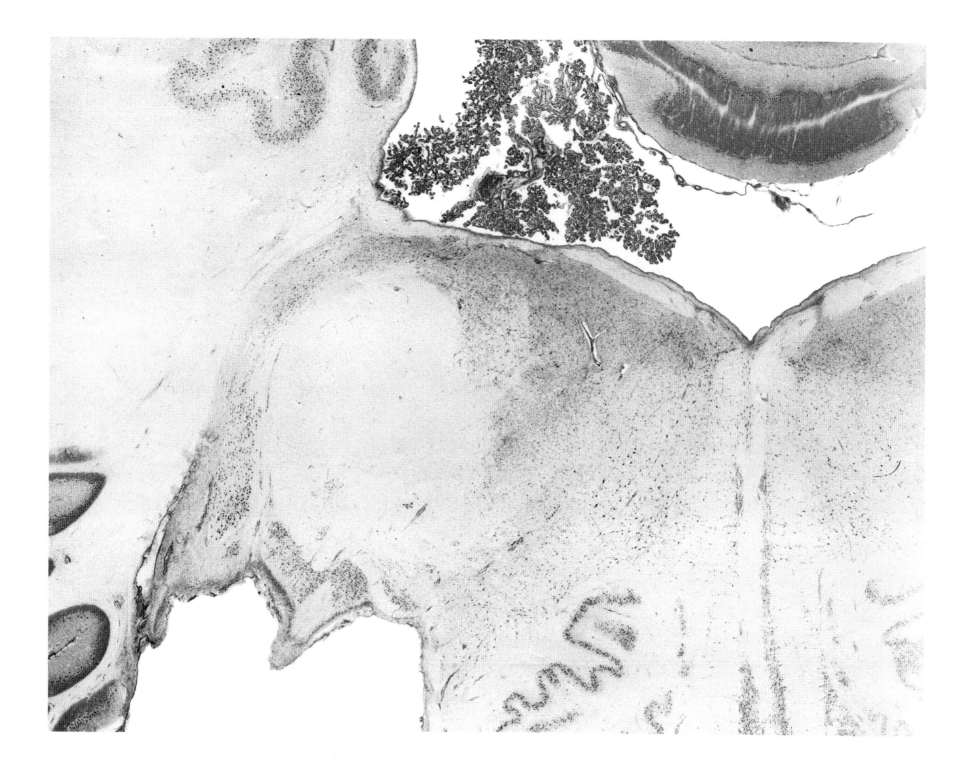

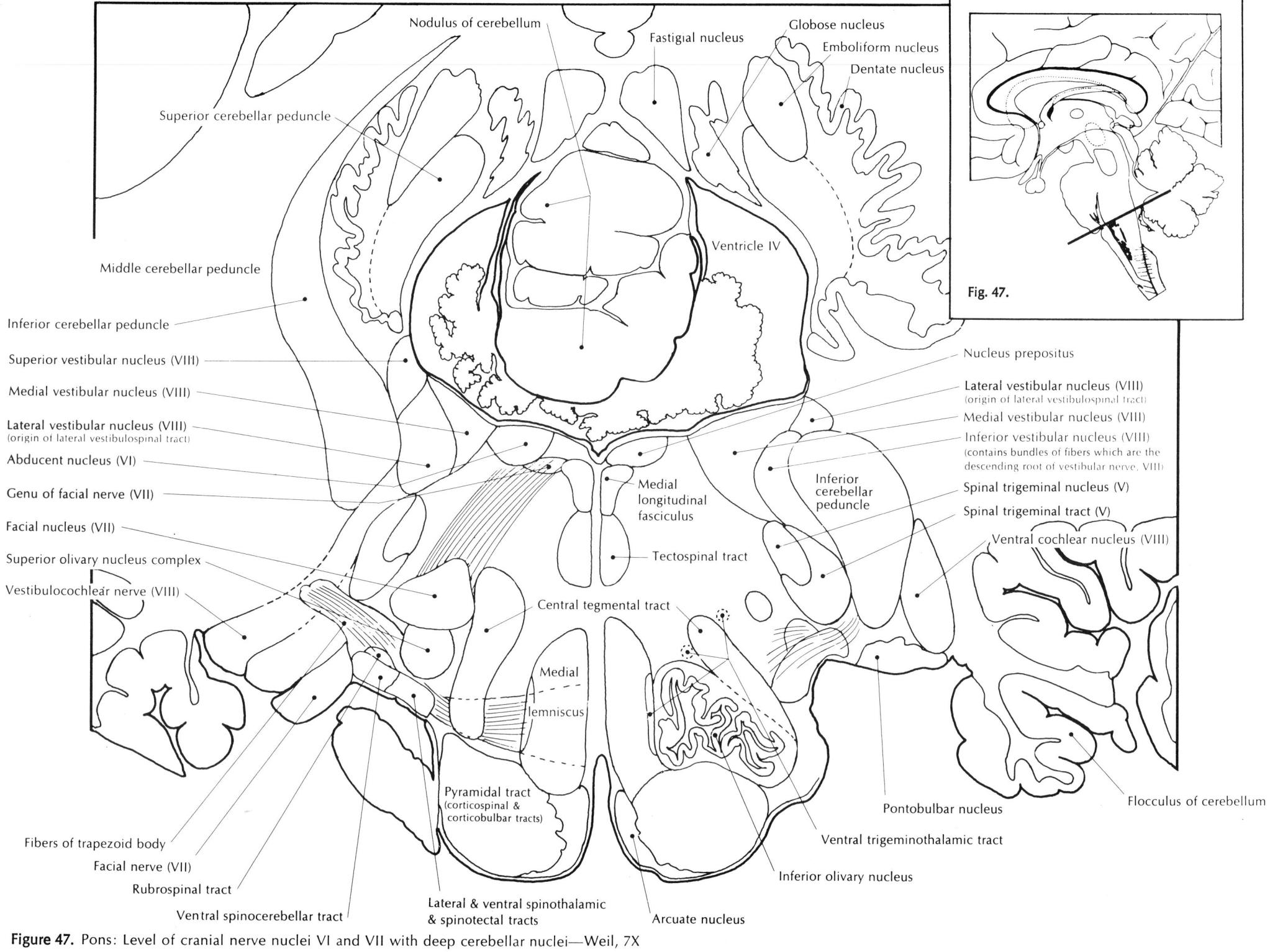

Figure 47. Pons: Level of cranial nerve nuclei VI and VII with deep cerebellar nuclei—Weil, 7X

Nodulus of cerebellum

Fastigial nucleus

Globose nucleus

Emboliform nucleus

Dentate nucleus

Superior cerebellar peduncle

Ventricle IV

Middle cerebellar peduncle

Inferior cerebellar peduncle

Nucleus prepositus

Superior vestibular nucleus (VIII)

Lateral vestibular nucleus (VIII)
(origin of lateral vestibulospinal tract)

Medial vestibular nucleus (VIII)

Medial vestibular nucleus (VIII)

Inferior vestibular nucleus (VIII)
(contains bundles of fibers which are the
descending root of vestibular nerve, VIII)

Lateral vestibular nucleus (VIII)
(origin of lateral vestibulospinal tract)

Abducent nucleus (VI)

Inferior
cerebellar
peduncle

Spinal trigeminal nucleus (V)

Genu of facial nerve (VII)

Medial
longitudinal
fasciculus

Spinal trigeminal tract (V)

Facial nucleus (VII)

Ventral cochlear nucleus (VIII)

Superior olivary nucleus complex

Tectospinal tract

Vestibulocochlear nerve (VIII)

Central tegmental tract

Medial
lemniscus

Fibers of trapezoid body

Pyramidal tract
(corticospinal &
corticobulbar tracts)

Pontobulbar nucleus

Facial nerve (VII)

Ventral trigeminothalamic tract

Rubrospinal tract

Inferior olivary nucleus

Ventral spinocerebellar tract

Lateral & ventral spinothalamic
& spinotectal tracts

Arcuate nucleus

Flocculus of cerebellum

Fig. 47.

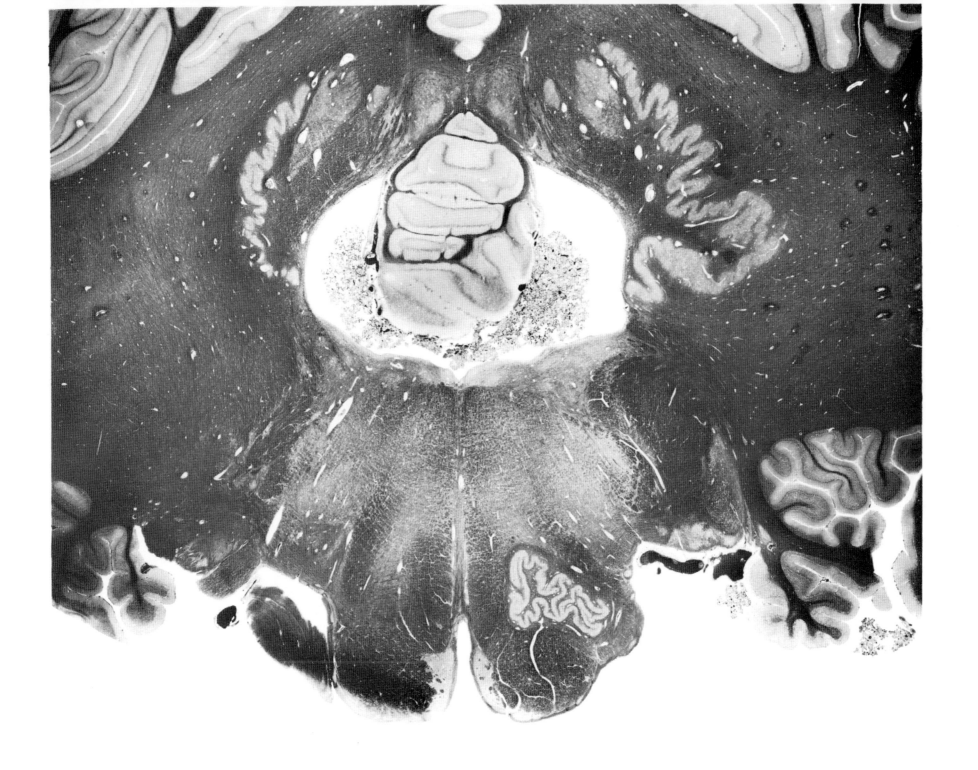

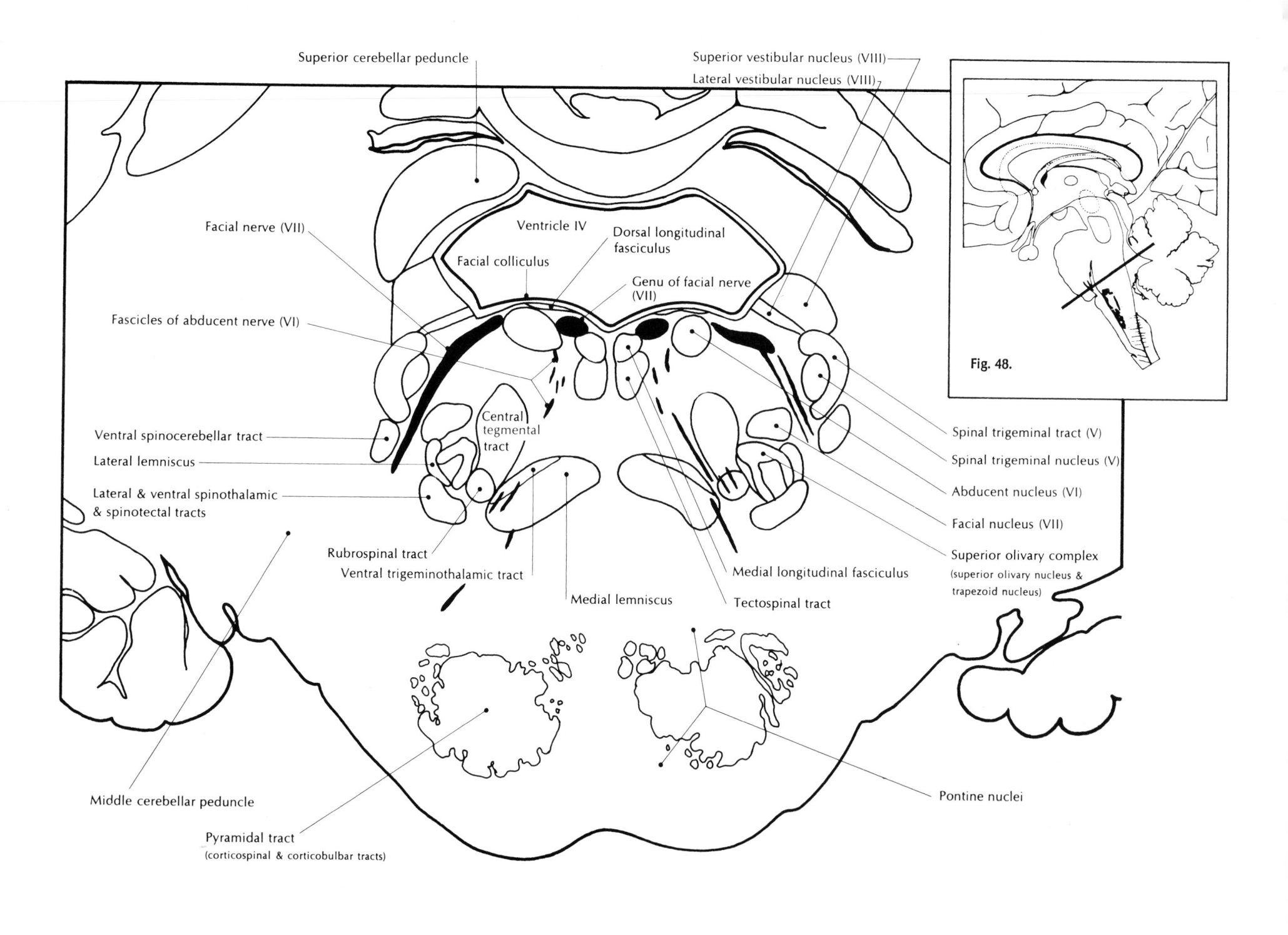

Superior cerebellar peduncle

Superior vestibular nucleus (VIII)

Lateral vestibular nucleus (VIII)

Facial nerve (VII)

Ventricle IV

Dorsal longitudinal fasciculus

Facial colliculus

Genu of facial nerve (VII)

Fascicles of abducent nerve (VI)

Fig. 48.

Central tegmental tract

Ventral spinocerebellar tract

Spinal trigeminal tract (V)

Lateral lemniscus

Spinal trigeminal nucleus (V)

Lateral & ventral spinothalamic & spinotectal tracts

Abducent nucleus (VI)

Facial nucleus (VII)

Rubrospinal tract

Superior olivary complex (superior olivary nucleus & trapezoid nucleus)

Ventral trigeminothalamic tract

Medial longitudinal fasciculus

Medial lemniscus

Tectospinal tract

Middle cerebellar peduncle

Pontine nuclei

Pyramidal tract (corticospinal & corticobulbar tracts)

Figure 48. Pons: Level of cranial nerve nuclei VI and VII—Weil, 6.5×

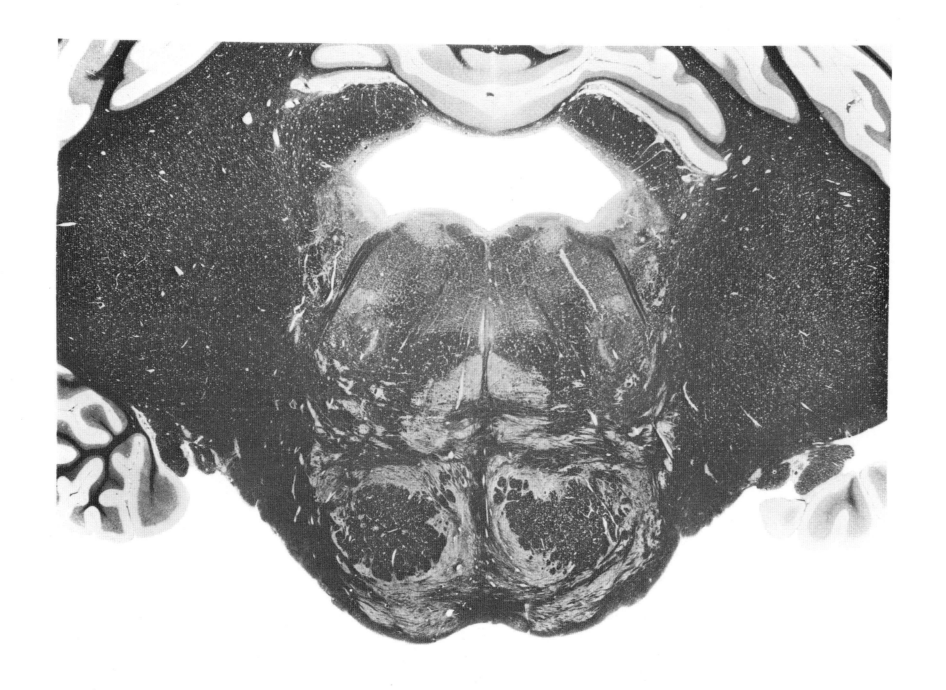

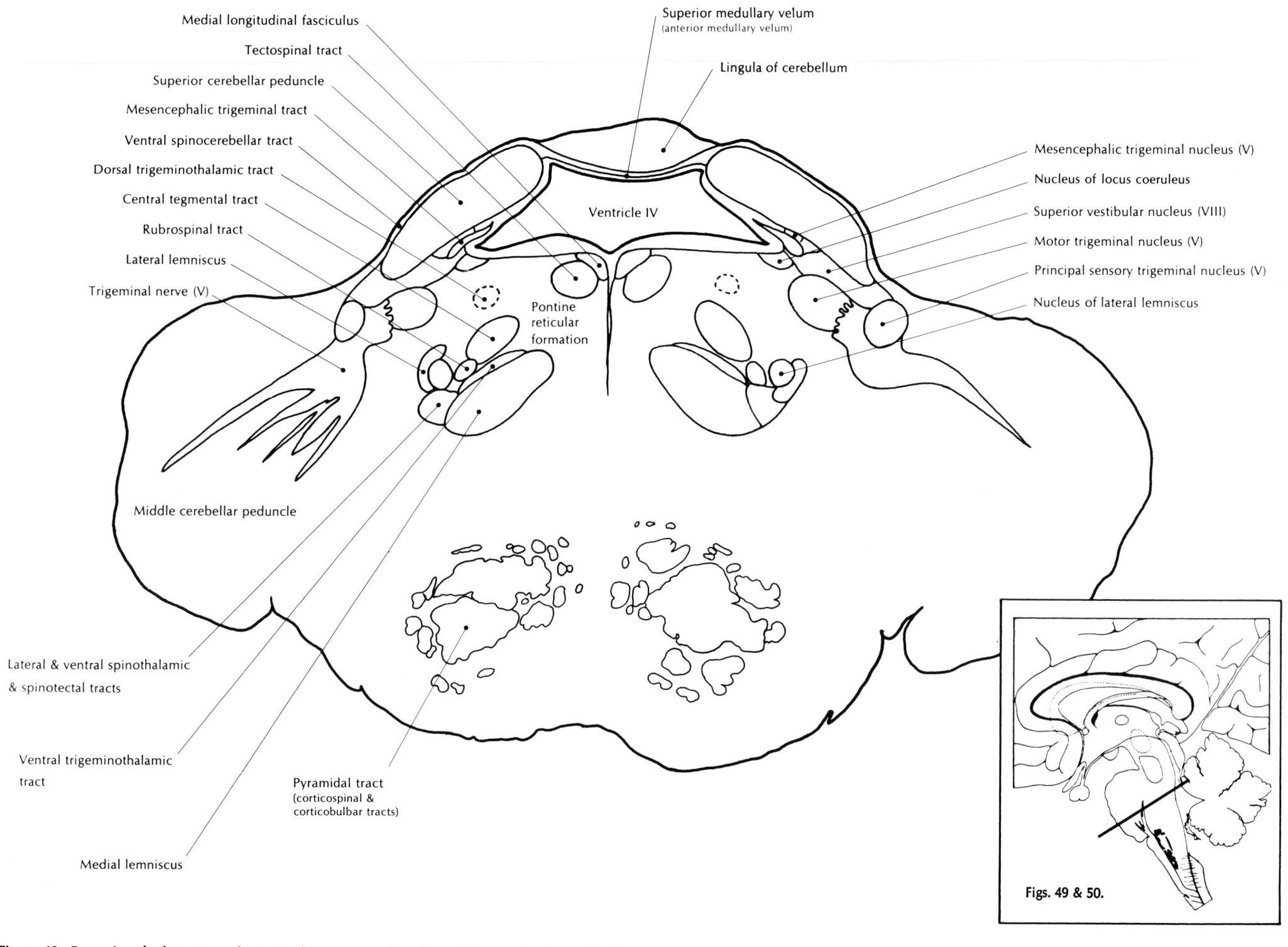

Medial longitudinal fasciculus

Tectospinal tract

Superior cerebellar peduncle

Mesencephalic trigeminal tract

Ventral spinocerebellar tract

Dorsal trigeminothalamic tract

Central tegmental tract

Rubrospinal tract

Lateral lemniscus

Trigeminal nerve (V)

Superior medullary velum
(anterior medullary velum)

Lingula of cerebellum

Mesencephalic trigeminal nucleus (V)

Nucleus of locus coeruleus

Superior vestibular nucleus (VIII)

Motor trigeminal nucleus (V)

Principal sensory trigeminal nucleus (V)

Nucleus of lateral lemniscus

Ventricle IV

Pontine
reticular
formation

Middle cerebellar peduncle

Lateral & ventral spinothalamic
& spinotectal tracts

Ventral trigeminothalamic
tract

Pyramidal tract
(corticospinal &
corticobulbar tracts)

Medial lemniscus

Figs. 49 & 50.

Figure 49. Pons: Level of motor and principal sensory nuclei of cranial nerve V—Weil, 6.5×

98

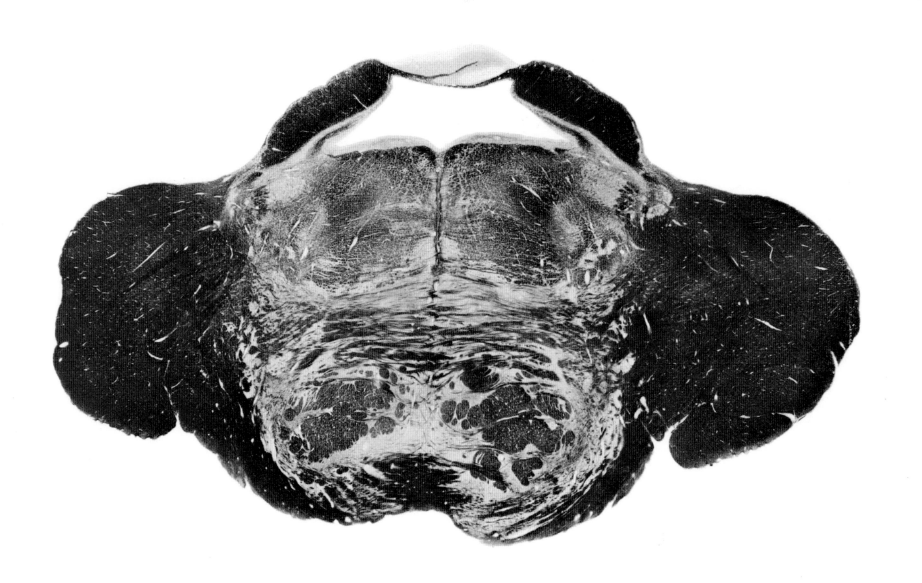

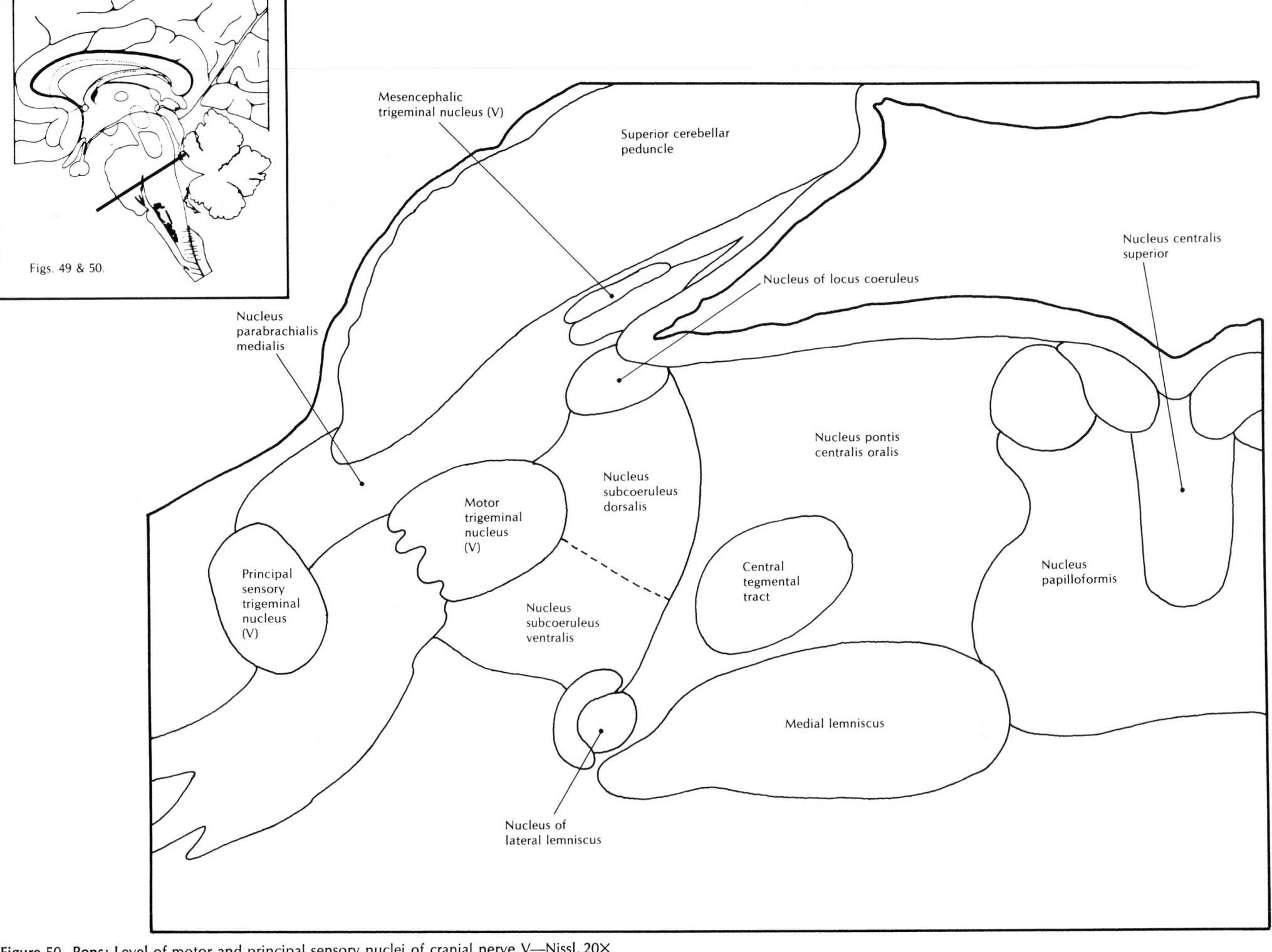

Figure 50. Pons: Level of motor and principal sensory nuclei of cranial nerve V—Nissl, 20X

Figs. 49 & 50.

Mesencephalic trigeminal nucleus (V)

Superior cerebellar peduncle

Nucleus centralis superior

Nucleus of locus coeruleus

Nucleus parabrachialis medialis

Nucleus pontis centralis oralis

Motor trigeminal nucleus (V)

Nucleus subcoeruleus dorsalis

Central tegmental tract

Nucleus papilloformis

Principal sensory trigeminal nucleus (V)

Nucleus subcoeruleus ventralis

Medial lemniscus

Nucleus of lateral lemniscus

100

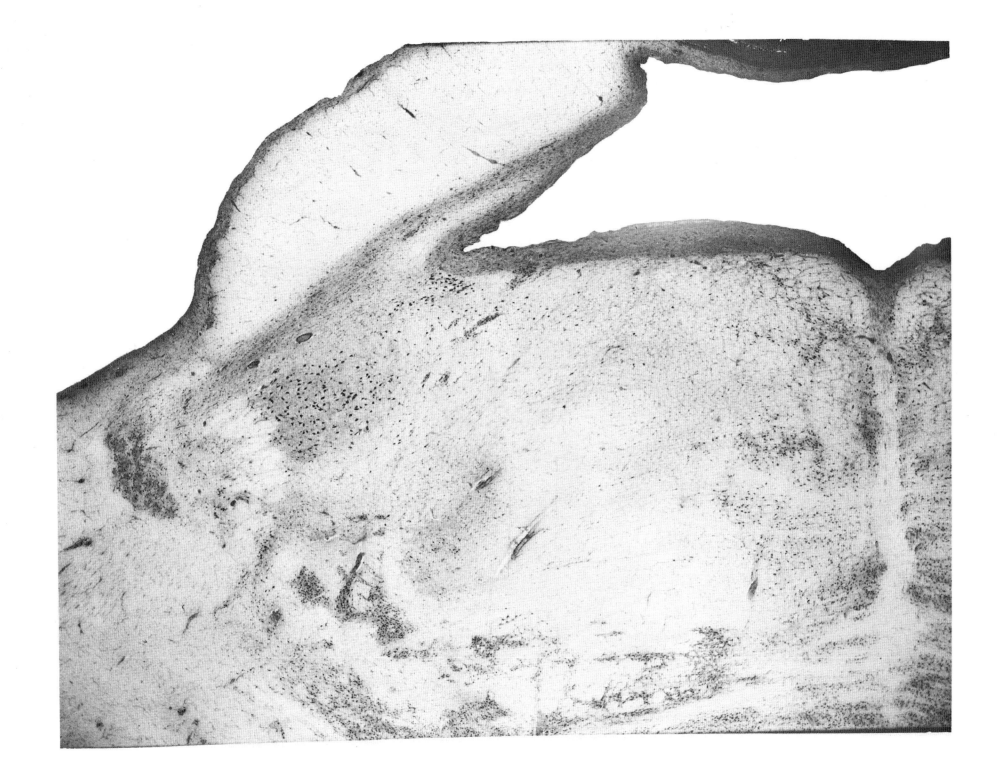

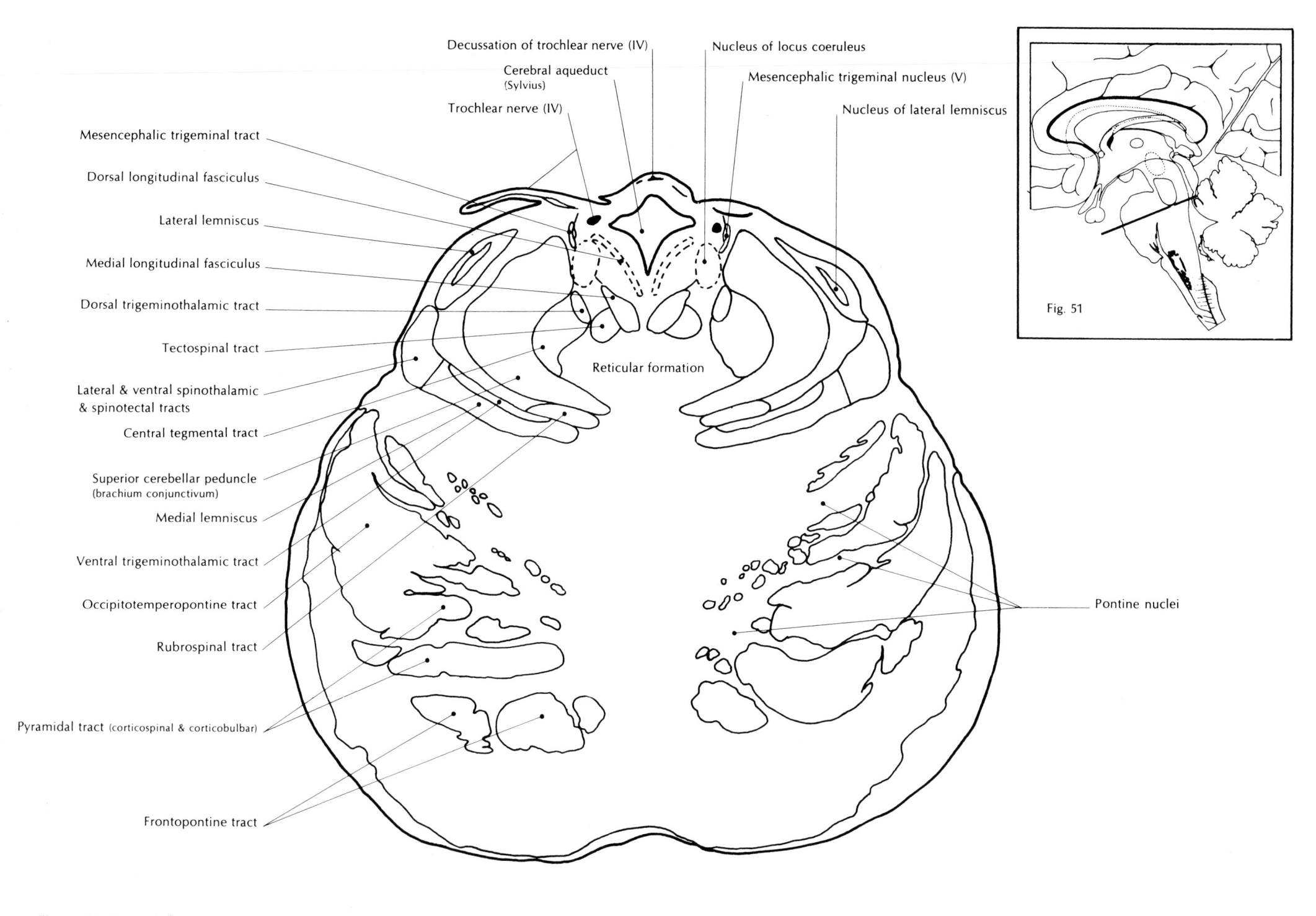

Decussation of trochlear nerve (IV)

Cerebral aqueduct (Sylvius)

Trochlear nerve (IV)

Nucleus of locus coeruleus

Mesencephalic trigeminal nucleus (V)

Nucleus of lateral lemniscus

Mesencephalic trigeminal tract

Dorsal longitudinal fasciculus

Lateral lemniscus

Medial longitudinal fasciculus

Dorsal trigeminothalamic tract

Tectospinal tract

Lateral & ventral spinothalamic & spinotectal tracts

Central tegmental tract

Superior cerebellar peduncle (brachium conjunctivum)

Medial lemniscus

Ventral trigeminothalamic tract

Occipitotemperopontine tract

Rubrospinal tract

Pyramidal tract (corticospinal & corticobulbar)

Frontopontine tract

Reticular formation

Pontine nuclei

Fig. 51

Figure 51. Pons: Isthmus, contains medial longitudinal fasciculus interconnecting the extraocular muscle motor nuclei, III, IV, and VI—Weil, 6.5×

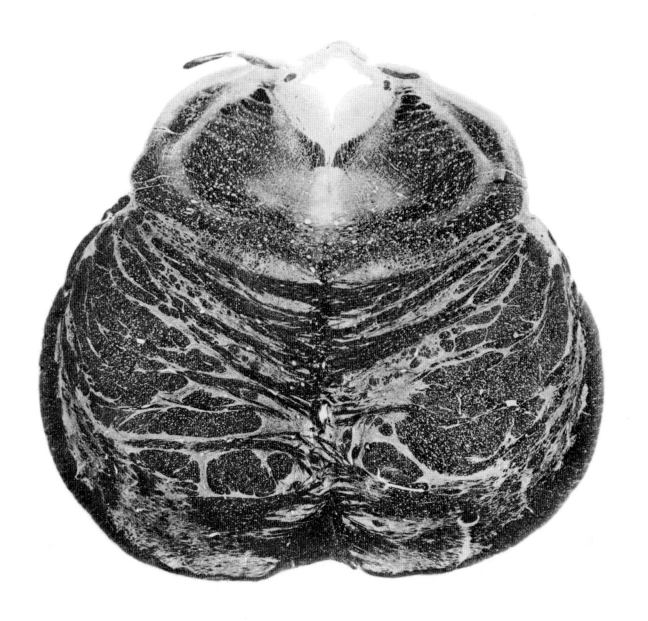

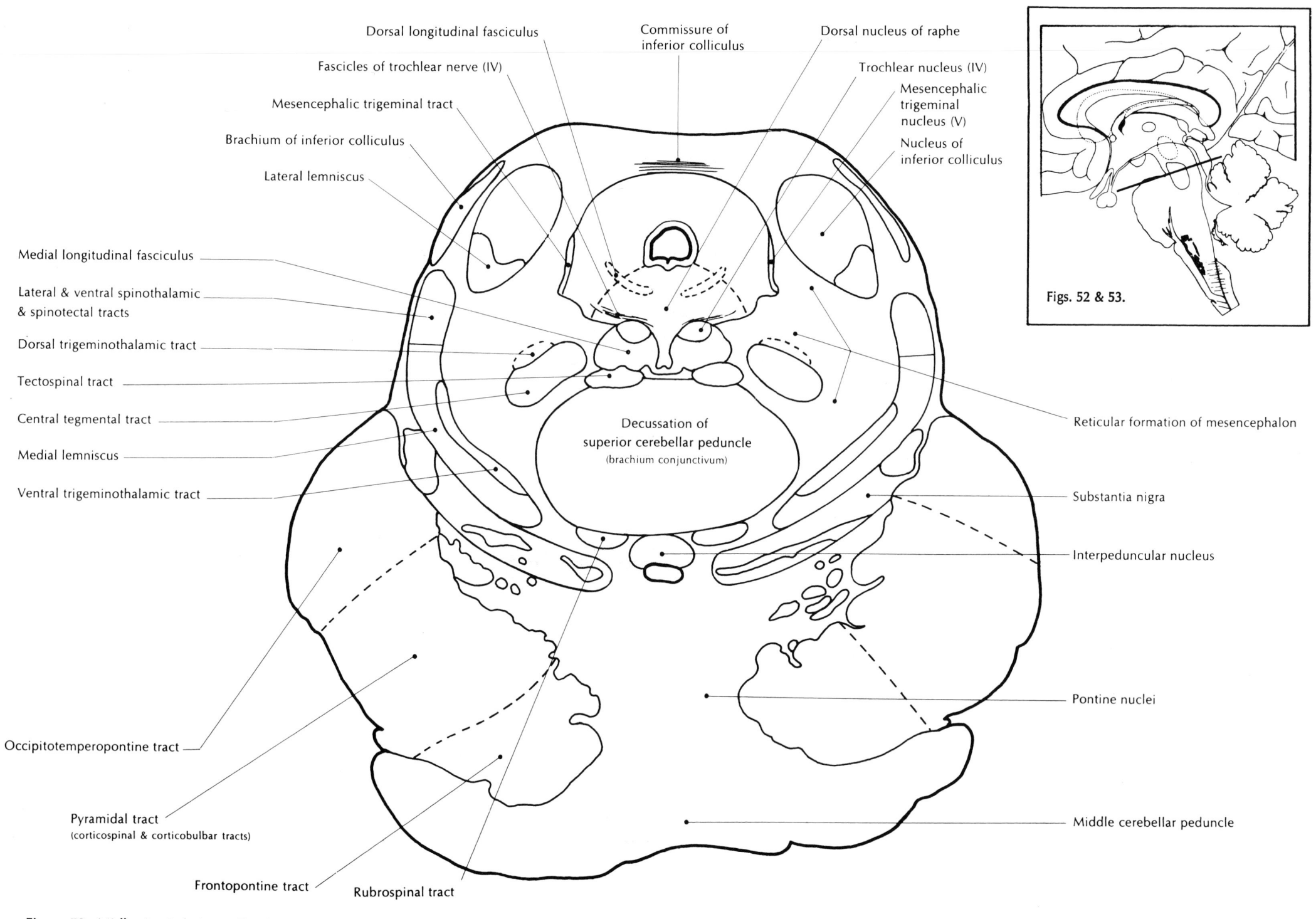

Dorsal longitudinal fasciculus

Fascicles of trochlear nerve (IV)

Mesencephalic trigeminal tract

Brachium of inferior colliculus

Lateral lemniscus

Commissure of inferior colliculus

Dorsal nucleus of raphe

Trochlear nucleus (IV)

Mesencephalic trigeminal nucleus (V)

Nucleus of inferior colliculus

Medial longitudinal fasciculus

Lateral & ventral spinothalamic & spinotectal tracts

Dorsal trigeminothalamic tract

Tectospinal tract

Central tegmental tract

Medial lemniscus

Ventral trigeminothalamic tract

Decussation of superior cerebellar peduncle (brachium conjunctivum)

Reticular formation of mesencephalon

Substantia nigra

Interpeduncular nucleus

Pontine nuclei

Middle cerebellar peduncle

Occipitotemperopontine tract

Pyramidal tract (corticospinal & corticobulbar tracts)

Frontopontine tract

Rubrospinal tract

Figs. 52 & 53.

Figure 52. Midbrain: Inferior colliculus—Weil, 6.5×

104

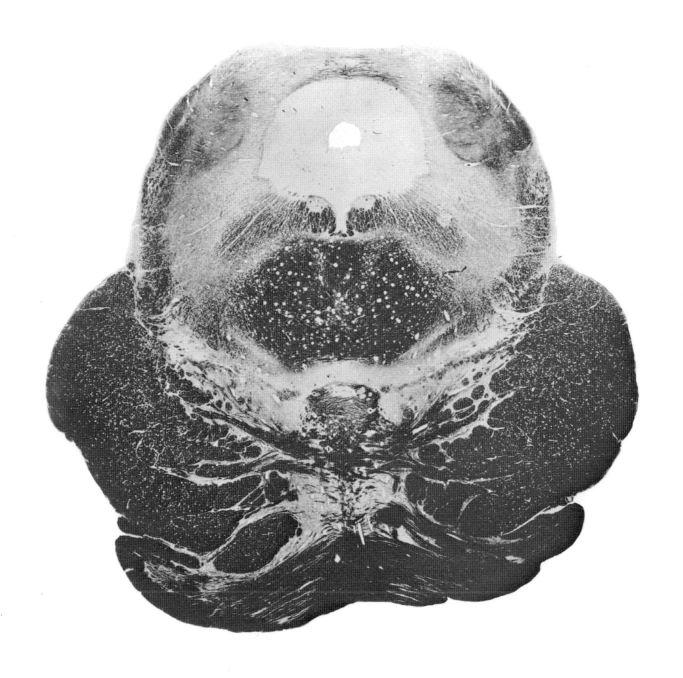

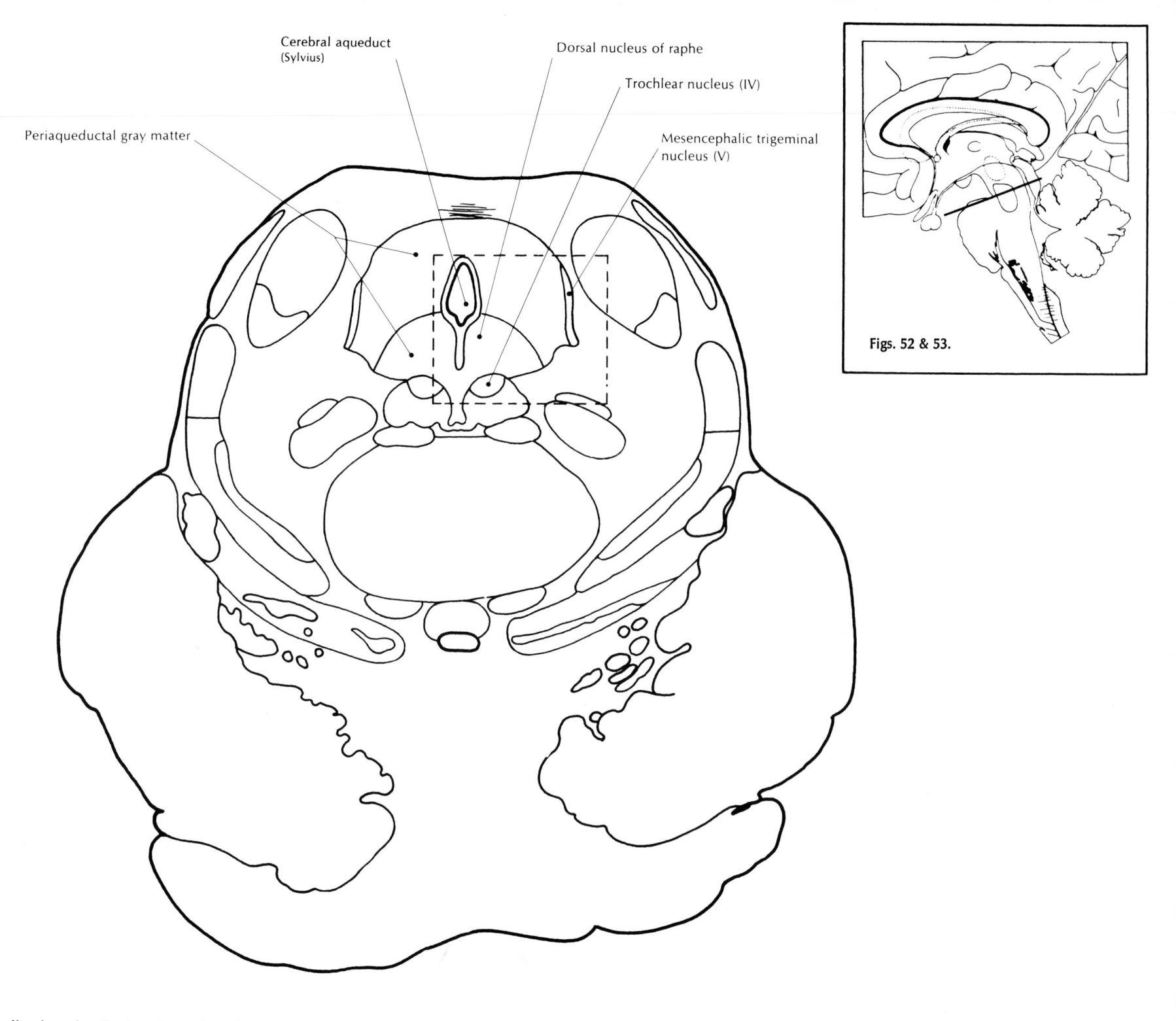

Cerebral aqueduct
(Sylvius)

Dorsal nucleus of raphe

Trochlear nucleus (IV)

Periaqueductal gray matter

Mesencephalic trigeminal
nucleus (V)

Figs. 52 & 53.

Figure 53. Midbrain: Inferior colliculus, detail of periaqueductal gray matter and trochlear nucleus—Nissl, 46×

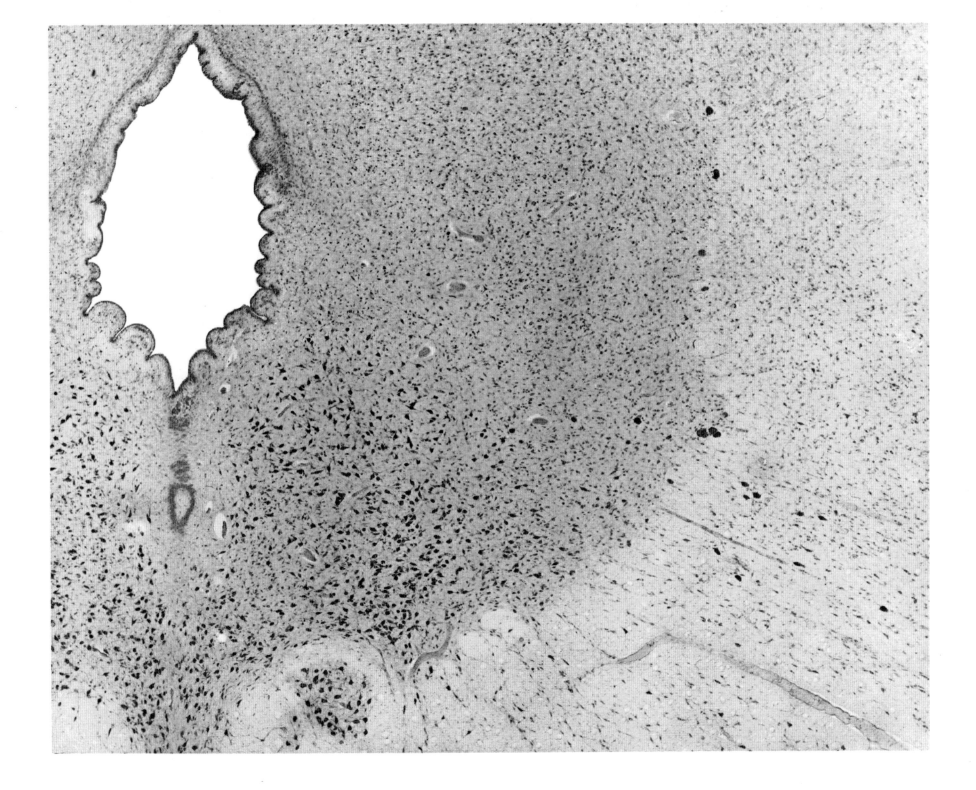

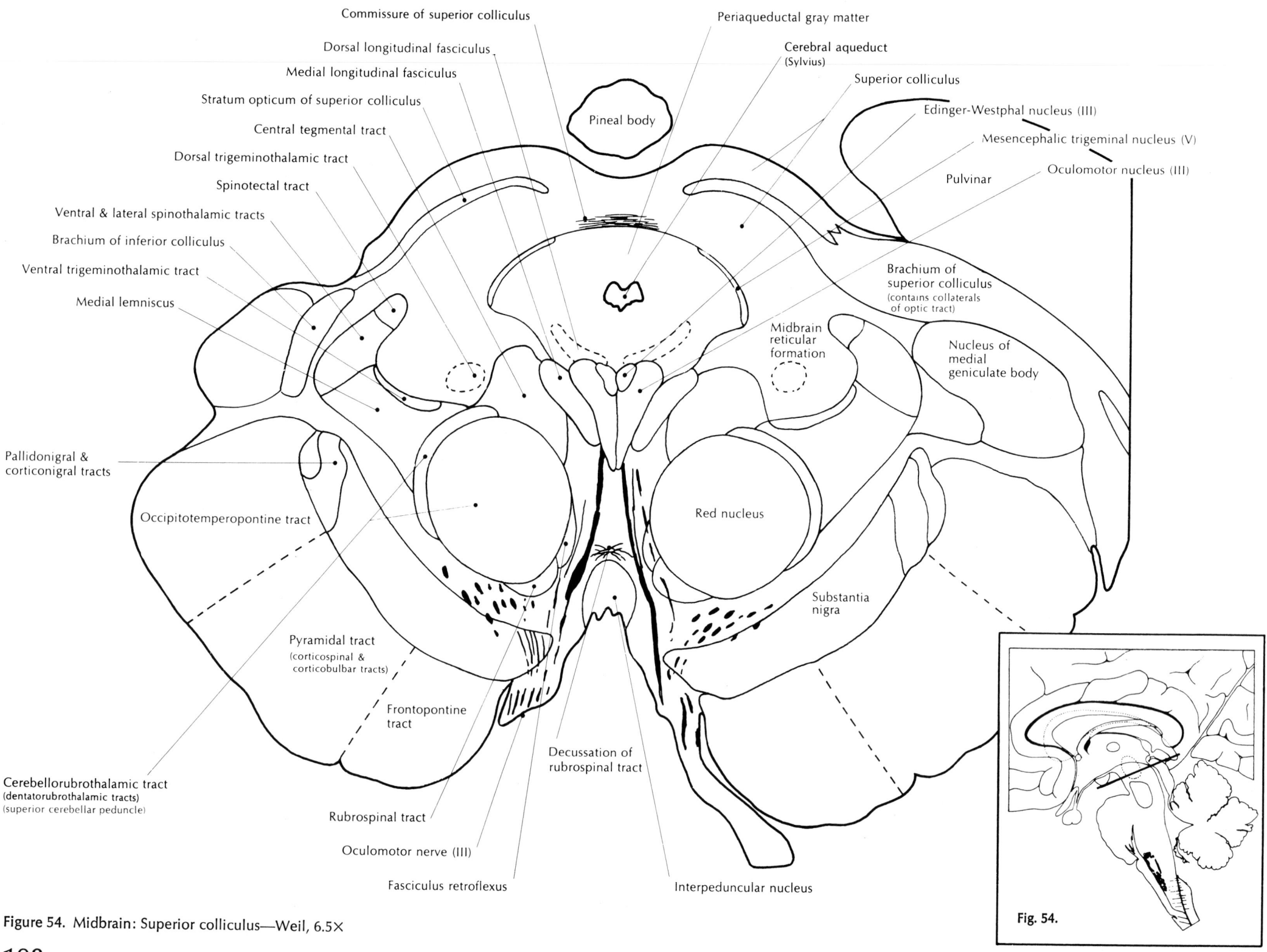

Commissure of superior colliculus

Dorsal longitudinal fasciculus

Medial longitudinal fasciculus

Stratum opticum of superior colliculus

Central tegmental tract

Dorsal trigeminothalamic tract

Spinotectal tract

Ventral & lateral spinothalamic tracts

Brachium of inferior colliculus

Ventral trigeminothalamic tract

Medial lemniscus

Pallidonigral & corticonigral tracts

Occipitotemperopontine tract

Pyramidal tract
(corticospinal &
corticobulbar tracts)

Frontopontine tract

Cerebellorubrothalamic tract
(dentatorubrothalamic tracts)
(superior cerebellar peduncle)

Rubrospinal tract

Oculomotor nerve (III)

Fasciculus retroflexus

Periaqueductal gray matter

Cerebral aqueduct
(Sylvius)

Superior colliculus

Edinger-Westphal nucleus (III)

Mesencephalic trigeminal nucleus (V)

Oculomotor nucleus (III)

Pulvinar

Pineal body

Brachium of
superior colliculus
(contains collaterals
of optic tract)

Midbrain
reticular
formation

Nucleus of
medial
geniculate body

Red nucleus

Substantia
nigra

Decussation of
rubrospinal tract

Interpeduncular nucleus

Fig. 54.

Figure 54. Midbrain: Superior colliculus—Weil, 6.5×

108

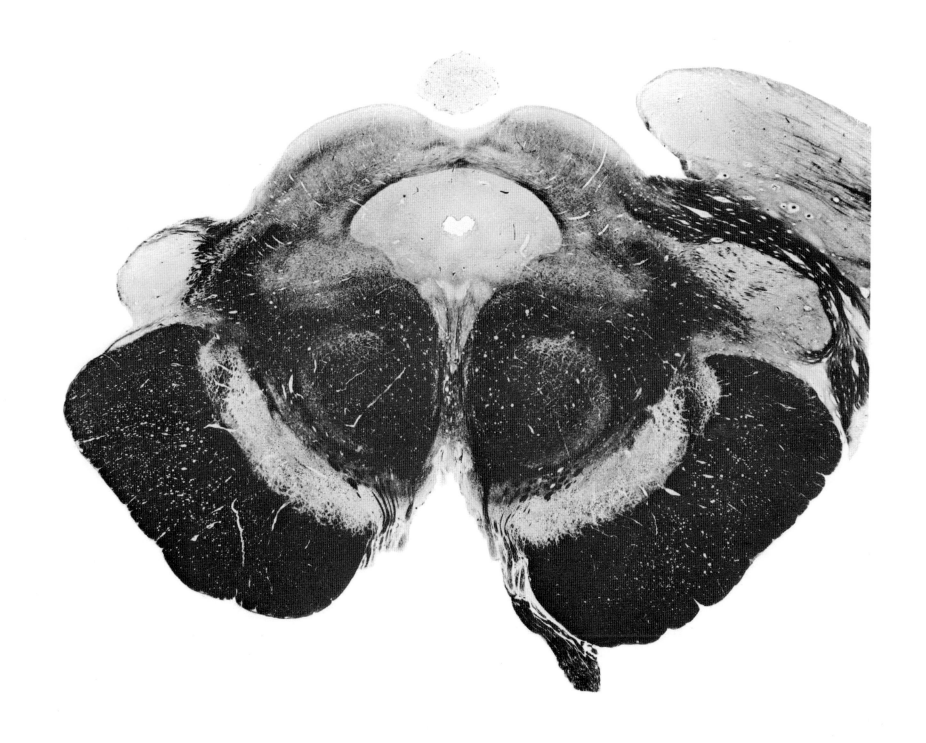

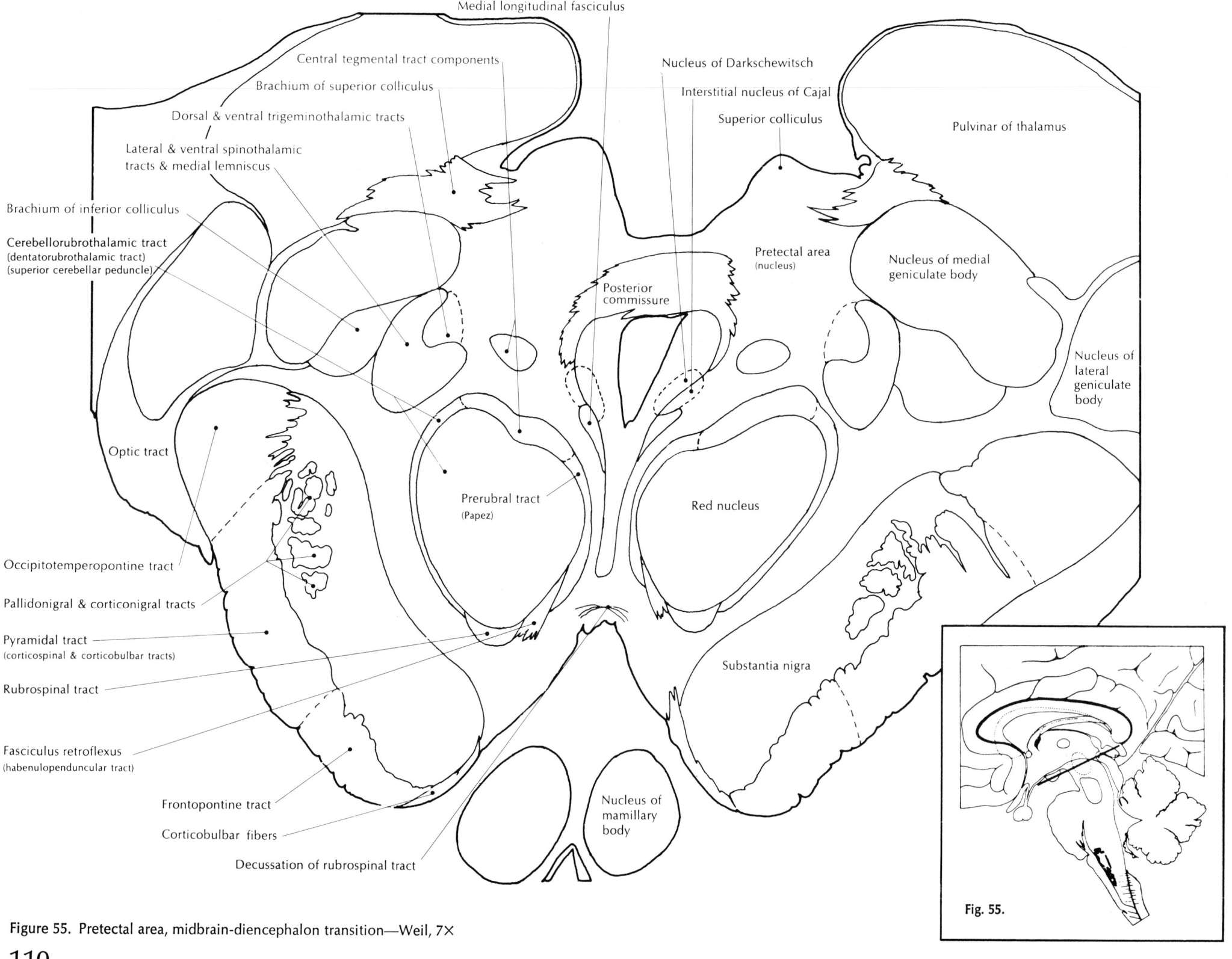

Figure 55. Pretectal area, midbrain-diencephalon transition—Weil, 7×

110

Medial longitudinal fasciculus

Central tegmental tract components

Brachium of superior colliculus

Dorsal & ventral trigeminothalamic tracts

Lateral & ventral spinothalamic tracts & medial lemniscus

Brachium of inferior colliculus

Cerebellorubrothalamic tract (dentatorubrothalamic tract) (superior cerebellar peduncle)

Optic tract

Occipitotemperopontine tract

Pallidonigral & corticonigral tracts

Pyramidal tract (corticospinal & corticobulbar tracts)

Rubrospinal tract

Fasciculus retroflexus (habenulopenduncular tract)

Frontopontine tract

Corticobulbar fibers

Decussation of rubrospinal tract

Nucleus of Darkschewitsch

Interstitial nucleus of Cajal

Superior colliculus

Pulvinar of thalamus

Pretectal area (nucleus)

Nucleus of medial geniculate body

Nucleus of lateral geniculate body

Posterior commissure

Prerubral tract (Papez)

Red nucleus

Substantia nigra

Nucleus of mamillary body

Fig. 55.

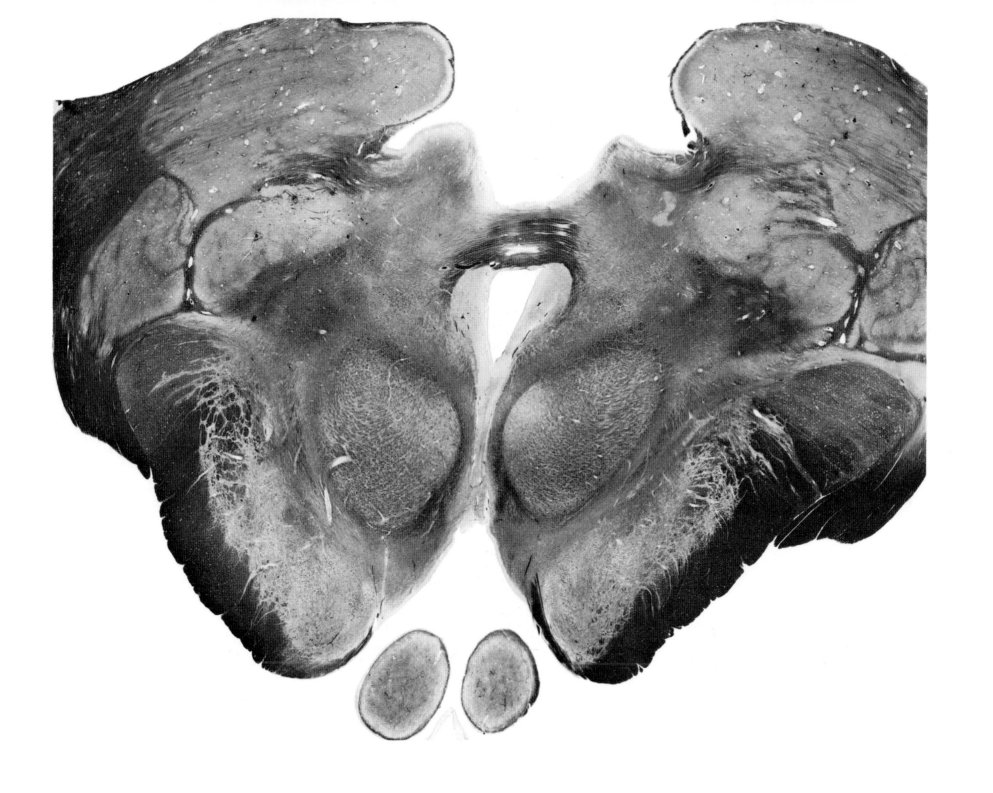

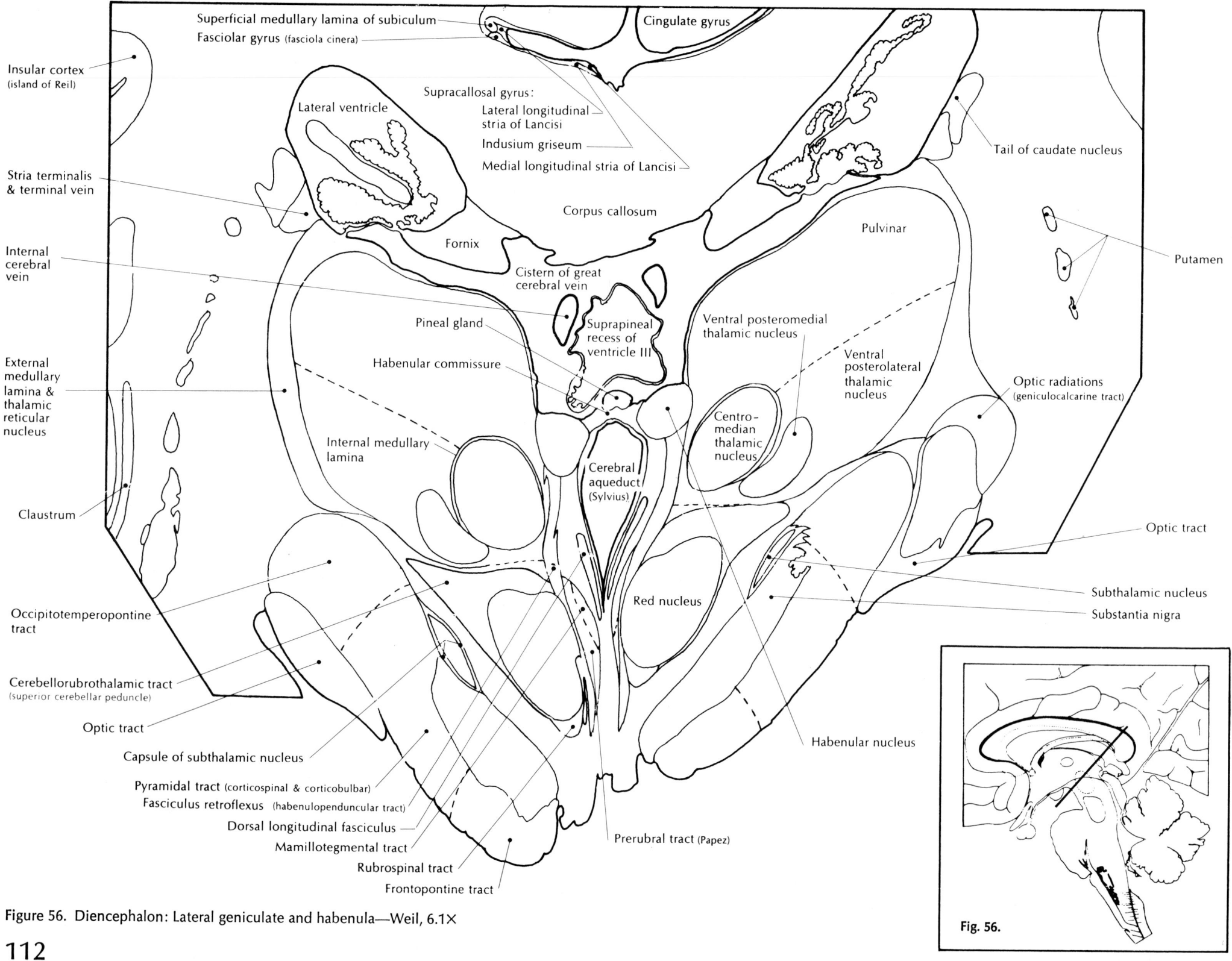

Insular cortex (island of Reil)

Superficial medullary lamina of subiculum

Fasciolar gyrus (fasciola cinera)

Cingulate gyrus

Supracallosal gyrus:

Lateral ventricle

Lateral longitudinal stria of Lancisi

Indusium griseum

Medial longitudinal stria of Lancisi

Tail of caudate nucleus

Stria terminalis & terminal vein

Corpus callosum

Pulvinar

Internal cerebral vein

Fornix

Cistern of great cerebral vein

Putamen

External medullary lamina & thalamic reticular nucleus

Pineal gland

Suprapineal recess of ventricle III

Ventral posteromedial thalamic nucleus

Ventral posterolateral thalamic nucleus

Habenular commissure

Optic radiations (geniculocalcarine tract)

Internal medullary lamina

Centro-median thalamic nucleus

Claustrum

Cerebral aqueduct (Sylvius)

Optic tract

Occipitotemperopontine tract

Red nucleus

Subthalamic nucleus

Substantia nigra

Cerebellorubrothalamic tract (superior cerebellar peduncle)

Optic tract

Capsule of subthalamic nucleus

Pyramidal tract (corticospinal & corticobulbar)

Fasciculus retroflexus (habenulopenduncular tract)

Dorsal longitudinal fasciculus

Mamillotegmental tract

Rubrospinal tract

Prerubral tract (Papez)

Habenular nucleus

Frontopontine tract

Figure 56. Diencephalon: Lateral geniculate and habenula—Weil, 6.1✕

112

Fig. 56.

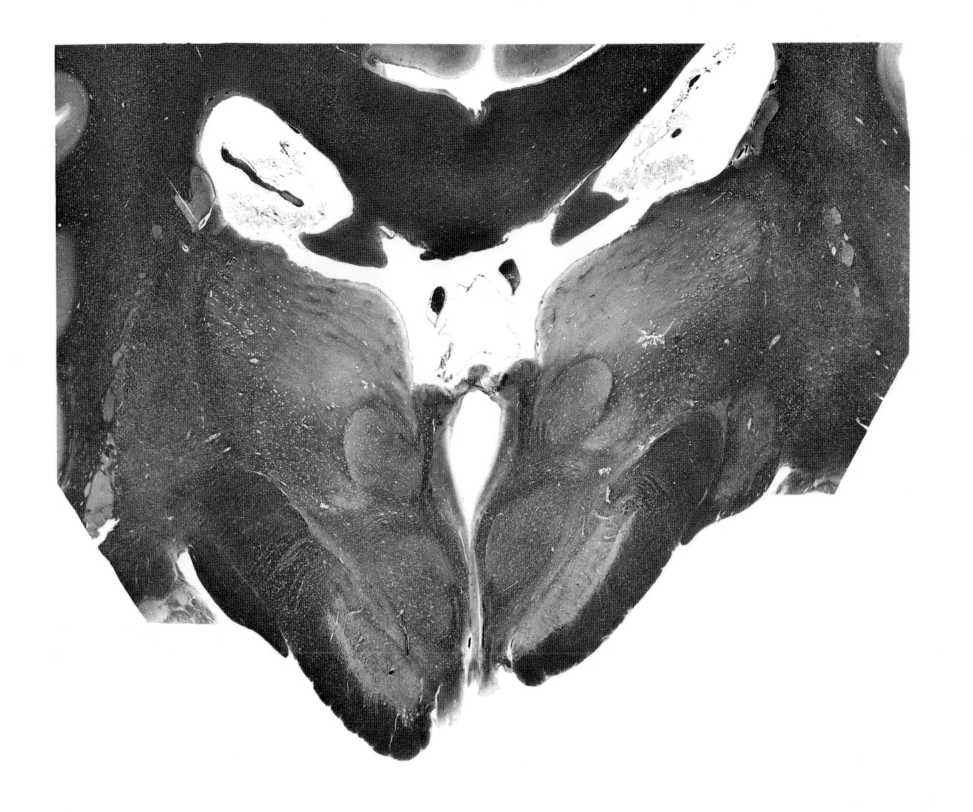

CORONAL MICROSCOPIC SECTIONS OF THE BASAL GANGLIA AND DIENCEPHALON, INCLUDING HORIZONTAL SECTIONS OF THE BRAIN STEM

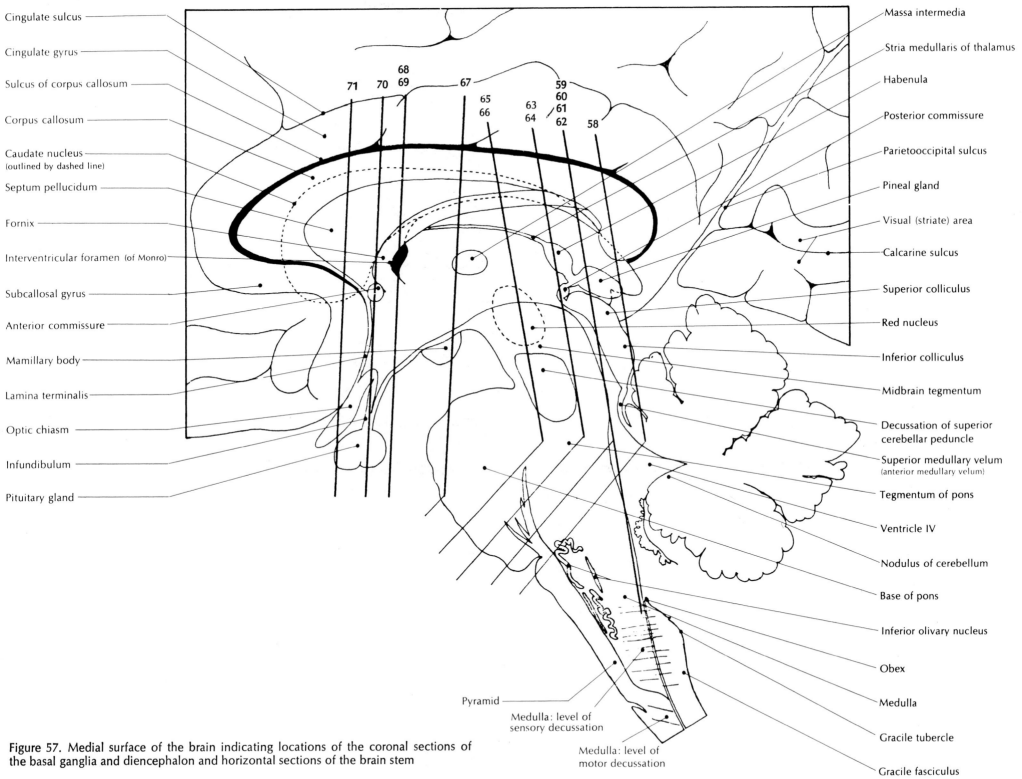

Cingulate sulcus

Cingulate gyrus

Sulcus of corpus callosum

Corpus callosum

Caudate nucleus
(outlined by dashed line)

Septum pellucidum

Fornix

Interventricular foramen (of Monro)

Subcallosal gyrus

Anterior commissure

Mamillary body

Lamina terminalis

Optic chiasm

Infundibulum

Pituitary gland

Massa intermedia

Stria medullaris of thalamus

Habenula

Posterior commissure

Parietooccipital sulcus

Pineal gland

Visual (striate) area

Calcarine sulcus

Superior colliculus

Red nucleus

Inferior colliculus

Midbrain tegmentum

Decussation of superior
cerebellar peduncle

Superior medullary velum
(anterior medullary velum)

Tegmentum of pons

Ventricle IV

Nodulus of cerebellum

Base of pons

Inferior olivary nucleus

Obex

Medulla

Gracile tubercle

Gracile fasciculus

Pyramid

Medulla: level of
sensory decussation

Medulla: level of
motor decussation

71 70 68 69 67 65 66 63 64 59 60 61 62 58

Figure 57. Medial surface of the brain indicating locations of the coronal sections of
the basal ganglia and diencephalon and horizontal sections of the brain stem

115

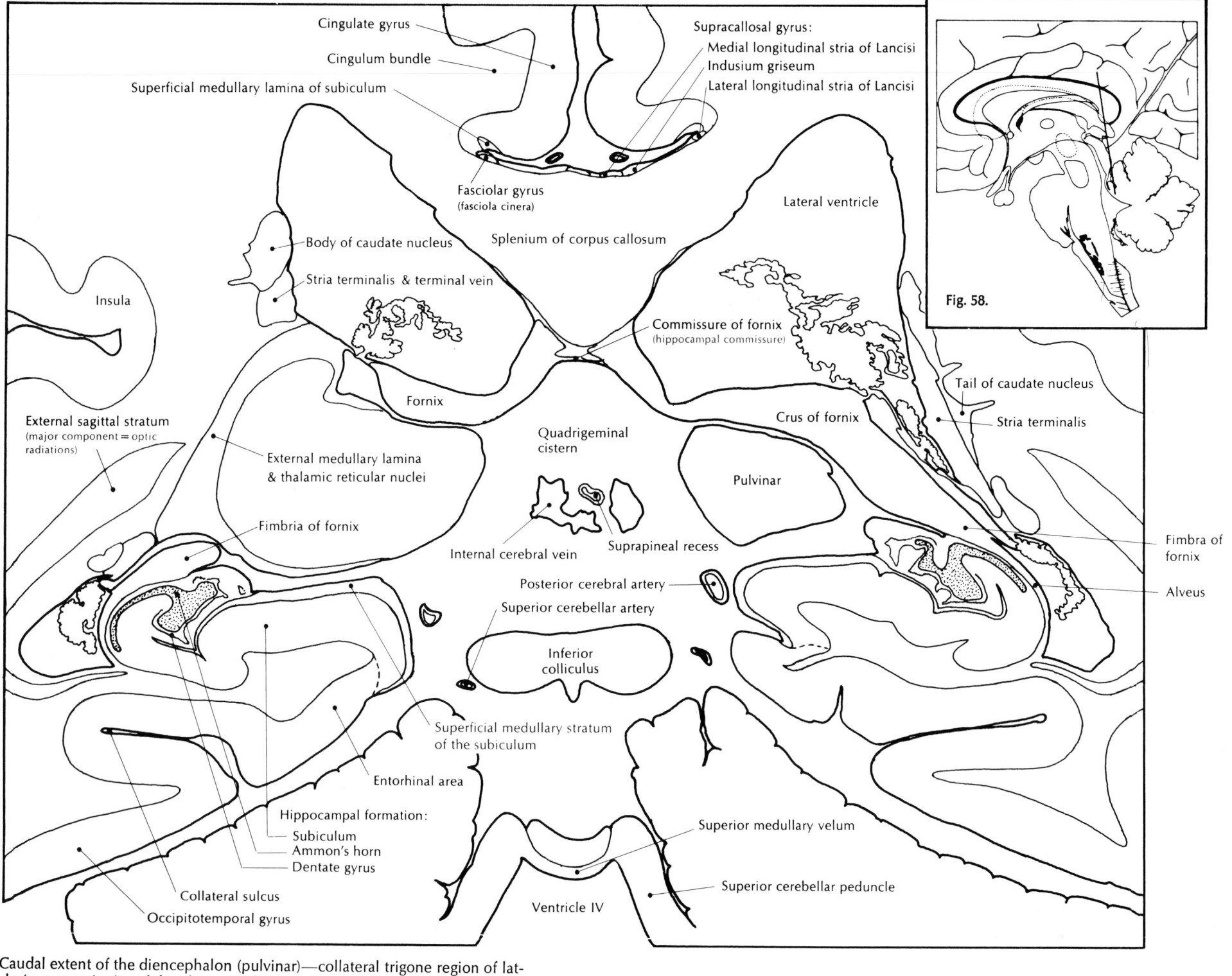

Cingulate gyrus

Cingulum bundle

Superficial medullary lamina of subiculum

Supracallosal gyrus:
Medial longitudinal stria of Lancisi
Indusium griseum
Lateral longitudinal stria of Lancisi

Fasciolar gyrus
(fasciola cinera)

Lateral ventricle

Body of caudate nucleus

Stria terminalis & terminal vein

Splenium of corpus callosum

Insula

Commissure of fornix
(hippocampal commissure)

Fig. 58.

Tail of caudate nucleus

Stria terminalis

Fornix

Crus of fornix

External sagittal stratum
(major component = optic
radiations)

External medullary lamina
& thalamic reticular nuclei

Quadrigeminal
cistern

Pulvinar

Fimbria of fornix

Internal cerebral vein

Suprapineal recess

Fimbra of
fornix

Posterior cerebral artery

Alveus

Superior cerebellar artery

Superficial medullary stratum
of the subiculum

Inferior
colliculus

Entorhinal area

Superior medullary velum

Hippocampal formation:
Subiculum
Ammon's horn
Dentate gyrus

Superior cerebellar peduncle

Collateral sulcus

Ventricle IV

Occipitotemporal gyrus

Figure 58. Caudal extent of the diencephalon (pulvinar)—collateral trigone region of lateral ventricle (note continuity of the alveus, fimbria, and fornix fiber system)—Weil, 4×

116

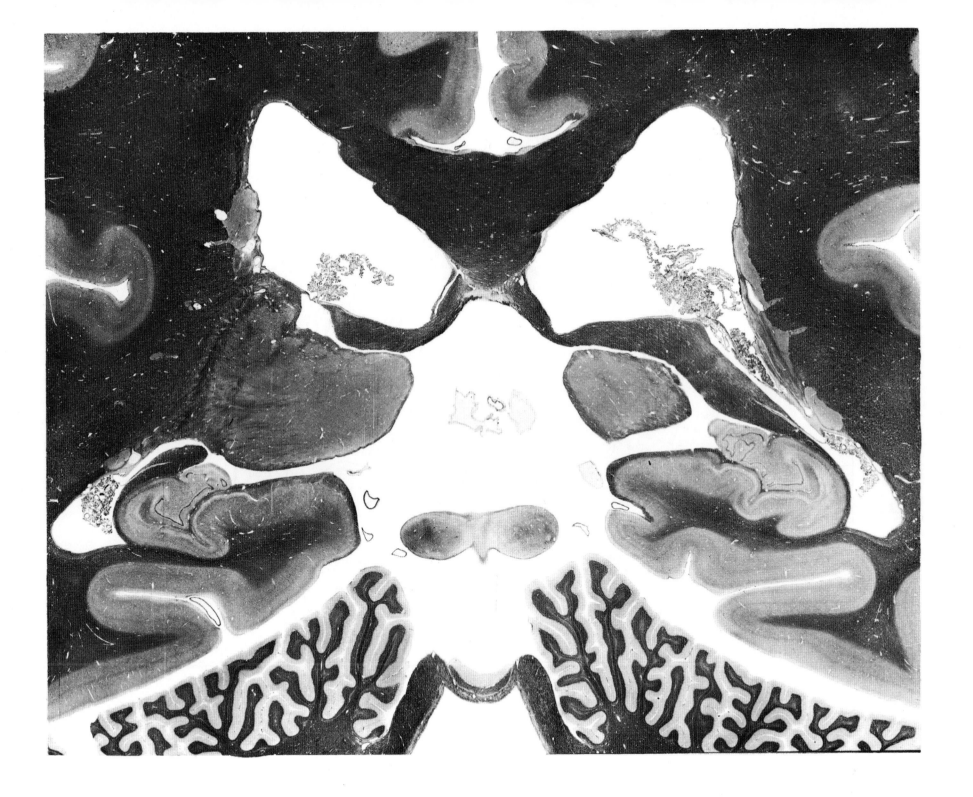

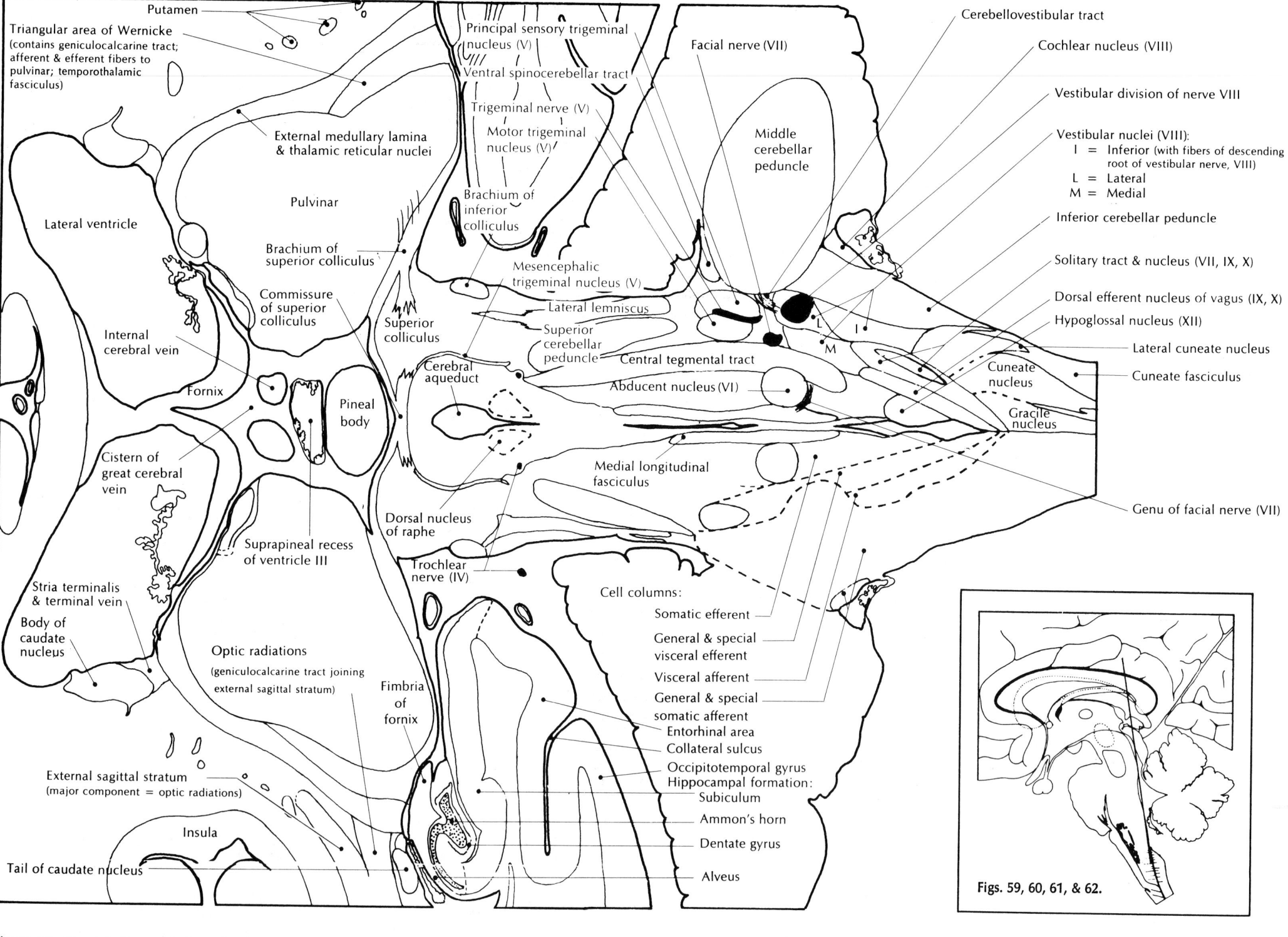

Figure 59. Caudal diencephalon plus horizontal section of brain stem—Weil, 2.3X

118

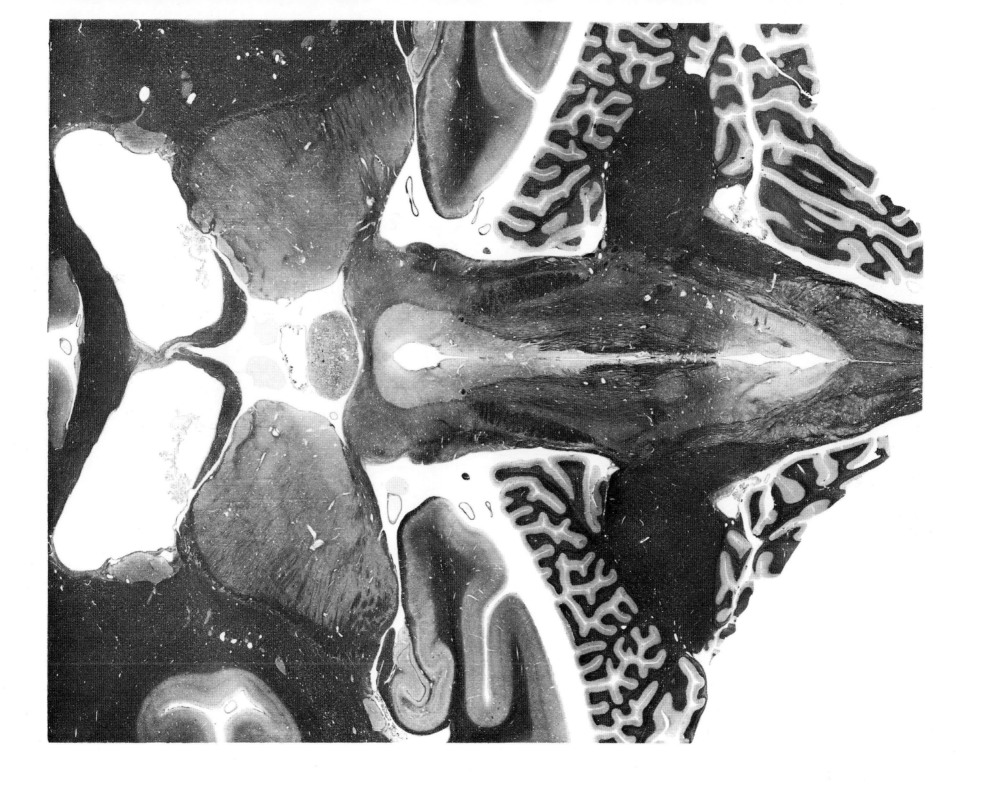

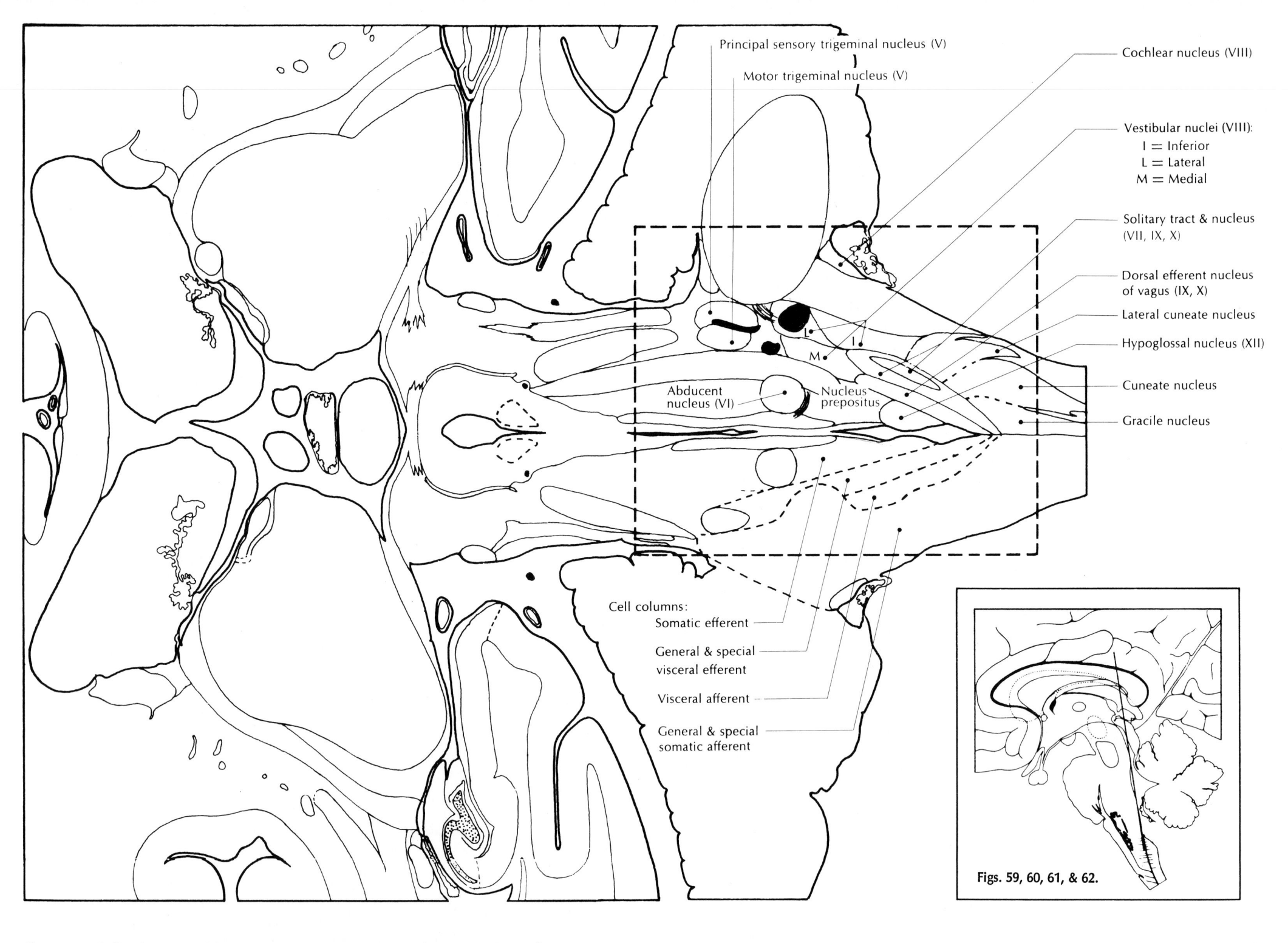

Figure 60. Cell columns and functional components of cranial nerve nuclei in the pons and medulla—Nissl, 10X

Principal sensory trigeminal nucleus (V)

Motor trigeminal nucleus (V)

Cochlear nucleus (VIII)

Vestibular nuclei (VIII):
I = Inferior
L = Lateral
M = Medial

Solitary tract & nucleus (VII, IX, X)

Dorsal efferent nucleus of vagus (IX, X)

Lateral cuneate nucleus

Hypoglossal nucleus (XII)

Cuneate nucleus

Gracile nucleus

Abducent nucleus (VI)

Nucleus prepositus

Cell columns:
Somatic efferent

General & special visceral efferent

Visceral afferent

General & special somatic afferent

Figs. 59, 60, 61, & 62.

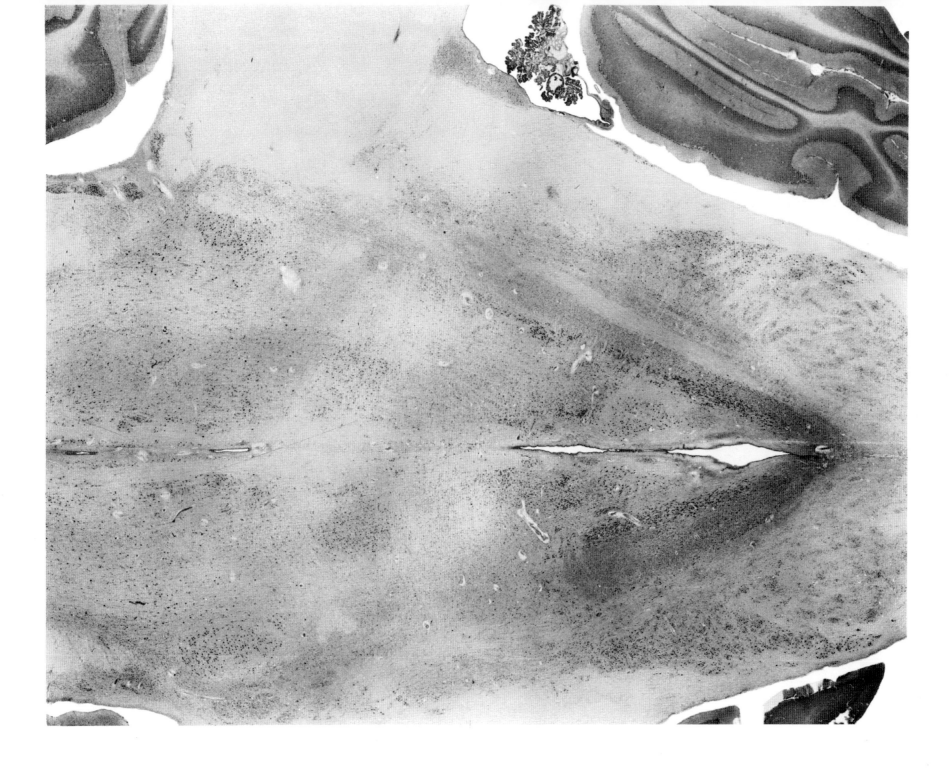

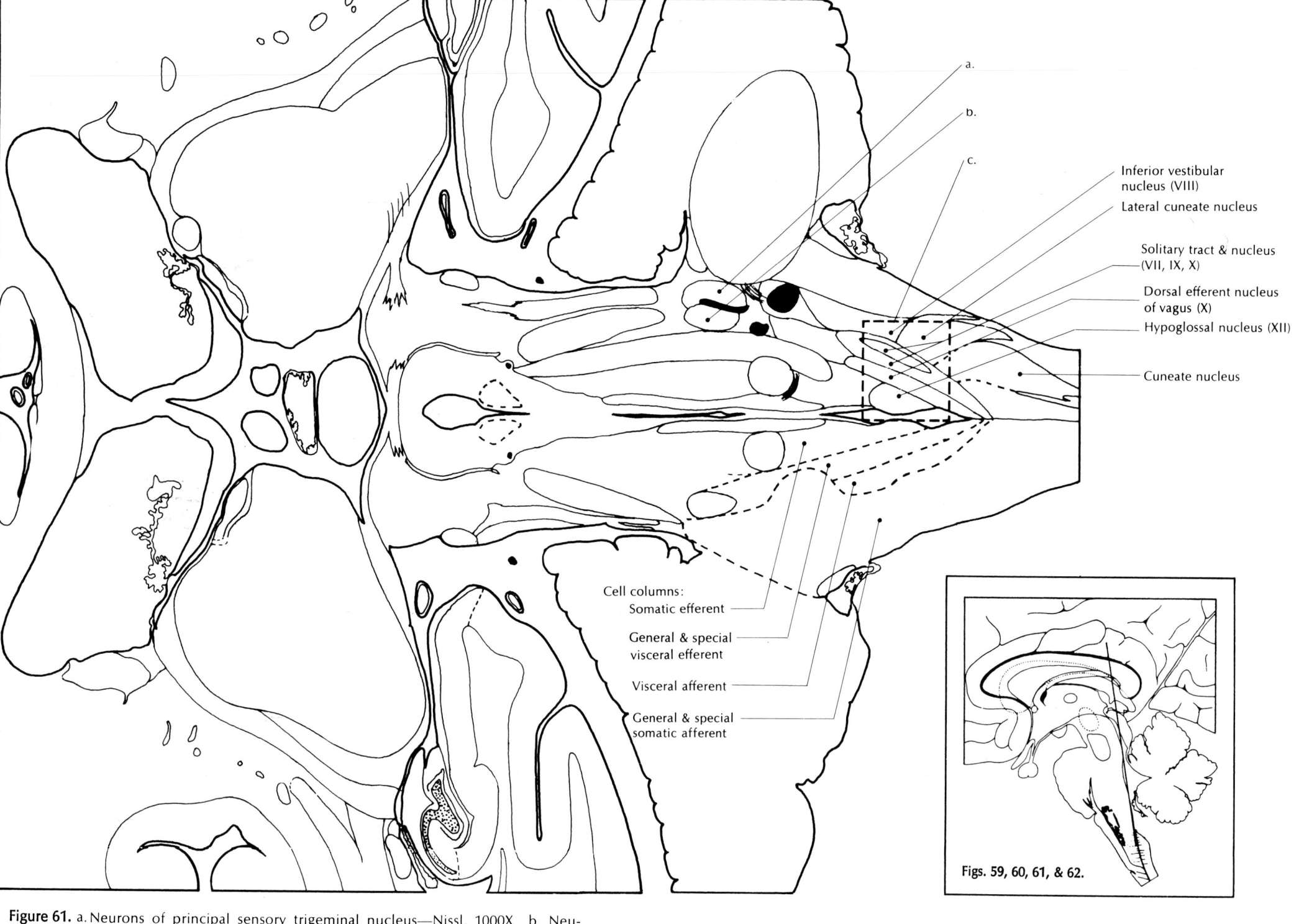

a.

b.

c.

Inferior vestibular
nucleus (VIII)

Lateral cuneate nucleus

Solitary tract & nucleus
(VII, IX, X)

Dorsal efferent nucleus
of vagus (X)

Hypoglossal nucleus (XII)

Cuneate nucleus

Cell columns:
 Somatic efferent

General & special
visceral efferent

Visceral afferent

General & special
somatic afferent

Figs. 59, 60, 61, & 62.

Figure 61. a. Neurons of principal sensory trigeminal nucleus—Nissl, 1000X   b. Neurons of motor trigeminal nucleus—Nissl, 1000X   c. Detail of cell columns and functional components of cranial nerve nuclei of the medulla—Nissl, 40X

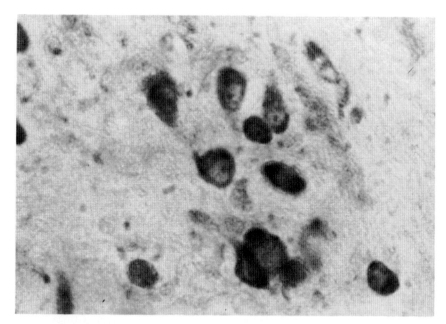

a.

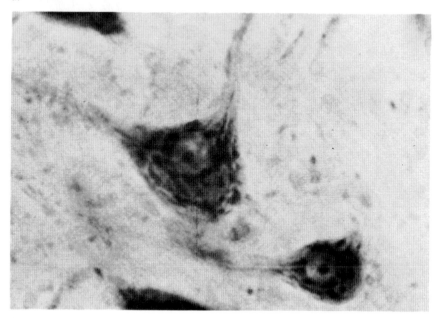

b.

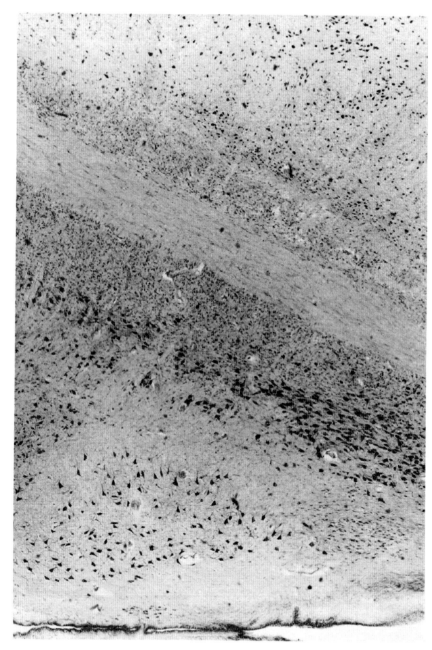

c.

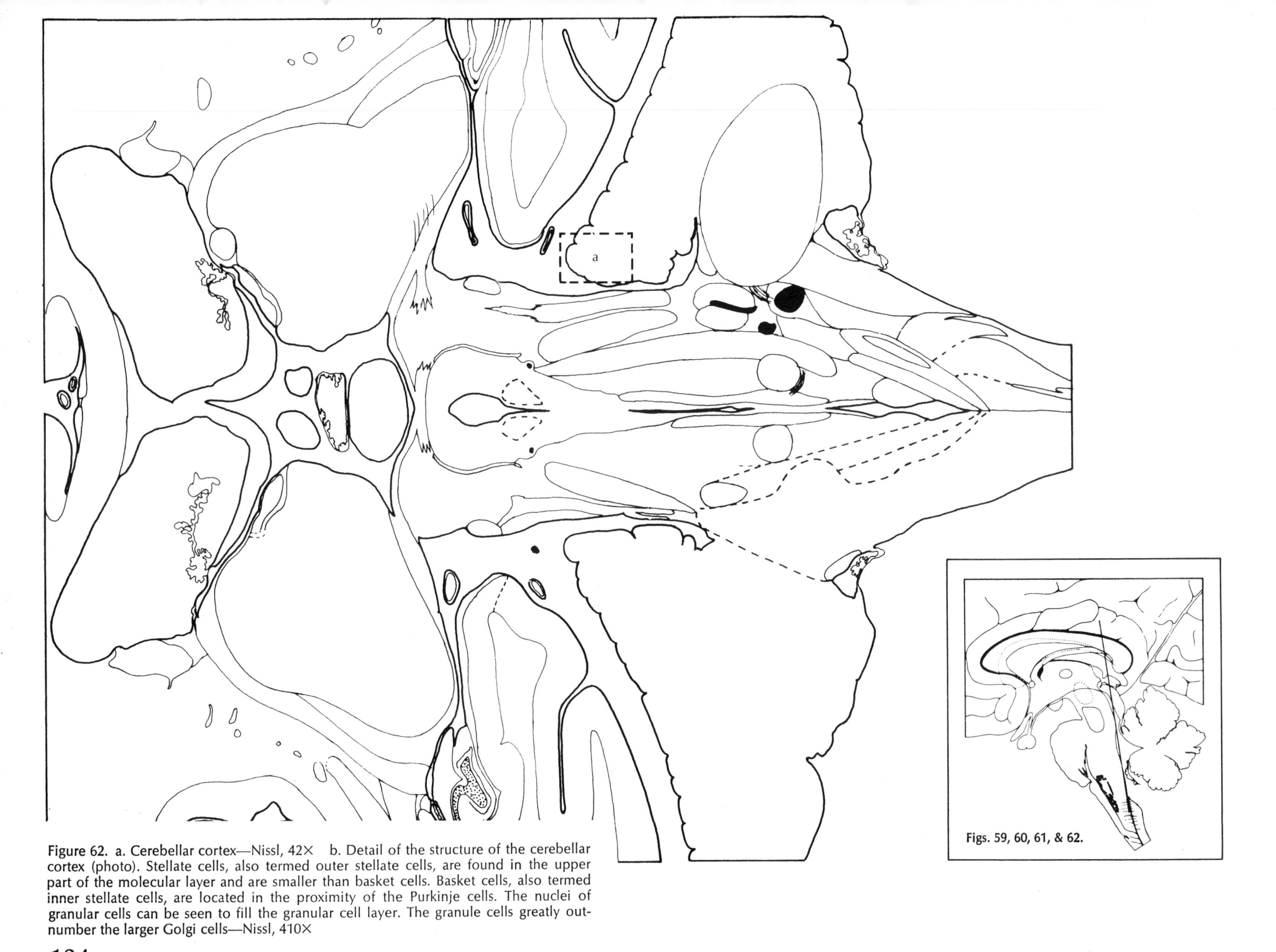

Figure 62. a. Cerebellar cortex—Nissl, 42× b. Detail of the structure of the cerebellar cortex (photo). Stellate cells, also termed outer stellate cells, are found in the upper part of the molecular layer and are smaller than basket cells. Basket cells, also termed inner stellate cells, are located in the proximity of the Purkinje cells. The nuclei of granular cells can be seen to fill the granular cell layer. The granule cells greatly outnumber the larger Golgi cells—Nissl, 410×

Figs. 59, 60, 61, & 62.

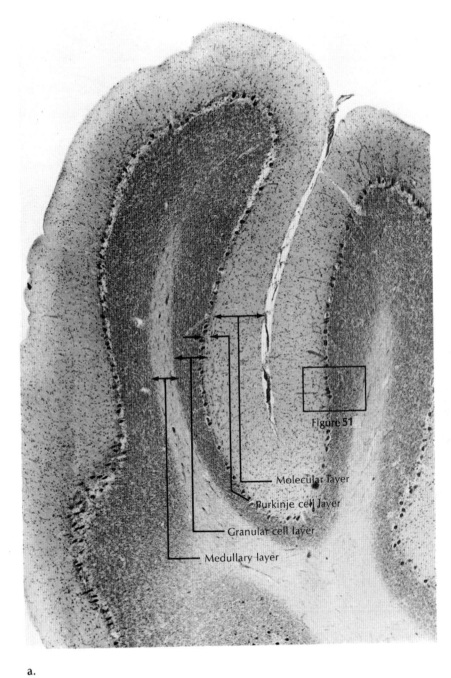

Molecular layer

Purkinje cell layer

Granular cell layer

Medullary layer

Figure 51

a.

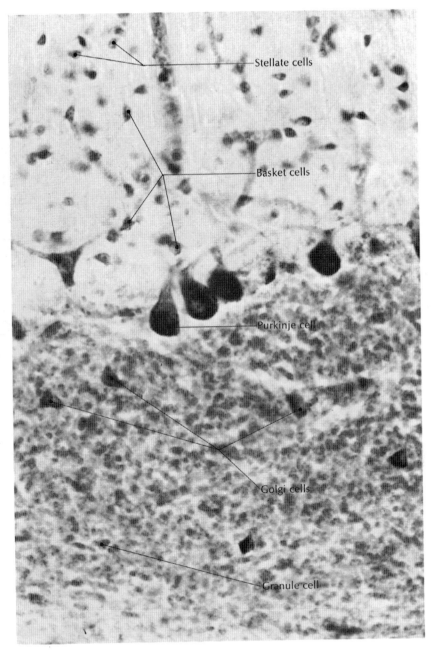

Stellate cells

Basket cells

Purkinje cell

Golgi cells

Granule cell

b.

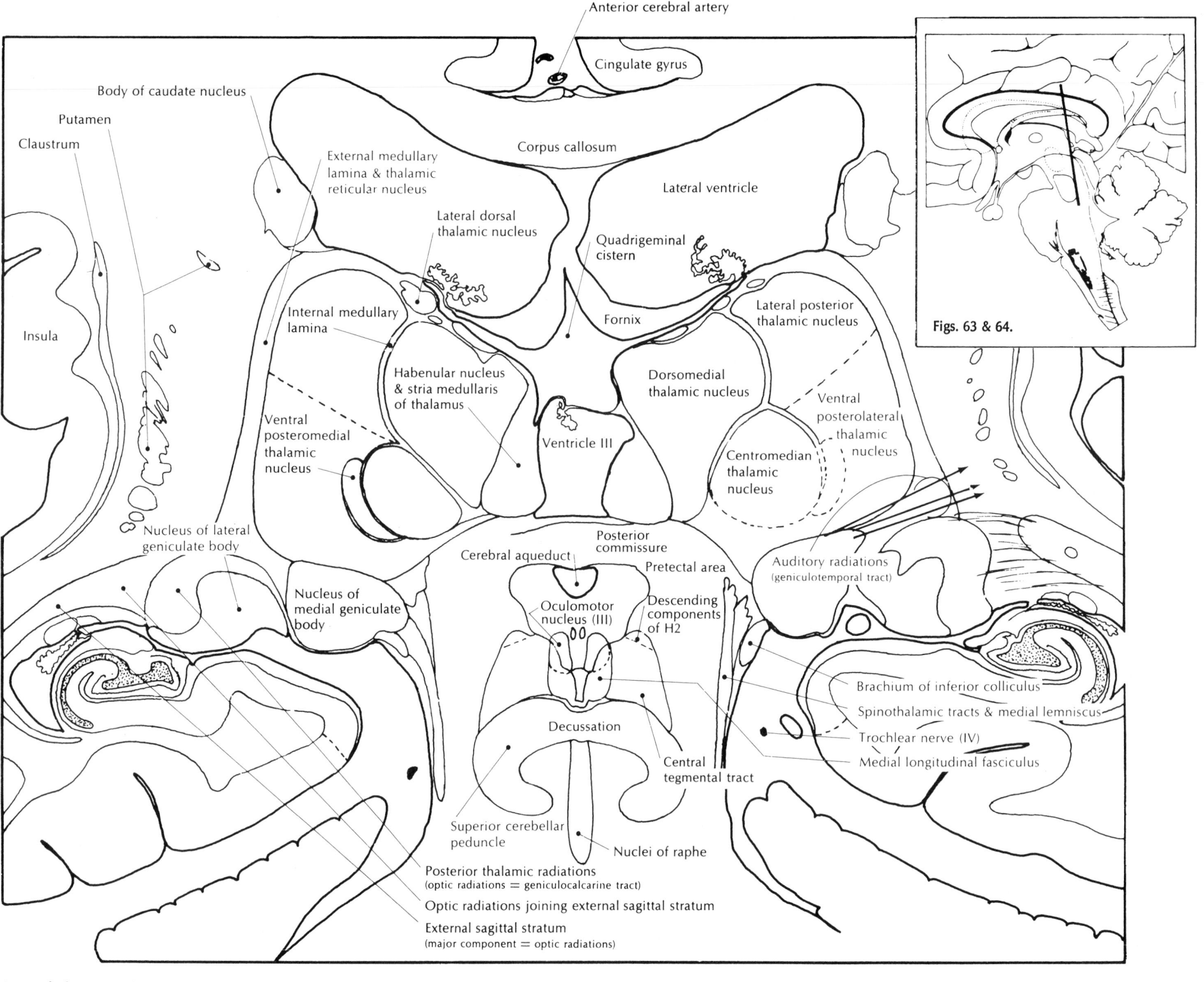

Figure 63. Diencephalon—caudal extent of lenticular nucleus at posterior commissure—Weil, 4×

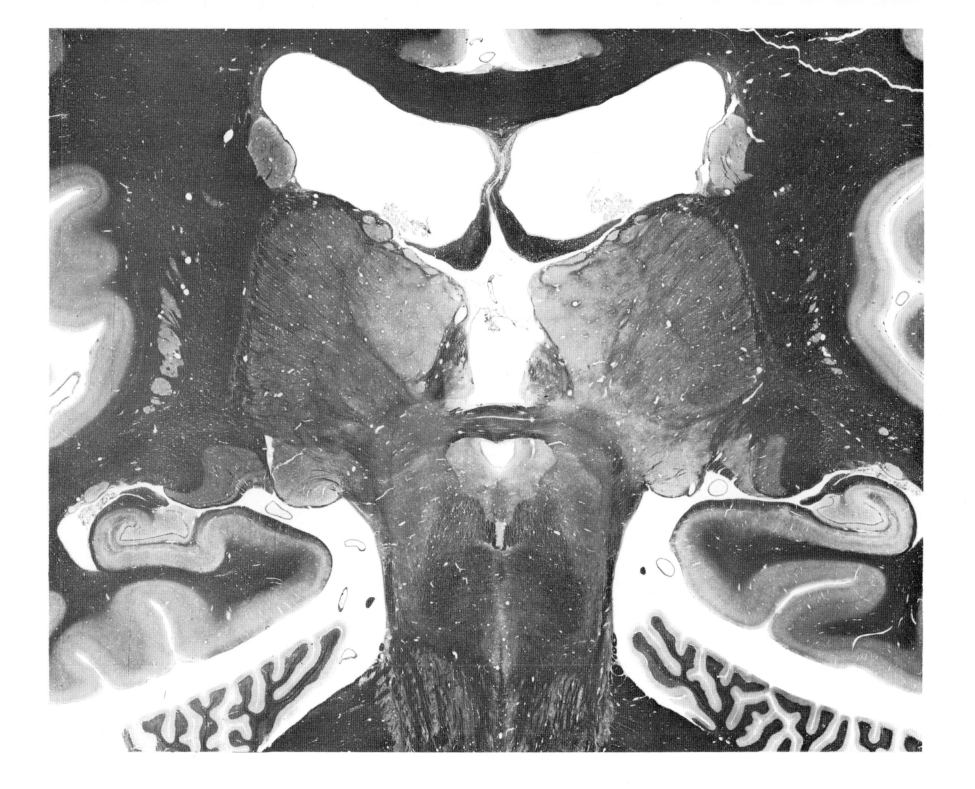

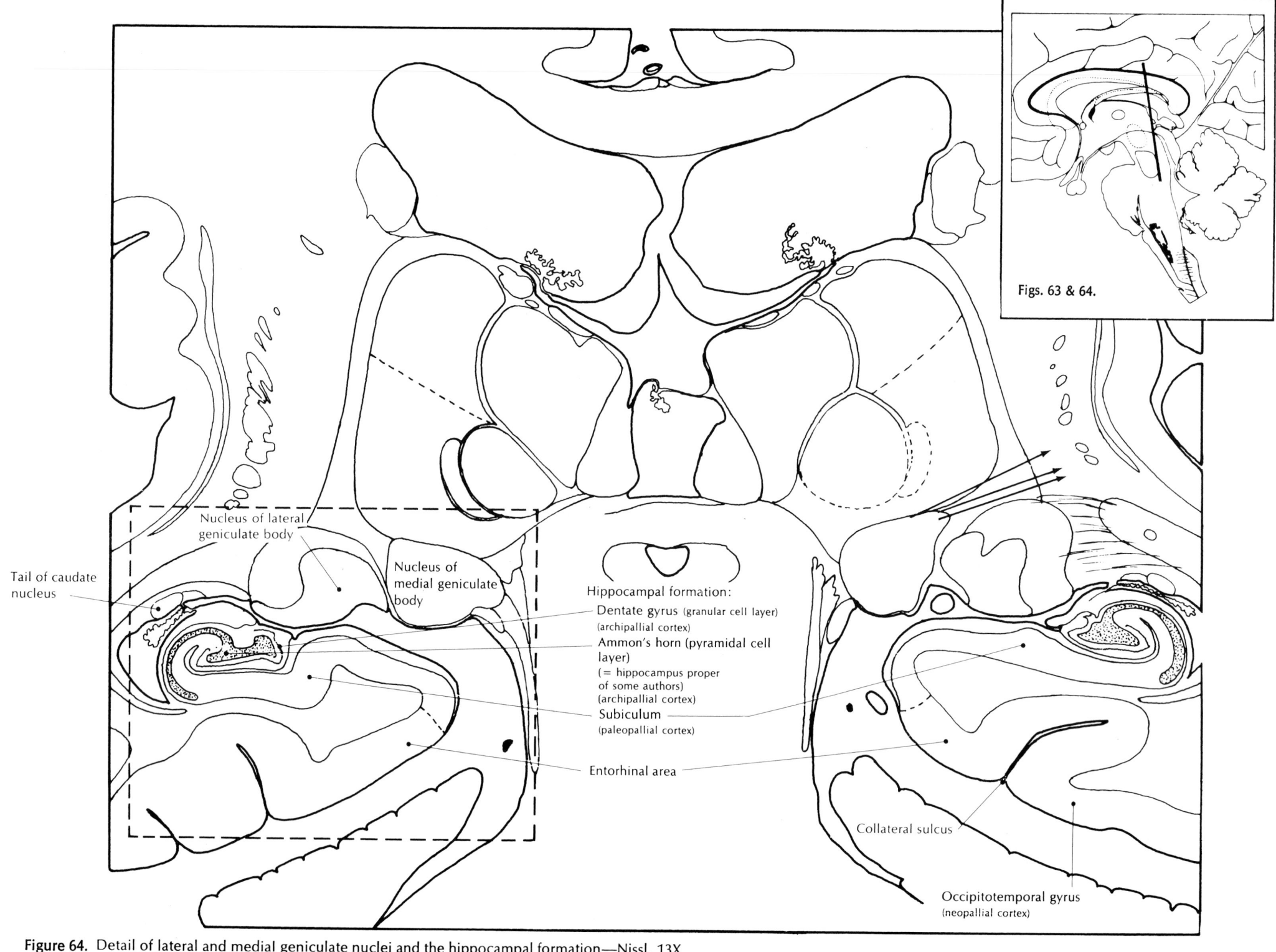

Figs. 63 & 64.

Nucleus of lateral geniculate body

Tail of caudate nucleus

Nucleus of medial geniculate body

Hippocampal formation:

Dentate gyrus (granular cell layer)
(archipallial cortex)

Ammon's horn (pyramidal cell layer)
(= hippocampus proper of some authors)
(archipallial cortex)

Subiculum
(paleopallial cortex)

Entorhinal area

Collateral sulcus

Occipitotemporal gyrus
(neopallial cortex)

Figure 64. Detail of lateral and medial geniculate nuclei and the hippocampal formation—Nissl, 13X

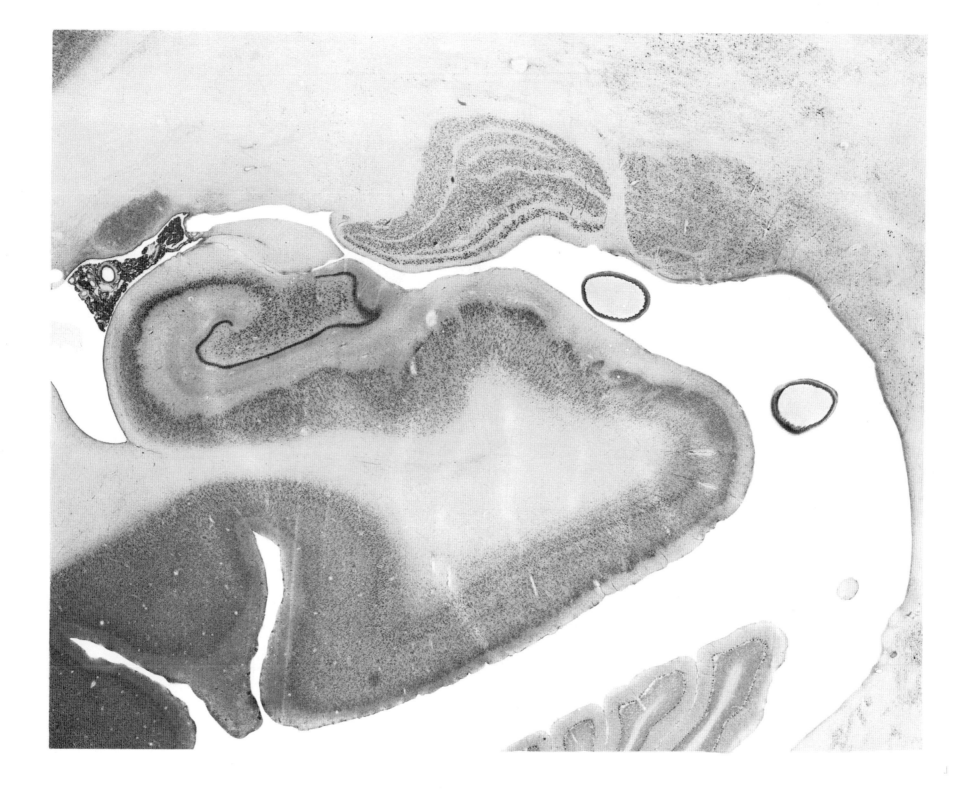

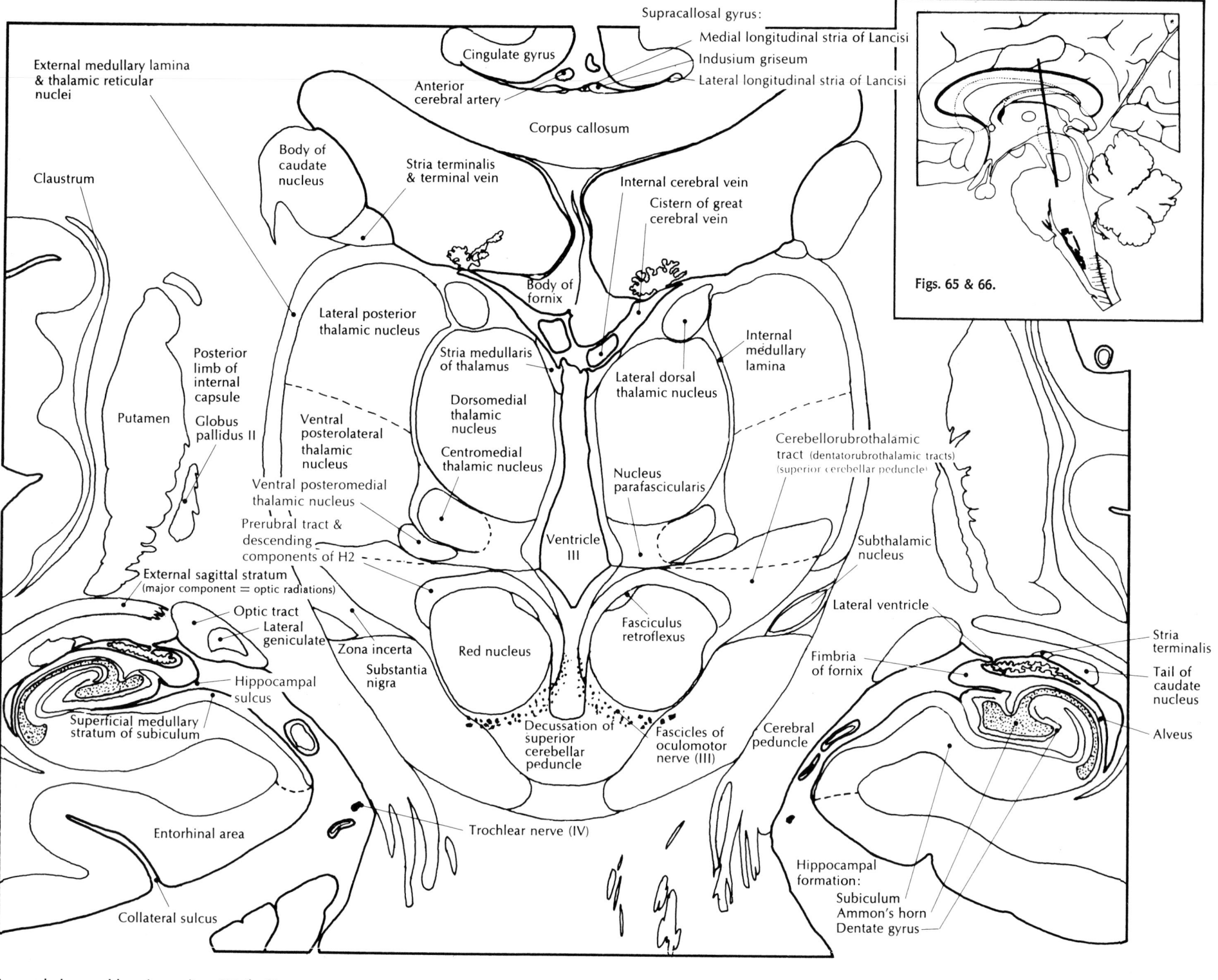

Figure 65. Diencephalon and basal ganglia—Weil, 4X

130

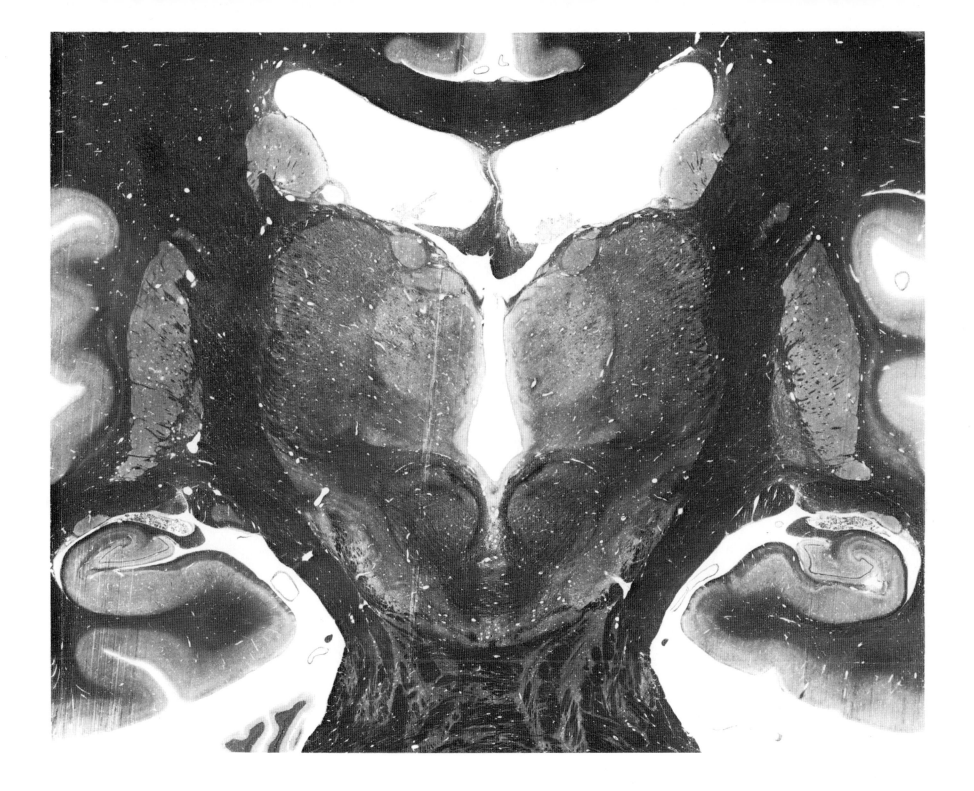

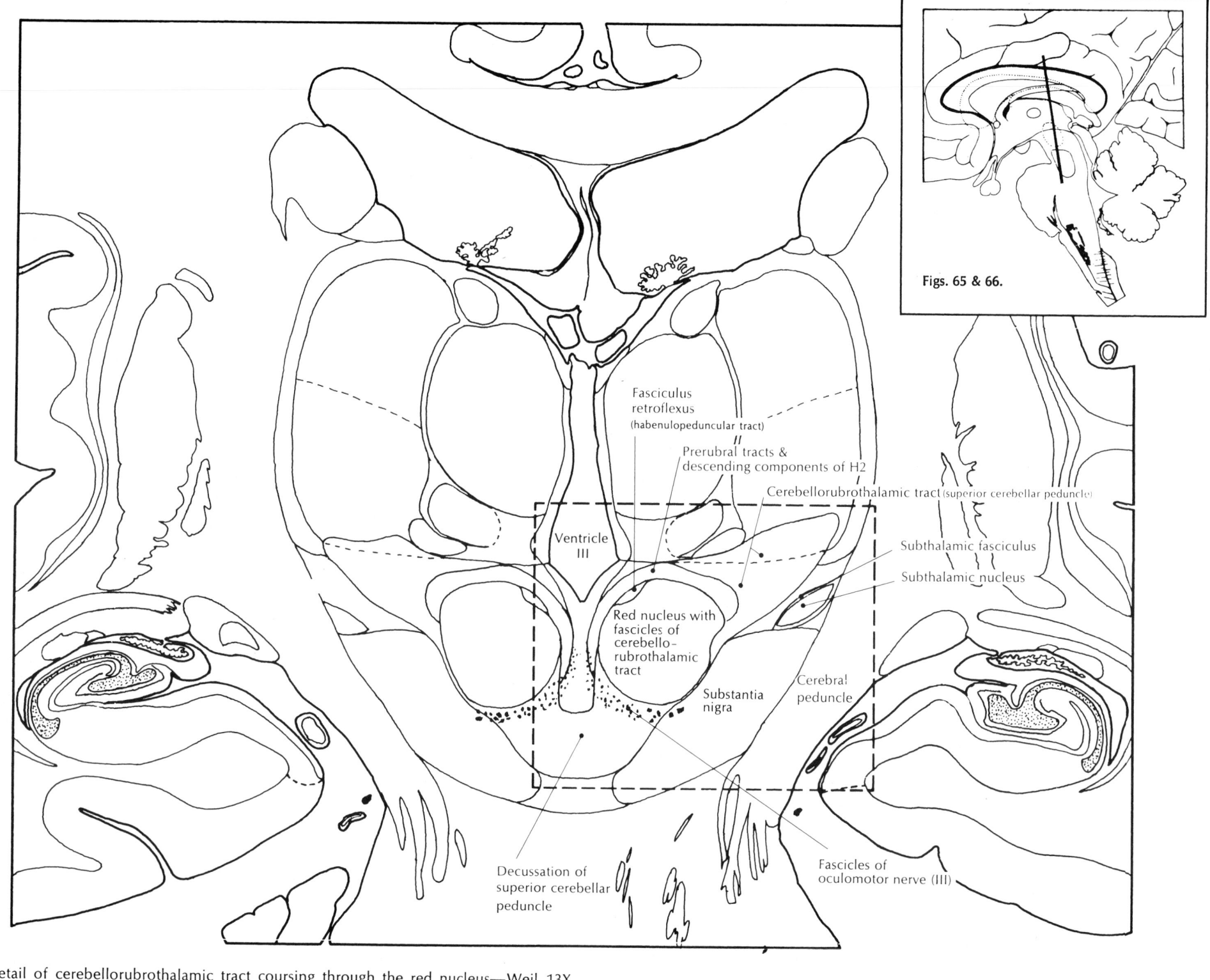

Figure 66. Detail of cerebellorubrothalamic tract coursing through the red nucleus—Weil, 13X

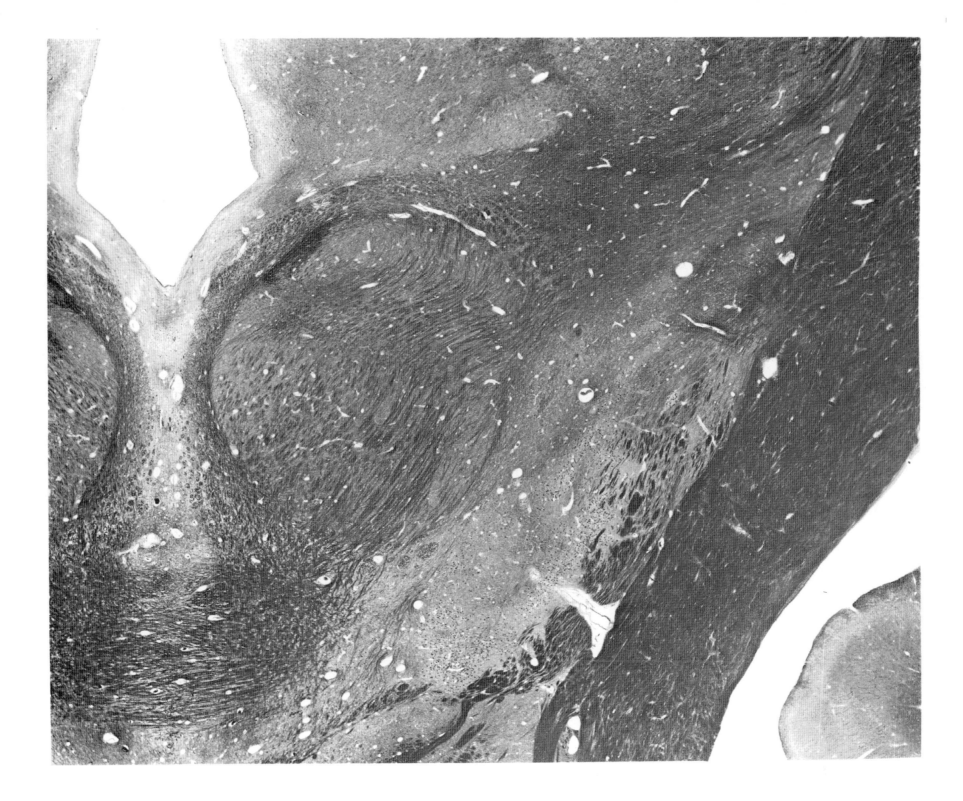

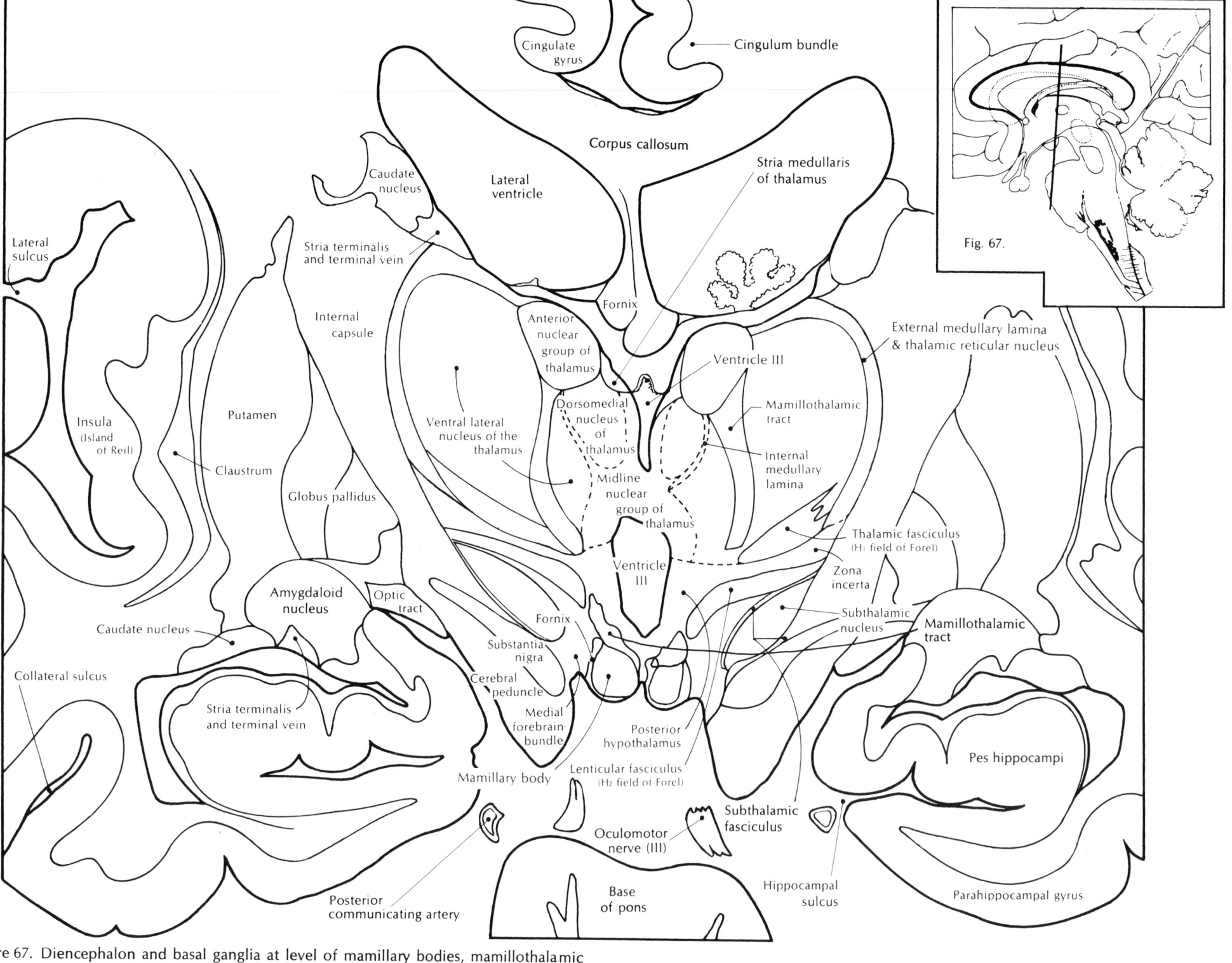

Figure 67. Diencephalon and basal ganglia at level of mamillary bodies, mamillothalamic tract, and anterior nuclear group of the thalamus—Weil, 4X

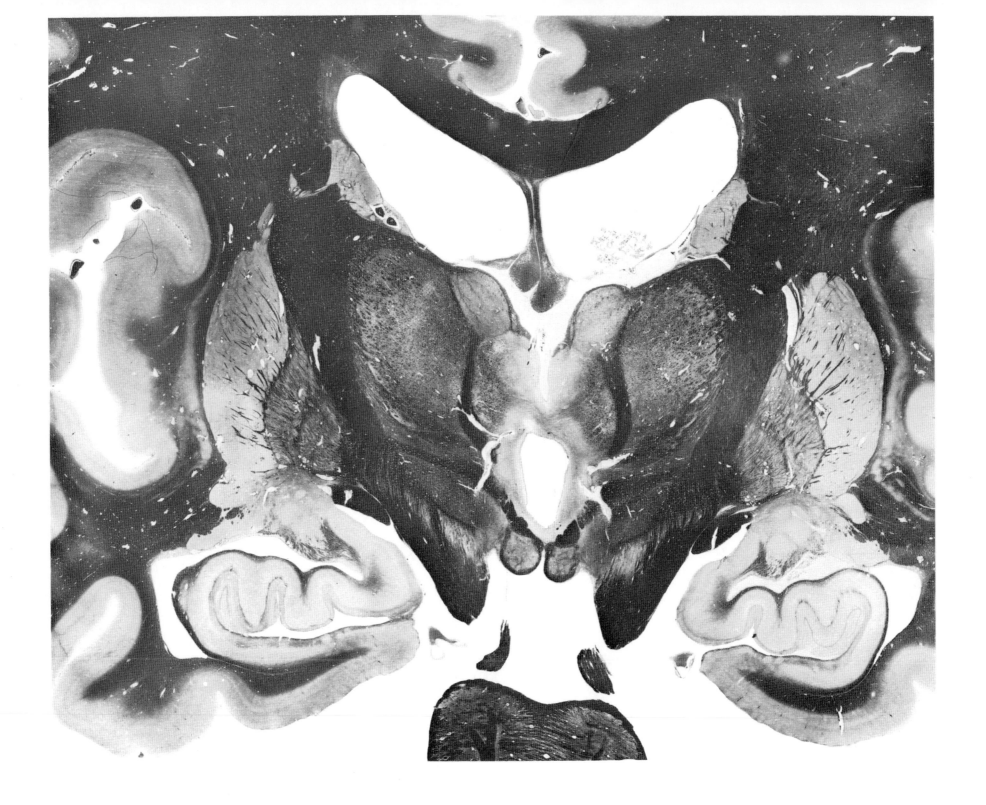

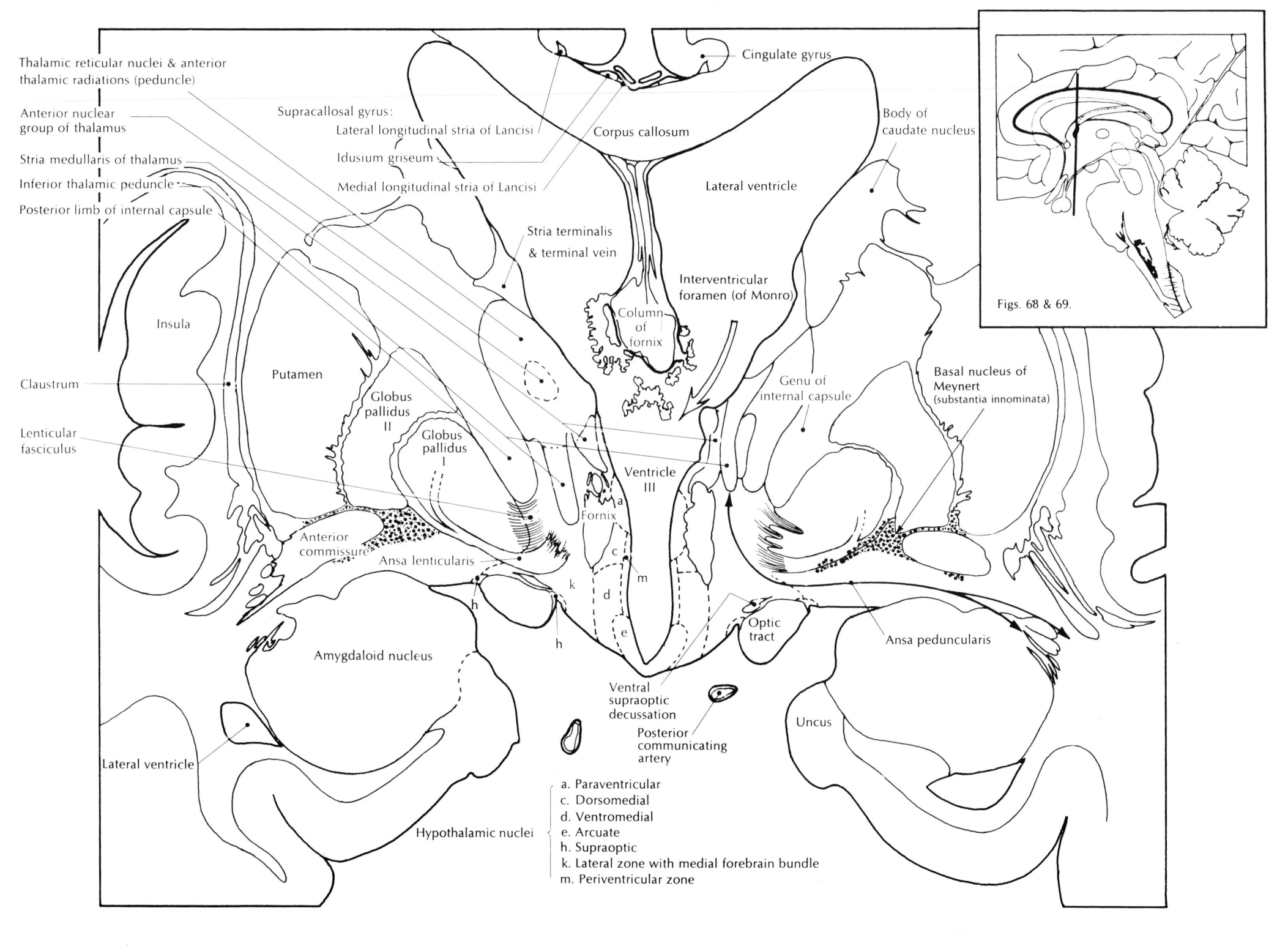

Figure 68. Basal ganglia and rostral diencephalon, tuberal region of hypothalamus—Weil, 4X

136

Labels (clockwise from top left):

Thalamic reticular nuclei & anterior thalamic radiations (peduncle)

Anterior nuclear group of thalamus

Stria medullaris of thalamus

Inferior thalamic peduncle

Posterior limb of internal capsule

Insula

Claustrum

Lenticular fasciculus

Putamen

Globus pallidus II

Globus pallidus I

Anterior commissure

Ansa lenticularis

Amygdaloid nucleus

Lateral ventricle

Hypothalamic nuclei

Supracallosal gyrus:
Lateral longitudinal stria of Lancisi
Idusium griseum
Medial longitudinal stria of Lancisi

Stria terminalis & terminal vein

Column of fornix

Fornix

Cingulate gyrus

Corpus callosum

Lateral ventricle

Interventricular foramen (of Monro)

Body of caudate nucleus

Genu of internal capsule

Basal nucleus of Meynert (substantia innominata)

Ventricle III

Optic tract

Ansa peduncularis

Ventral supraoptic decussation

Posterior communicating artery

Uncus

a. Paraventricular
c. Dorsomedial
d. Ventromedial
e. Arcuate
h. Supraoptic
k. Lateral zone with medial forebrain bundle
m. Periventricular zone

Figs. 68 & 69.

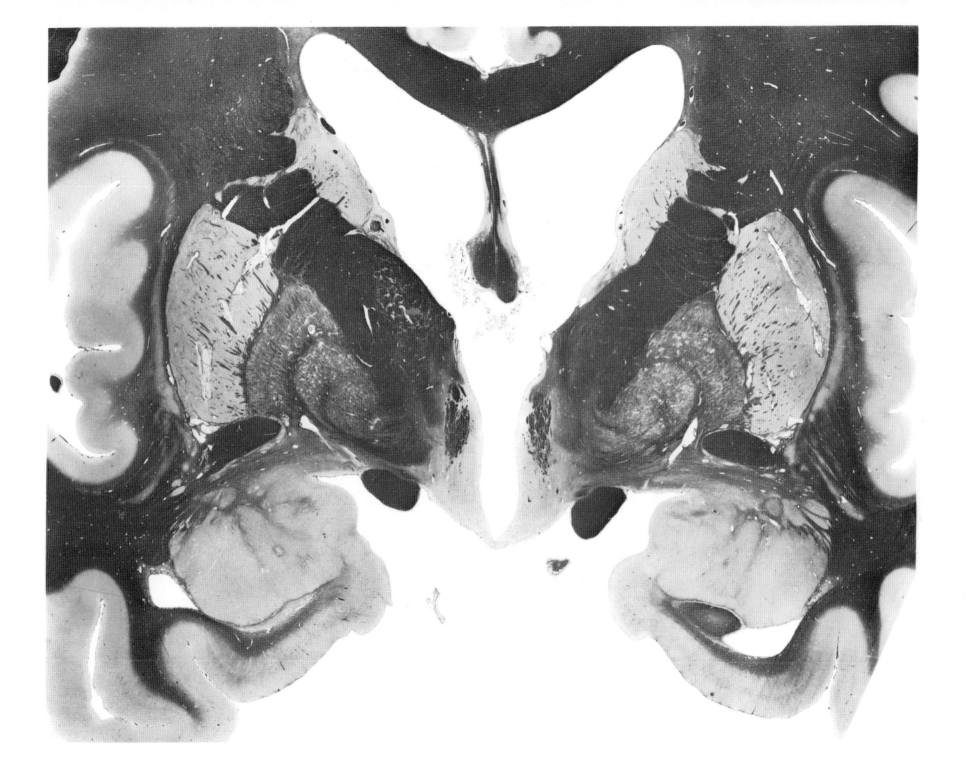

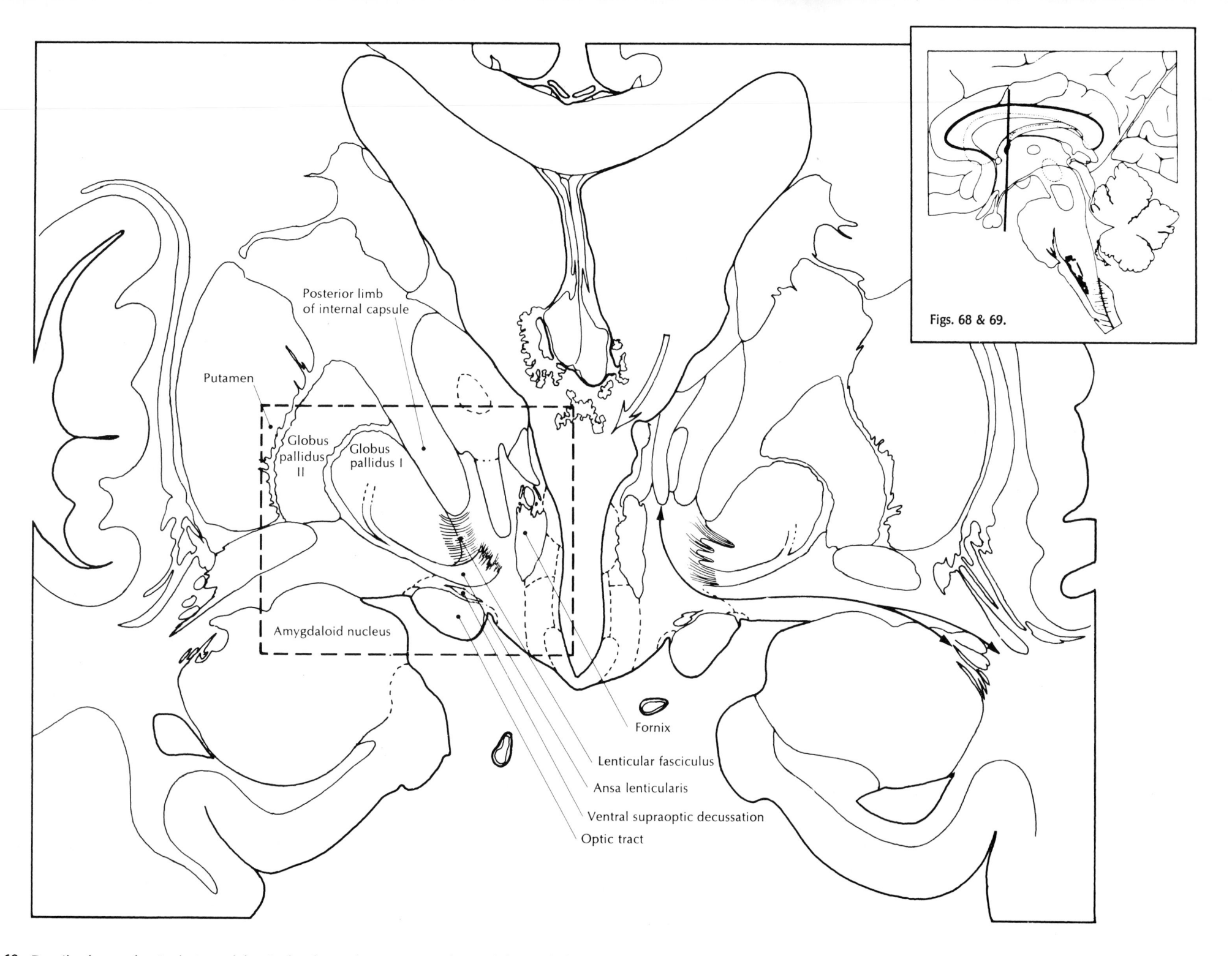

Figure 69. Detail of ansa lenticularis and lenticular fasciculus emerging from globus pallidus—Weil, 12X

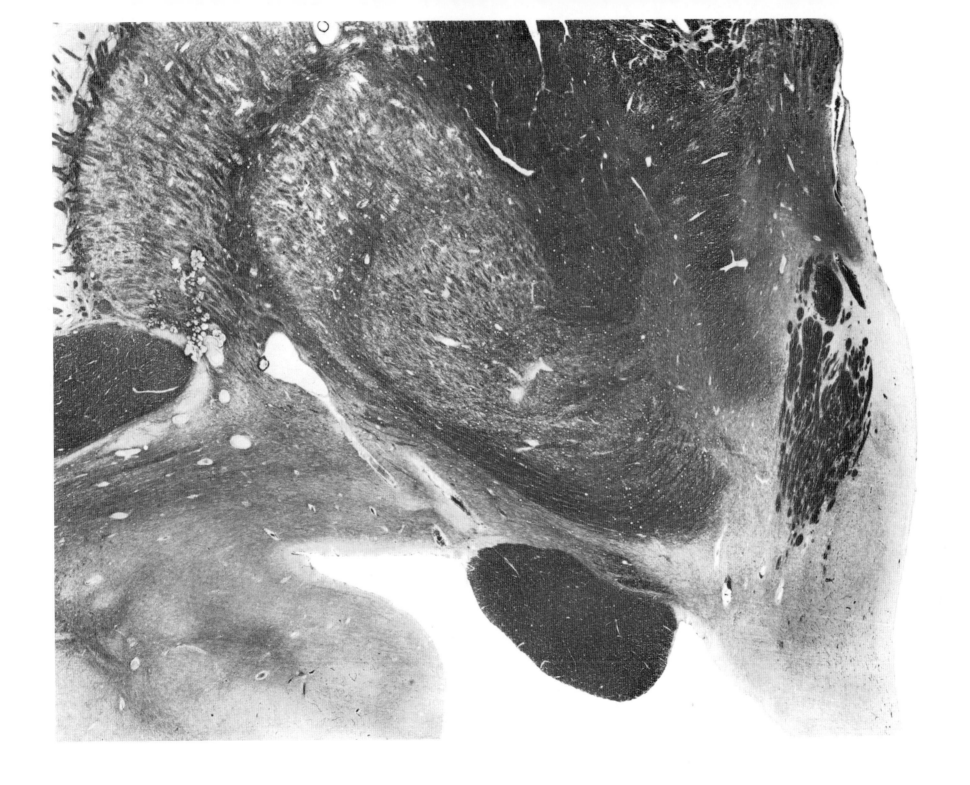

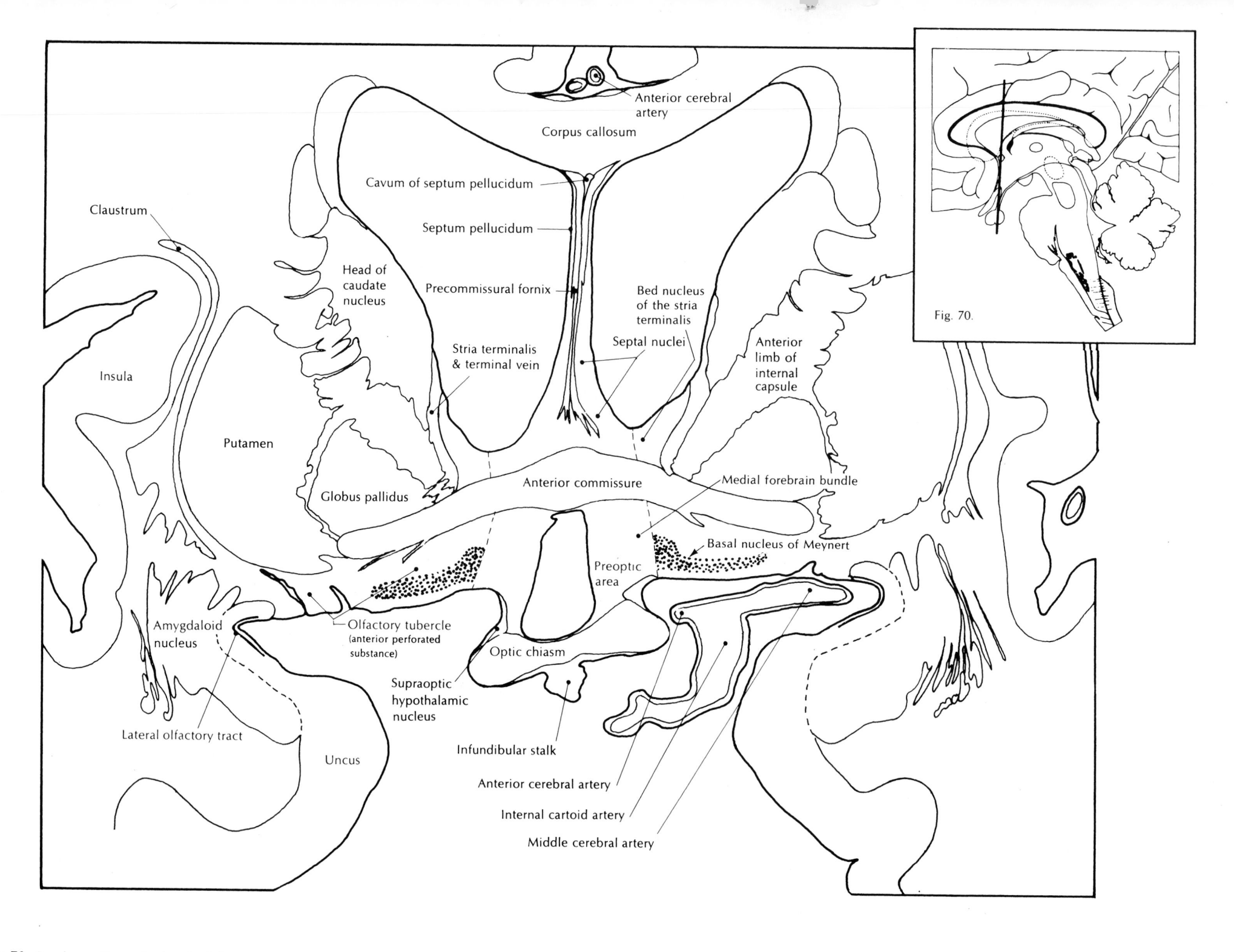

Figure 70. Basal ganglia at the level of the anterior commissure—Weil, 4X

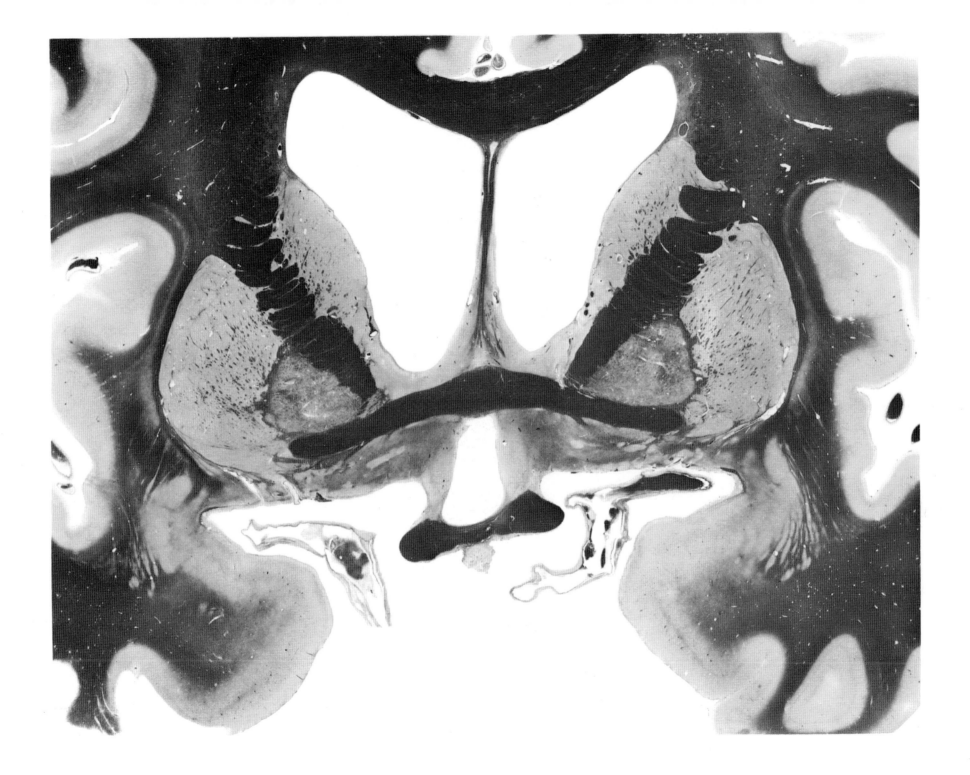

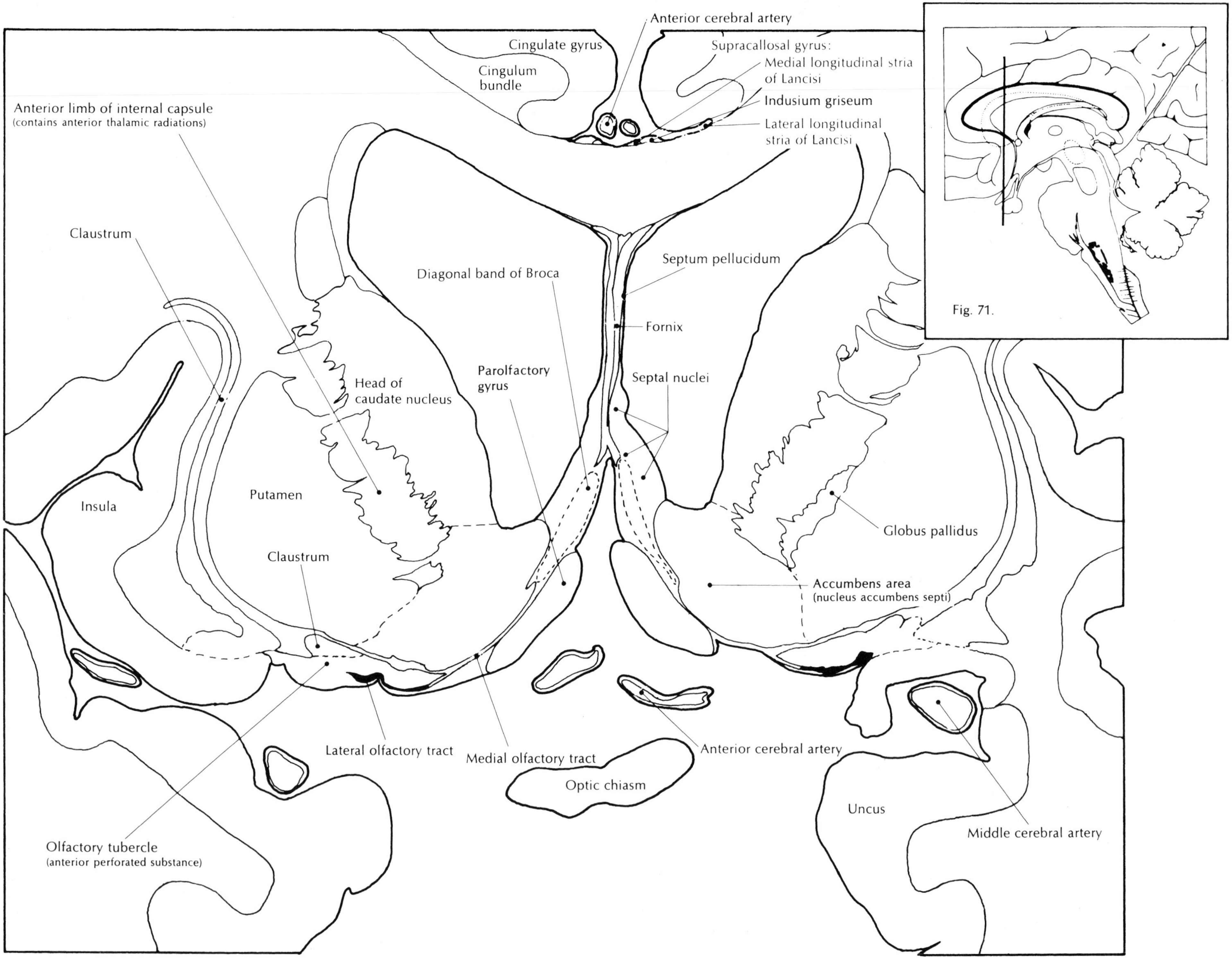
Anterior cerebral artery
Cingulate gyrus
Cingulum bundle
Supracallosal gyrus:
Medial longitudinal stria of Lancisi
Indusium griseum
Lateral longitudinal stria of Lancisi
Anterior limb of internal capsule
(contains anterior thalamic radiations)
Claustrum
Diagonal band of Broca
Septum pellucidum
Fornix
Fig. 71.
Head of caudate nucleus
Parolfactory gyrus
Septal nuclei
Putamen
Insula
Globus pallidus
Claustrum
Accumbens area
(nucleus accumbens septi)
Lateral olfactory tract
Medial olfactory tract
Anterior cerebral artery
Optic chiasm
Uncus
Middle cerebral artery
Olfactory tubercle
(anterior perforated substance)

Figure 71. Basal ganglia rostral to anterior commissure, head of the caudate nucleus—Weil, 4X

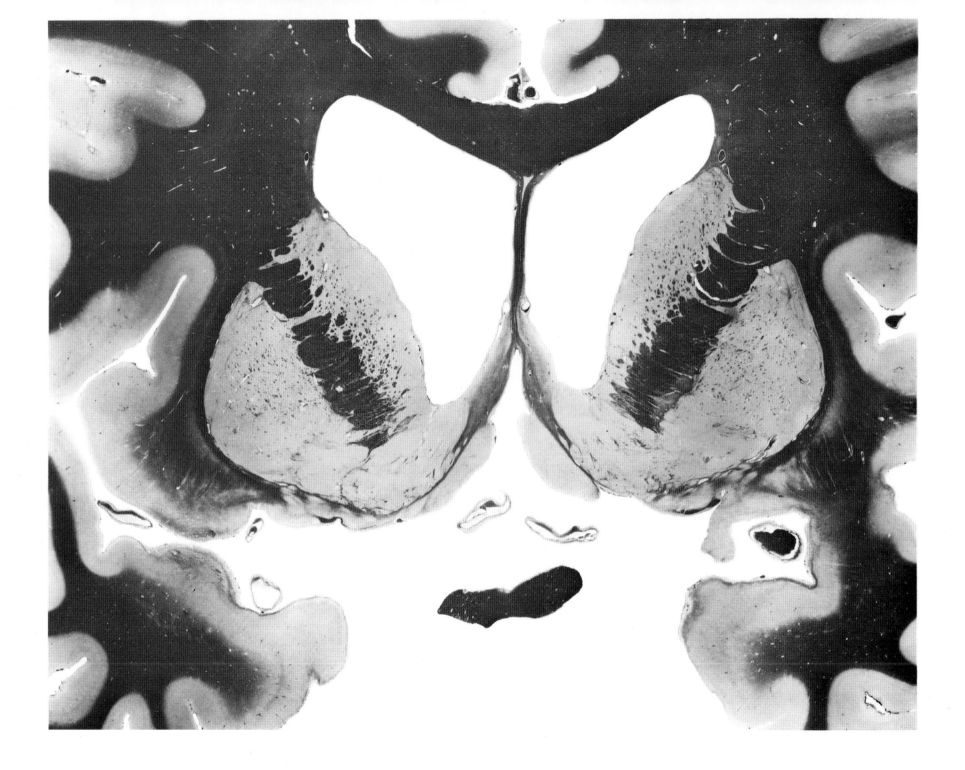

SAGITTAL MICROSCOPIC SECTIONS OF THE BRAIN STEM, DIENCEPHALON, AND BASAL GANGLIA

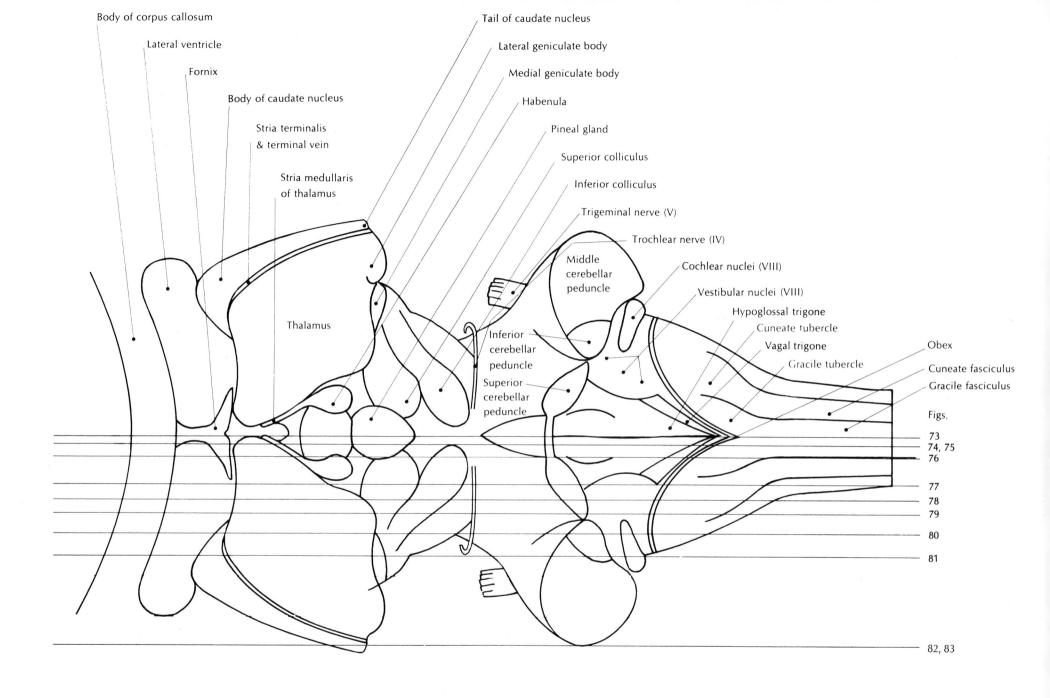

Body of corpus callosum

Lateral ventricle

Fornix

Body of caudate nucleus

Stria terminalis
& terminal vein

Stria medullaris
of thalamus

Tail of caudate nucleus

Lateral geniculate body

Medial geniculate body

Habenula

Pineal gland

Superior colliculus

Inferior colliculus

Trigeminal nerve (V)

Trochlear nerve (IV)

Cochlear nuclei (VIII)

Vestibular nuclei (VIII)

Hypoglossal trigone

Cuneate tubercle

Vagal trigone

Gracile tubercle

Obex

Cuneate fasciculus

Gracile fasciculus

Middle
cerebellar
peduncle

Inferior
cerebellar
peduncle

Superior
cerebellar
peduncle

Thalamus

Figs.

73

74, 75

76

77

78

79

80

81

82, 83

Figure 72. Dorsal surface of the brain stem and diencephalon indicating the locations
of the sagittal sections of the brain stem, diencephalon, and basal ganglia

145

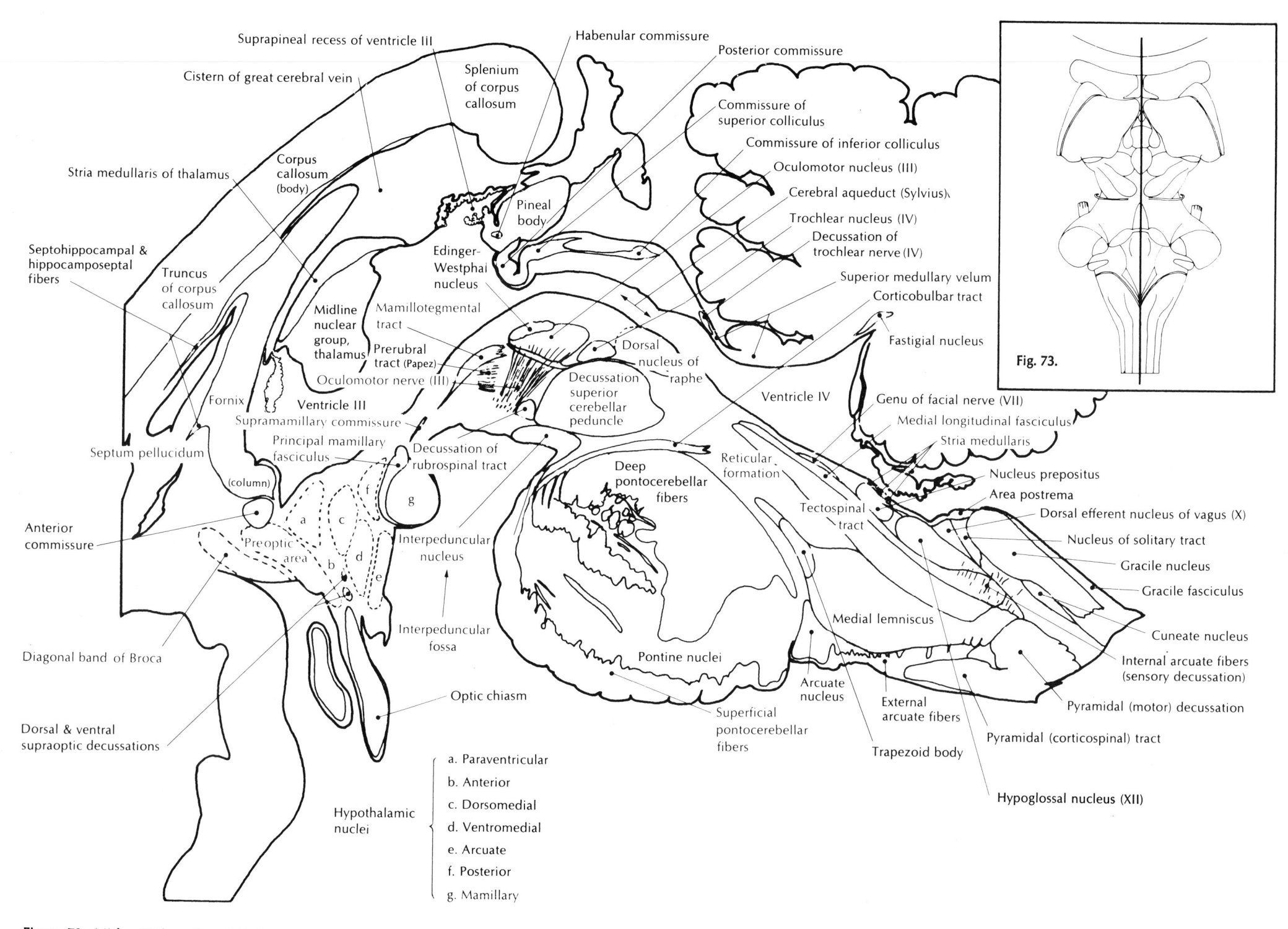

Figure 73. Midsagittal section—Weil, 3.5×

146

Suprapineal recess of ventricle III

Habenular commissure

Posterior commissure

Cistern of great cerebral vein

Splenium of corpus callosum

Commissure of superior colliculus

Commissure of inferior colliculus

Oculomotor nucleus (III)

Cerebral aqueduct (Sylvius)

Stria medullaris of thalamus

Corpus callosum (body)

Pineal body

Trochlear nucleus (IV)

Decussation of trochlear nerve (IV)

Edinger-Westphal nucleus

Superior medullary velum

Corticobulbar tract

Septohippocampal & hippocamposeptal fibers

Truncus of corpus callosum

Midline nuclear group, thalamus

Mamillotegmental tract

Dorsal nucleus of raphe

Fastigial nucleus

Prerubral tract (Papez)

Decussation superior cerebellar peduncle

Ventricle IV

Genu of facial nerve (VII)

Fornix

Oculomotor nerve (III)

Medial longitudinal fasciculus

Ventricle III

Stria medullaris

Septum pellucidum

Supramamillary commissure

Principal mamillary fasciculus

Decussation of rubrospinal tract

Reticular formation

Nucleus prepositus

Area postrema

(column)

Deep pontocerebellar fibers

Tectospinal tract

Dorsal efferent nucleus of vagus (X)

Anterior commissure

Interpeduncular nucleus

Nucleus of solitary tract

Gracile nucleus

Preoptic area

Gracile fasciculus

Diagonal band of Broca

Interpeduncular fossa

Cuneate nucleus

Medial lemniscus

Internal arcuate fibers (sensory decussation)

Optic chiasm

Pontine nuclei

Arcuate nucleus

External arcuate fibers

Pyramidal (motor) decussation

Dorsal & ventral supraoptic decussations

Superficial pontocerebellar fibers

Pyramidal (corticospinal) tract

Trapezoid body

Hypoglossal nucleus (XII)

Hypothalamic nuclei

a. Paraventricular
b. Anterior
c. Dorsomedial
d. Ventromedial
e. Arcuate
f. Posterior
g. Mamillary

Fig. 73.

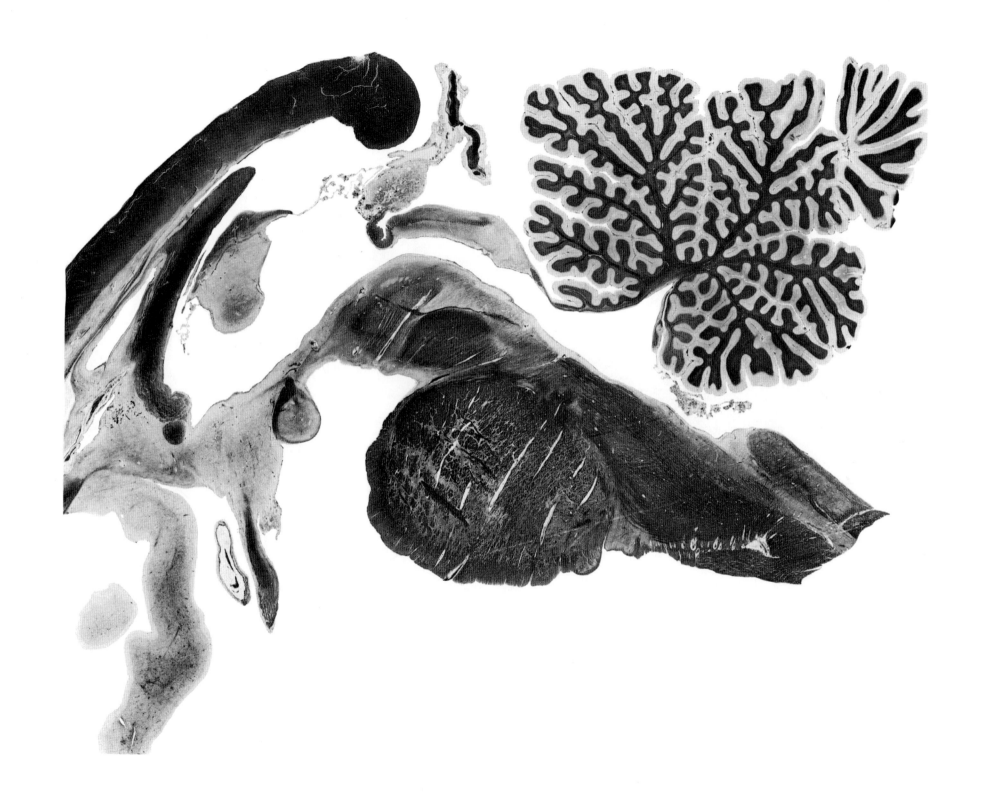

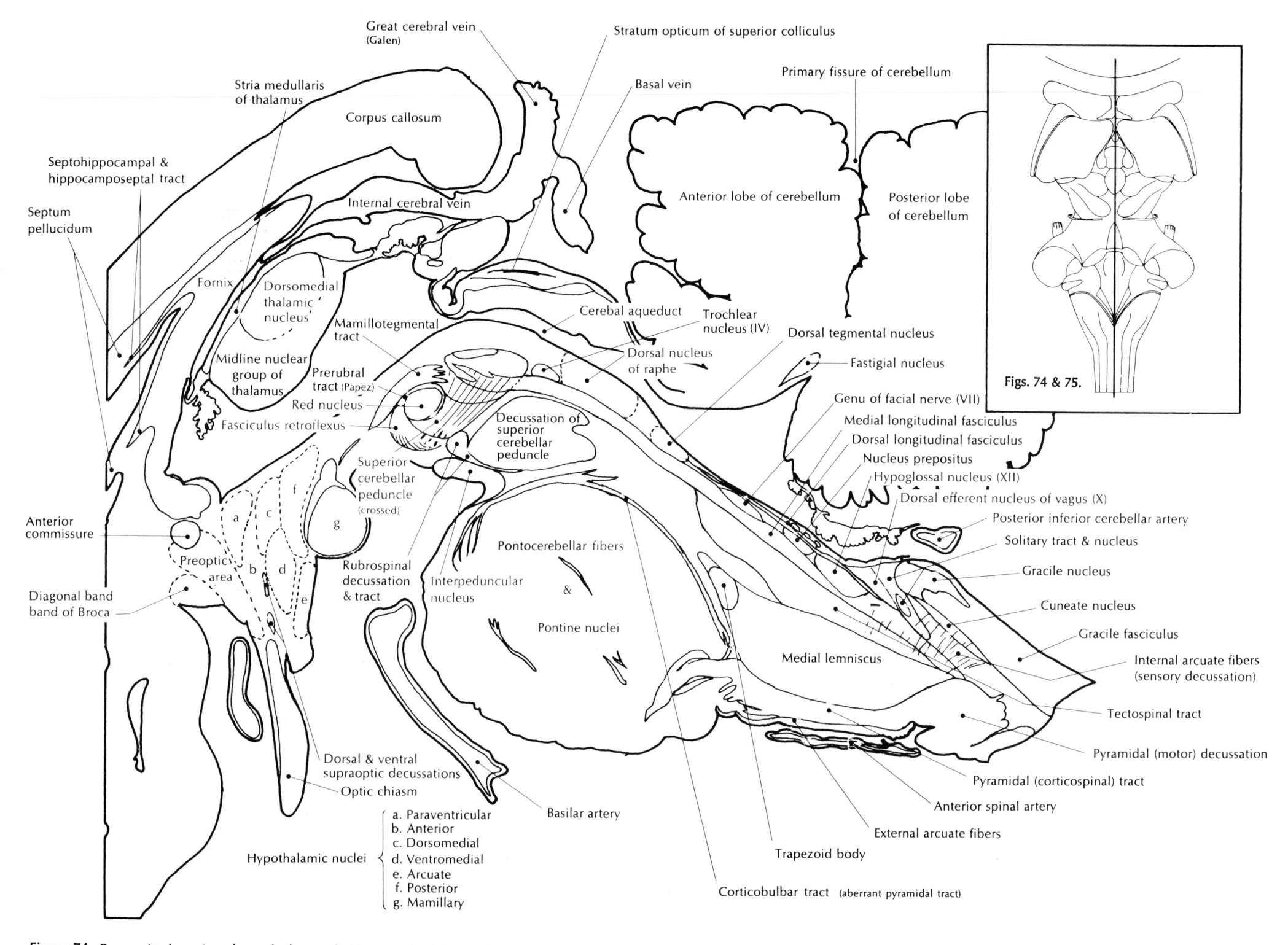

Figure 74. Parasagittal section through the medial longitudinal fasciculus—Weil, 3.5X

148

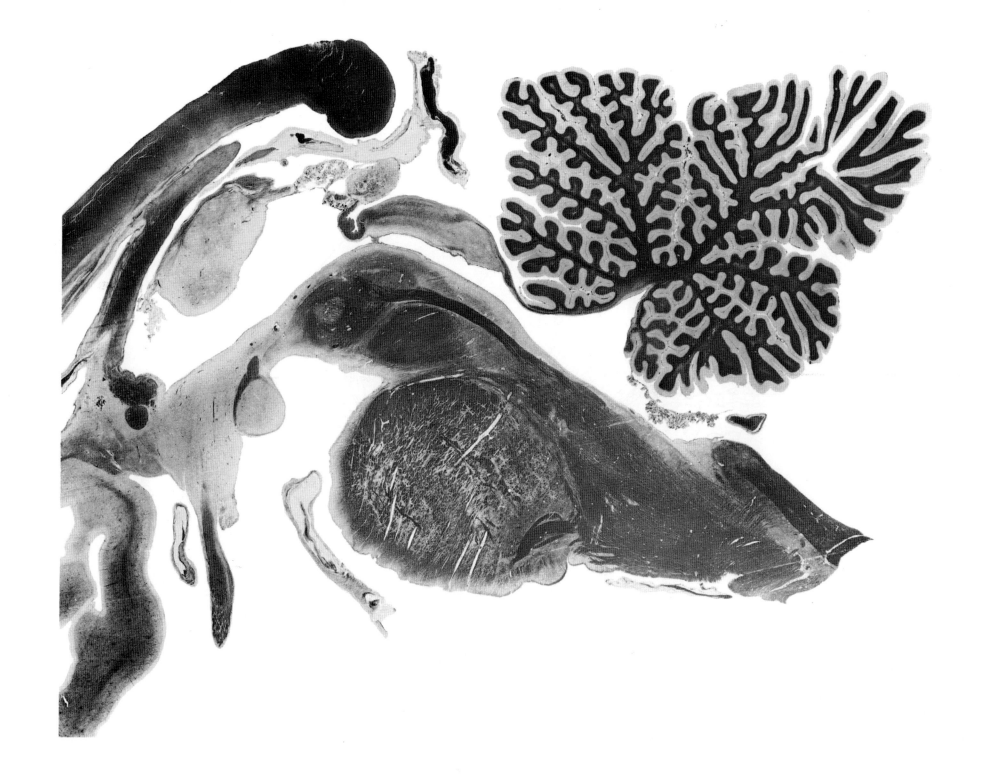

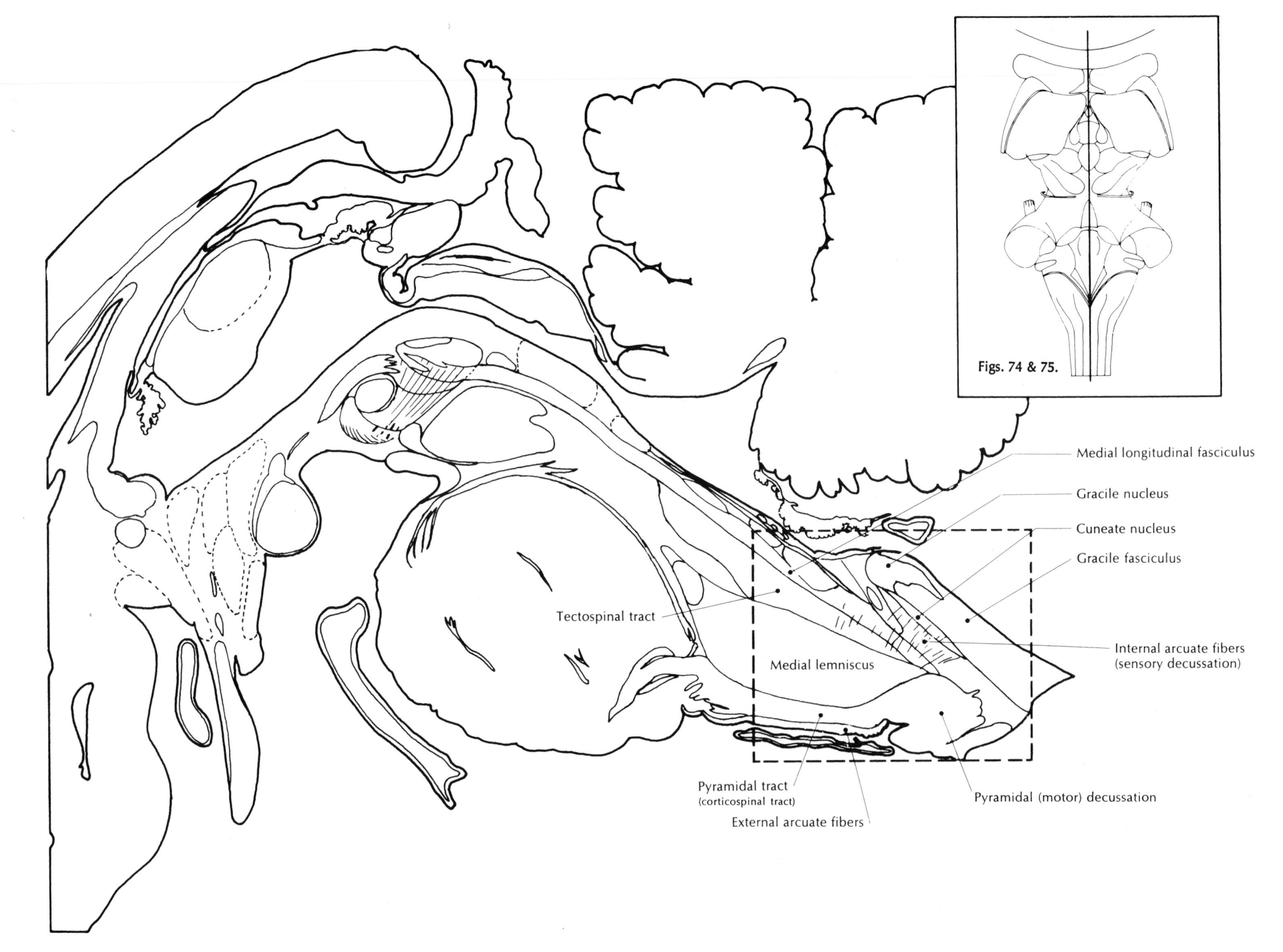

Figure 75. Detail of the motor and sensory decussations in the caudal half of the medulla—Weil, 14X

Figs. 74 & 75.

Medial longitudinal fasciculus

Gracile nucleus

Cuneate nucleus

Gracile fasciculus

Internal arcuate fibers
(sensory decussation)

Pyramidal (motor) decussation

Tectospinal tract

Medial lemniscus

Pyramidal tract
(corticospinal tract)

External arcuate fibers

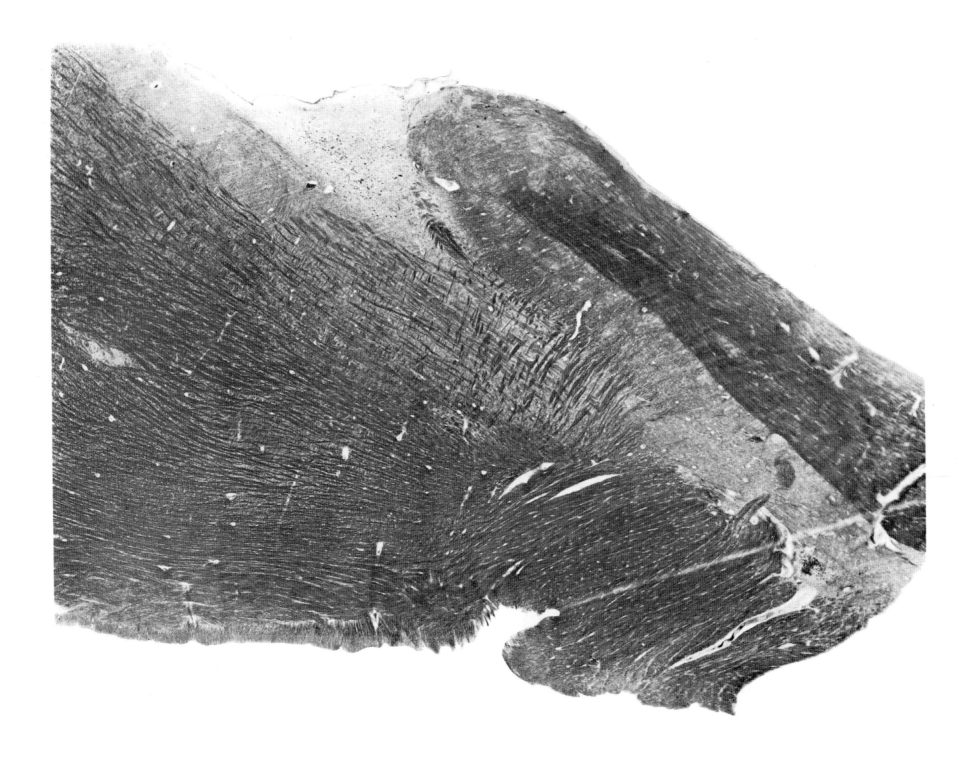

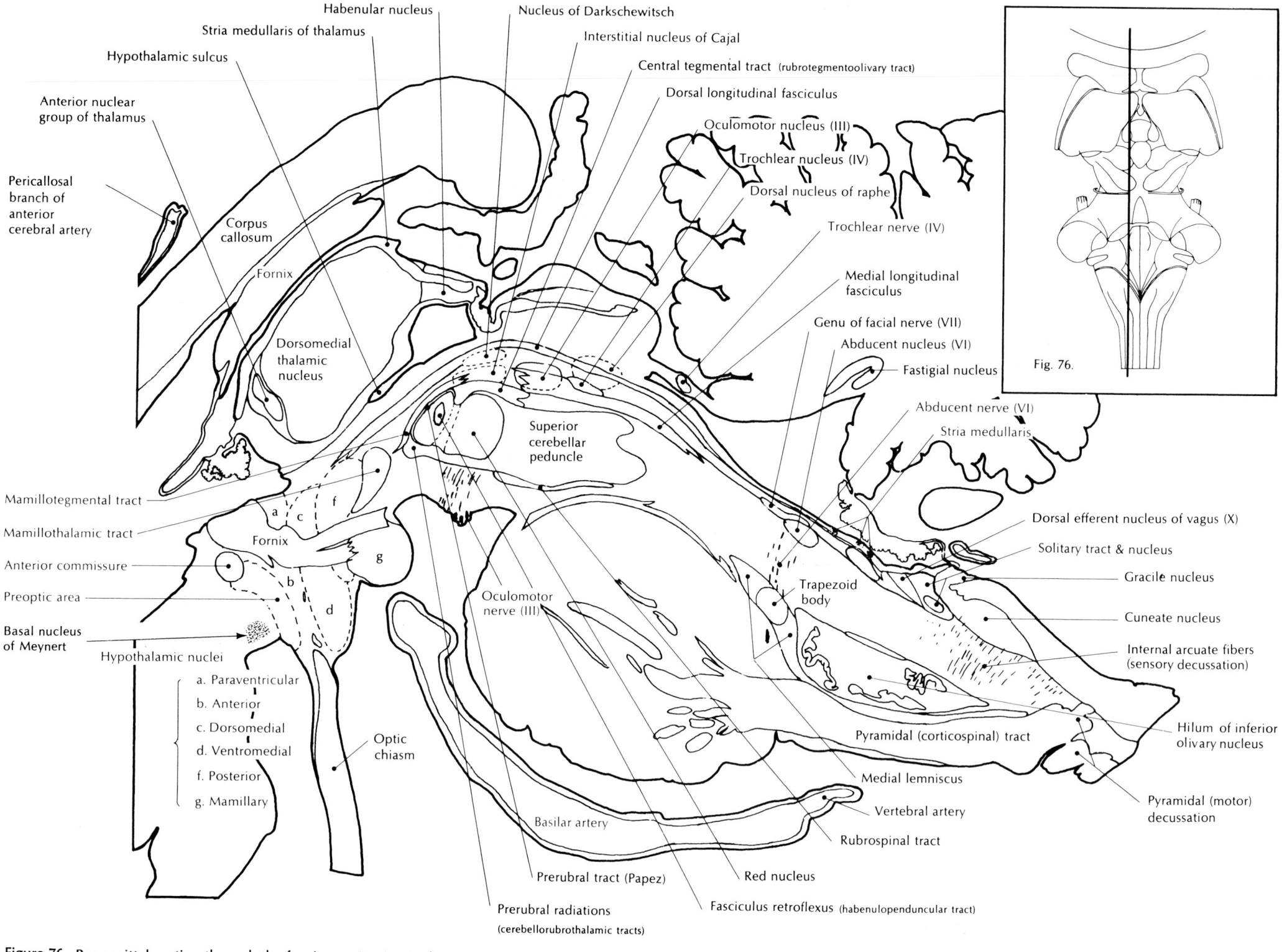

Figure 76. Parasagittal section through the fornix terminating in the mamillary nucleus—Weil, 3.5X

152

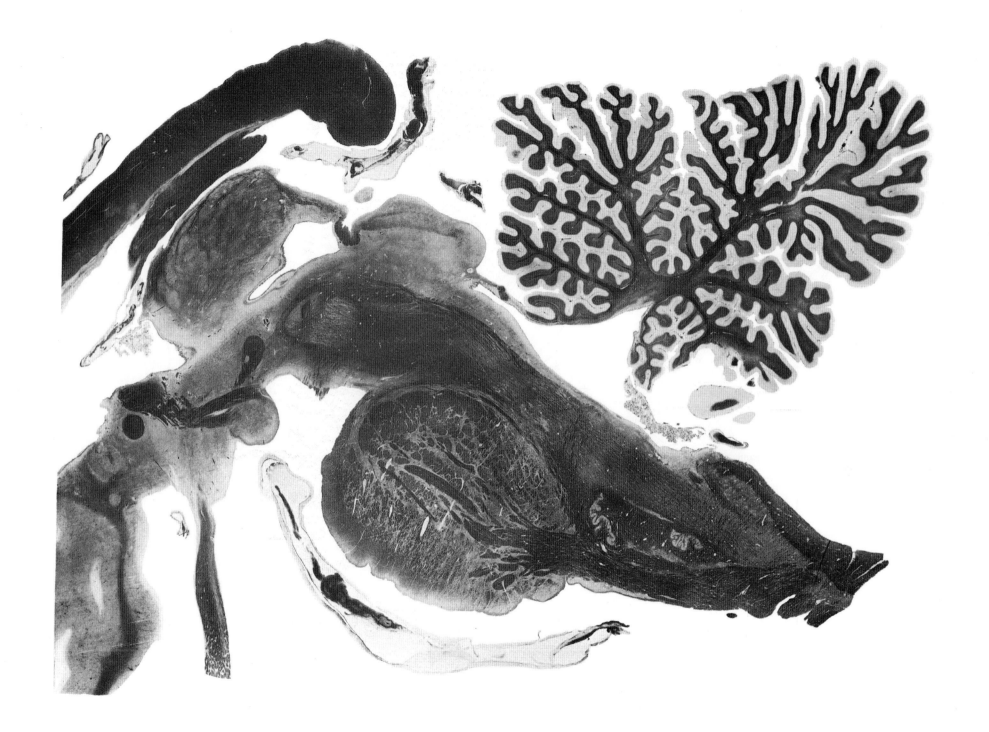

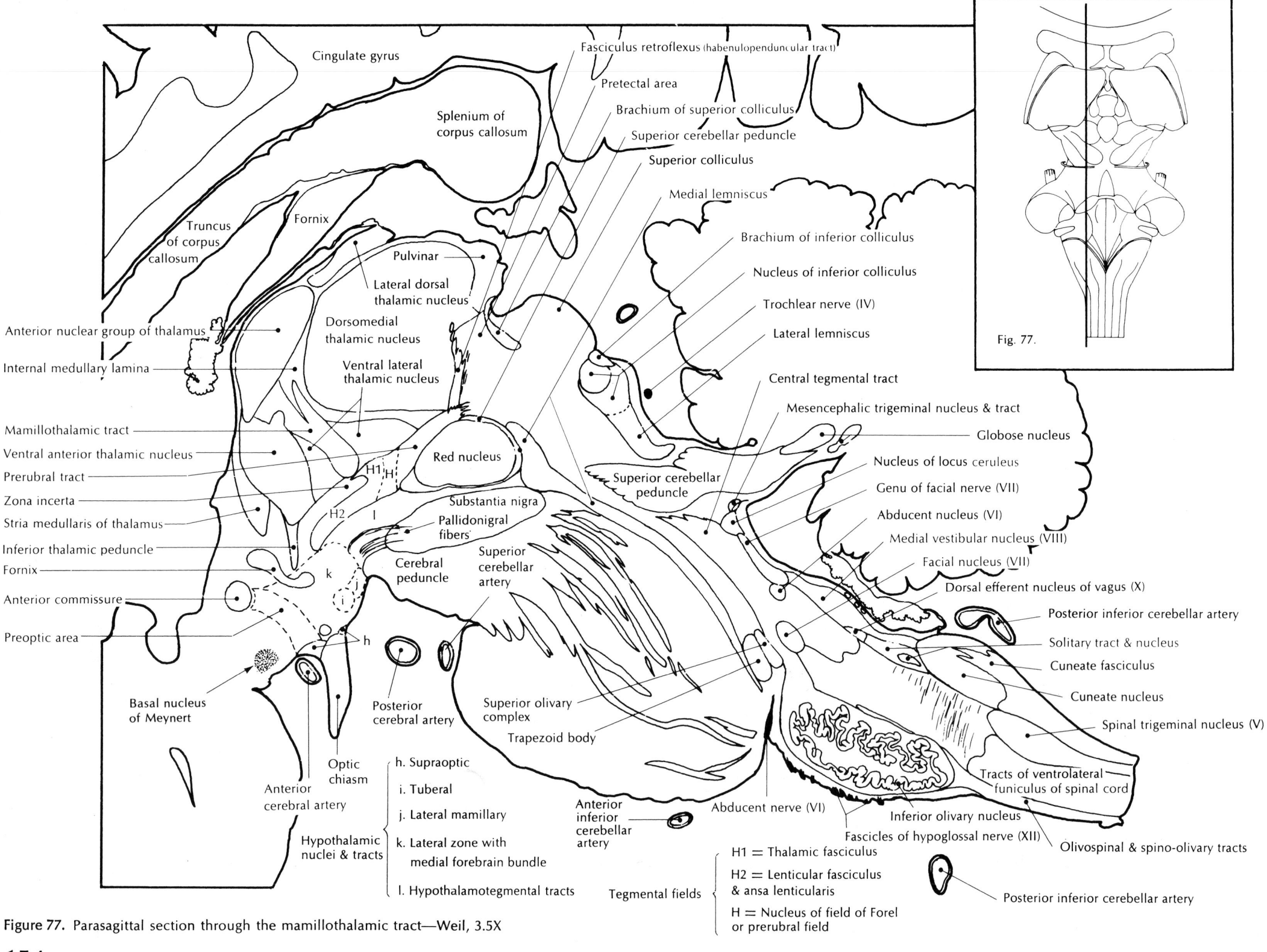

Cingulate gyrus

Fasciculus retroflexus (habenulopenduncular tract)

Pretect area

Brachium of superior colliculus

Splenium of corpus callosum

Superior cerebellar peduncle

Superior colliculus

Truncus of corpus callosum

Fornix

Medial lemniscus

Brachium of inferior colliculus

Pulvinar

Nucleus of inferior colliculus

Lateral dorsal thalamic nucleus

Trochlear nerve (IV)

Anterior nuclear group of thalamus

Dorsomedial thalamic nucleus

Lateral lemniscus

Internal medullary lamina

Ventral lateral thalamic nucleus

Central tegmental tract

Mesencephalic trigeminal nucleus & tract

Red nucleus

Globose nucleus

Mamillothalamic tract

Nucleus of locus ceruleus

Ventral anterior thalamic nucleus

Superior cerebellar peduncle

Genu of facial nerve (VII)

Prerubral tract

Substantia nigra

Abducent nucleus (VI)

Zona incerta

Pallidonigral fibers

Medial vestibular nucleus (VIII)

Stria medullaris of thalamus

Superior cerebellar artery

Facial nucleus (VII)

Inferior thalamic peduncle

Superior cerebellar peduncle

Cerebral peduncle

Dorsal efferent nucleus of vagus (X)

Fornix

Anterior commissure

Posterior inferior cerebellar artery

Solitary tract & nucleus

Preoptic area

Cuneate fasciculus

Cuneate nucleus

Basal nucleus of Meynert

Posterior cerebral artery

Superior olivary complex

Spinal trigeminal nucleus (V)

Trapezoid body

Optic chiasm

Anterior cerebral artery

h. Supraoptic

Anterior inferior cerebellar artery

Tracts of ventrolateral funiculus of spinal cord

Abducent nerve (VI)

Inferior olivary nucleus

i. Tuberal

Anterior cerebral artery

j. Lateral mamillary

Fascicles of hypoglossal nerve (XII)

Olivospinal & spino-olivary tracts

k. Lateral zone with medial forebrain bundle

Hypothalamic nuclei & tracts

H1 = Thalamic fasciculus

l. Hypothalamotegmental tracts

Tegmental fields

H2 = Lenticular fasciculus & ansa lenticularis

Posterior inferior cerebellar artery

H = Nucleus of field of Forel or prerubral field

Figure 77. Parasagittal section through the mamillothalamic tract—Weil, 3.5X

Fig. 77.

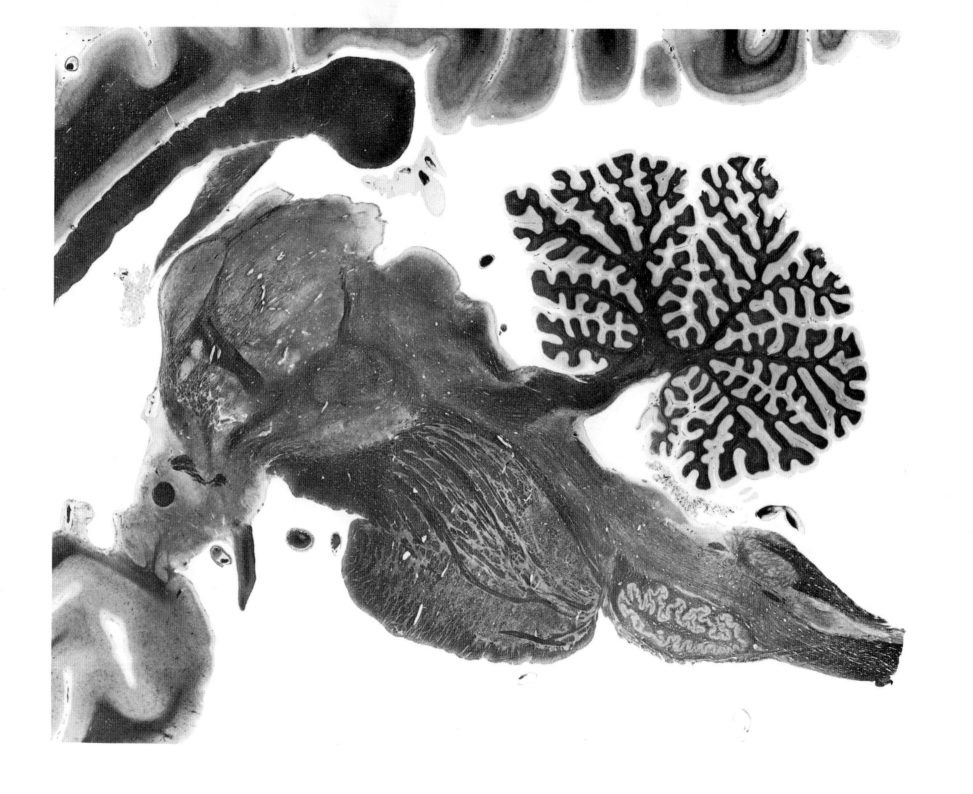

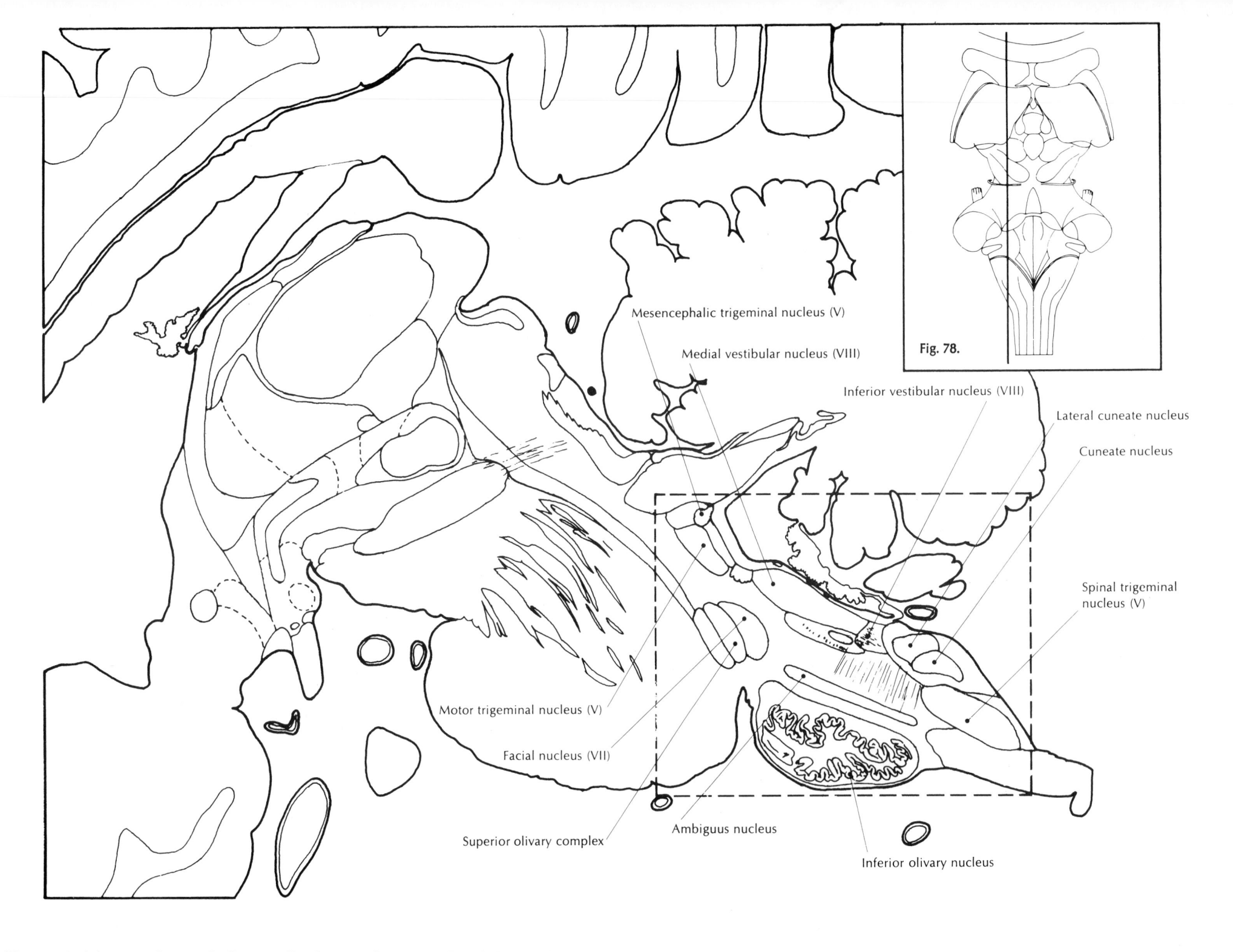

Mesencephalic trigeminal nucleus (V)

Medial vestibular nucleus (VIII)

Inferior vestibular nucleus (VIII)

Lateral cuneate nucleus

Cuneate nucleus

Spinal trigeminal nucleus (V)

Fig. 78.

Motor trigeminal nucleus (V)

Facial nucleus (VII)

Superior olivary complex

Ambiguus nucleus

Inferior olivary nucleus

Figure 78. Detail of the special visceral efferent cell column in the pons and medulla—Nissl, 11X

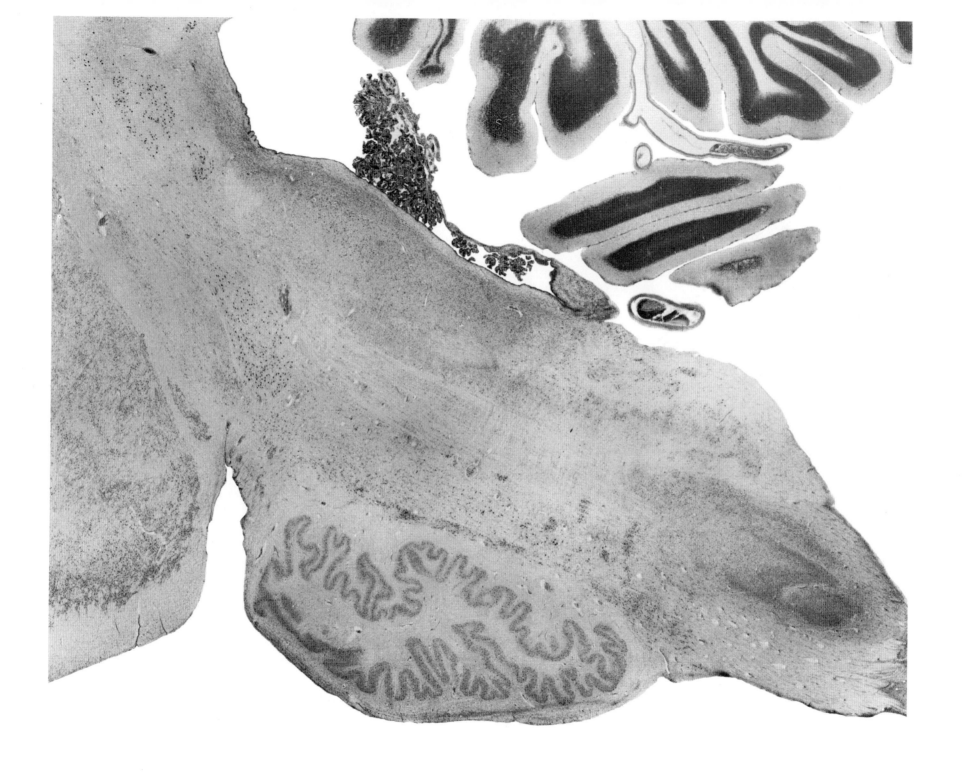

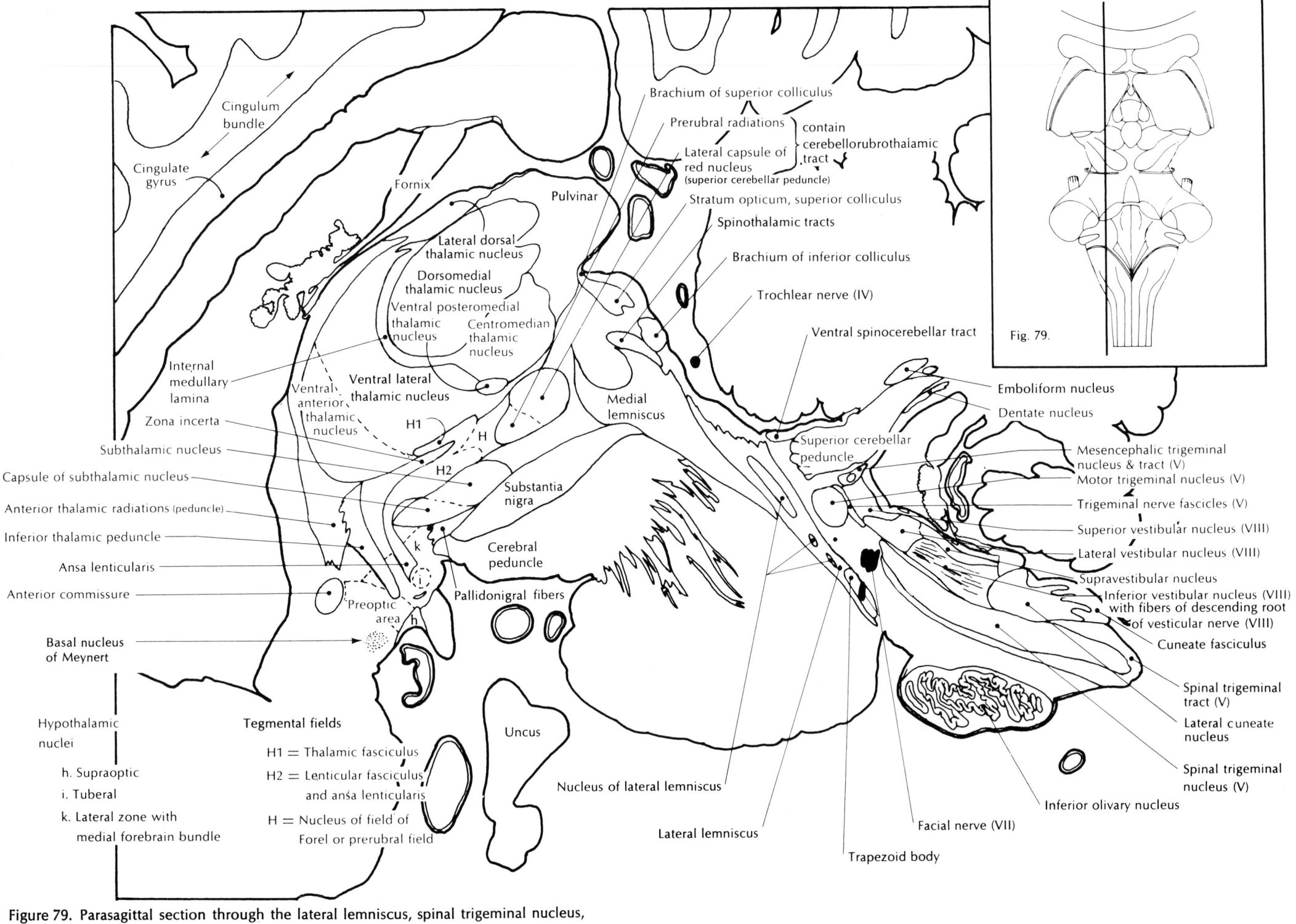

Cingulum bundle

Cingulate gyrus

Fornix

Pulvinar

Brachium of superior colliculus

Prerubral radiations — contain cerebellorubrothalamic tract

Lateral capsule of red nucleus (superior cerebellar peduncle)

Stratum opticum, superior colliculus

Spinothalamic tracts

Brachium of inferior colliculus

Trochlear nerve (IV)

Ventral spinocerebellar tract

Fig. 79.

Lateral dorsal thalamic nucleus

Dorsomedial thalamic nucleus

Ventral posteromedial thalamic nucleus

Centromedian thalamic nucleus

Emboliform nucleus

Dentate nucleus

Internal medullary lamina

Ventral lateral thalamic nucleus

Medial lemniscus

Ventral anterior thalamic nucleus

Zona incerta

H1

H

Superior cerebellar peduncle

Mesencephalic trigeminal nucleus & tract (V)

Subthalamic nucleus

H2

Substantia nigra

Motor trigeminal nucleus (V)

Capsule of subthalamic nucleus

Trigeminal nerve fascicles (V)

Anterior thalamic radiations (peduncle)

Superior vestibular nucleus (VIII)

Inferior thalamic peduncle

Cerebral peduncle

Lateral vestibular nucleus (VIII)

k

Supravestibular nucleus

Ansa lenticularis

Pallidonigral fibers

Inferior vestibular nucleus (VIII) with fibers of descending root of vesticular nerve (VIII)

Anterior commissure

Preoptic area

h

Basal nucleus of Meynert

Cuneate fasciculus

Spinal trigeminal tract (V)

Lateral cuneate nucleus

Hypothalamic nuclei

Tegmental fields

Uncus

Spinal trigeminal nucleus (V)

h. Supraoptic

i. Tuberal

k. Lateral zone with medial forebrain bundle

H1 = Thalamic fasciculus

H2 = Lenticular fasciculus and ansa lenticularis

H = Nucleus of field of Forel or prerubral field

Nucleus of lateral lemniscus

Lateral lemniscus

Trapezoid body

Facial nerve (VII)

Inferior olivary nucleus

Figure 79. Parasagittal section through the lateral lemniscus, spinal trigeminal nucleus, and lateral vestibulospinal tract—Weil, 3.5X

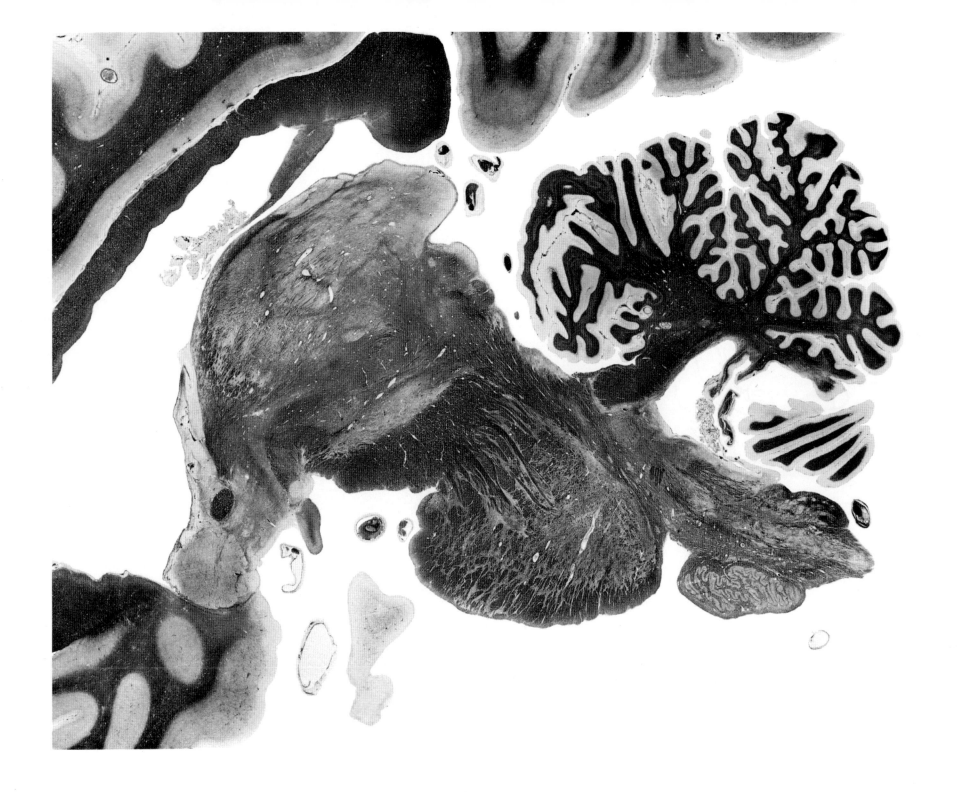

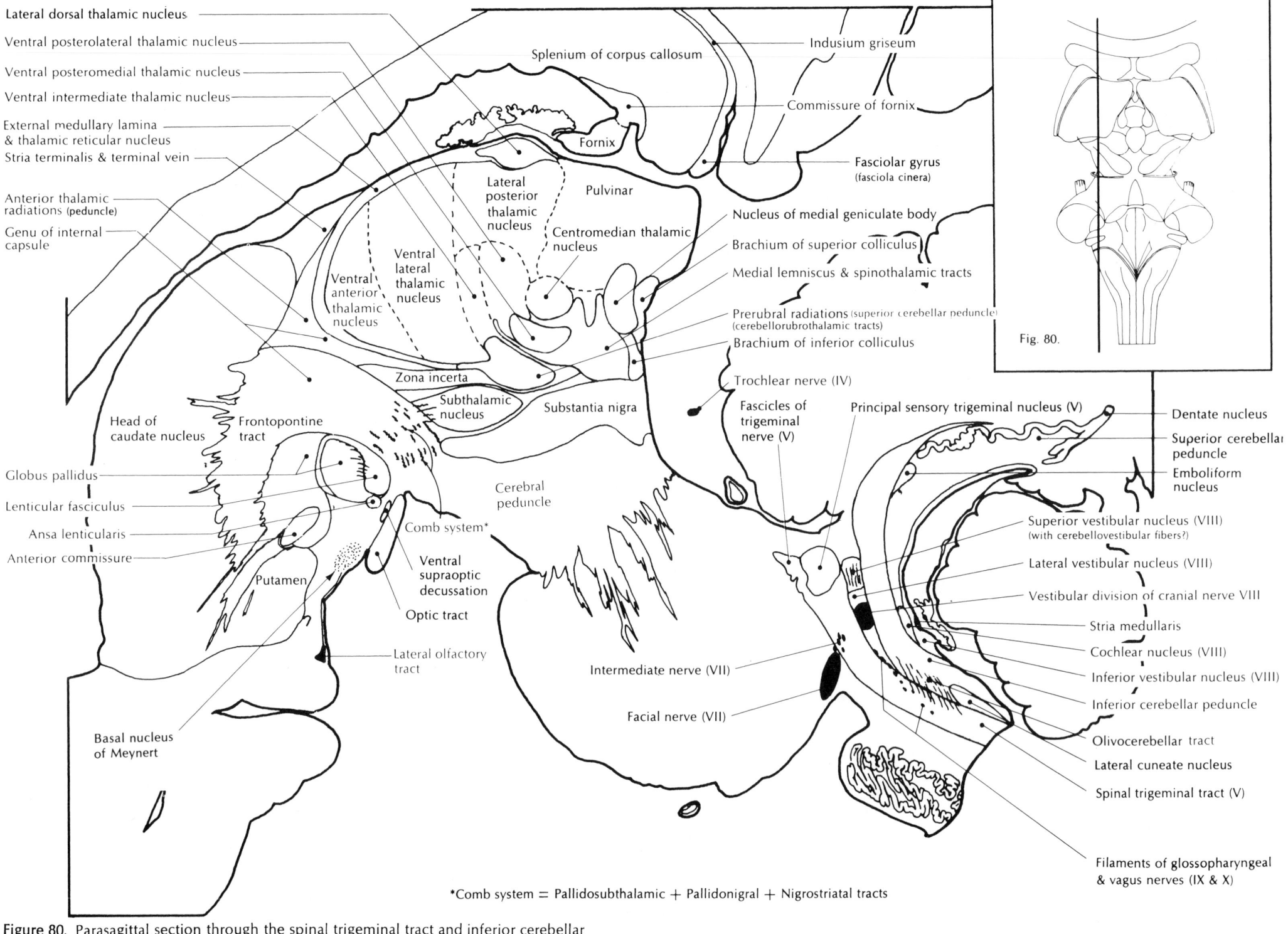

Lateral dorsal thalamic nucleus

Ventral posterolateral thalamic nucleus

Ventral posteromedial thalamic nucleus

Ventral intermediate thalamic nucleus

External medullary lamina & thalamic reticular nucleus

Stria terminalis & terminal vein

Anterior thalamic radiations (peduncle)

Genu of internal capsule

Head of caudate nucleus

Frontopontine tract

Globus pallidus

Lenticular fasciculus

Ansa lenticularis

Anterior commissure

Putamen

Basal nucleus of Meynert

Splenium of corpus callosum

Indusium griseum

Commissure of fornix

Fornix

Fasciolar gyrus (fasciola cinera)

Lateral posterior thalamic nucleus

Pulvinar

Nucleus of medial geniculate body

Centromedian thalamic nucleus

Brachium of superior colliculus

Medial lemniscus & spinothalamic tracts

Ventral lateral thalamic nucleus

Ventral anterior thalamic nucleus

Prerubral radiations (superior cerebellar peduncle) (cerebellorubrothalamic tracts)

Brachium of inferior colliculus

Zona incerta

Subthalamic nucleus

Substantia nigra

Trochlear nerve (IV)

Fascicles of trigeminal nerve (V)

Principal sensory trigeminal nucleus (V)

Dentate nucleus

Superior cerebellar peduncle

Emboliform nucleus

Cerebral peduncle

Comb system*

Ventral supraoptic decussation

Optic tract

Superior vestibular nucleus (VIII) (with cerebellovestibular fibers?)

Lateral vestibular nucleus (VIII)

Vestibular division of cranial nerve VIII

Stria medullaris

Lateral olfactory tract

Cochlear nucleus (VIII)

Inferior vestibular nucleus (VIII)

Intermediate nerve (VII)

Inferior cerebellar peduncle

Olivocerebellar tract

Facial nerve (VII)

Lateral cuneate nucleus

Spinal trigeminal tract (V)

Filaments of glossopharyngeal & vagus nerves (IX & X)

Fig. 80.

*Comb system = Pallidosubthalamic + Pallidonigral + Nigrostriatal tracts

Figure 80. Parasagittal section through the spinal trigeminal tract and inferior cerebellar peduncle—Weil, 3.5X

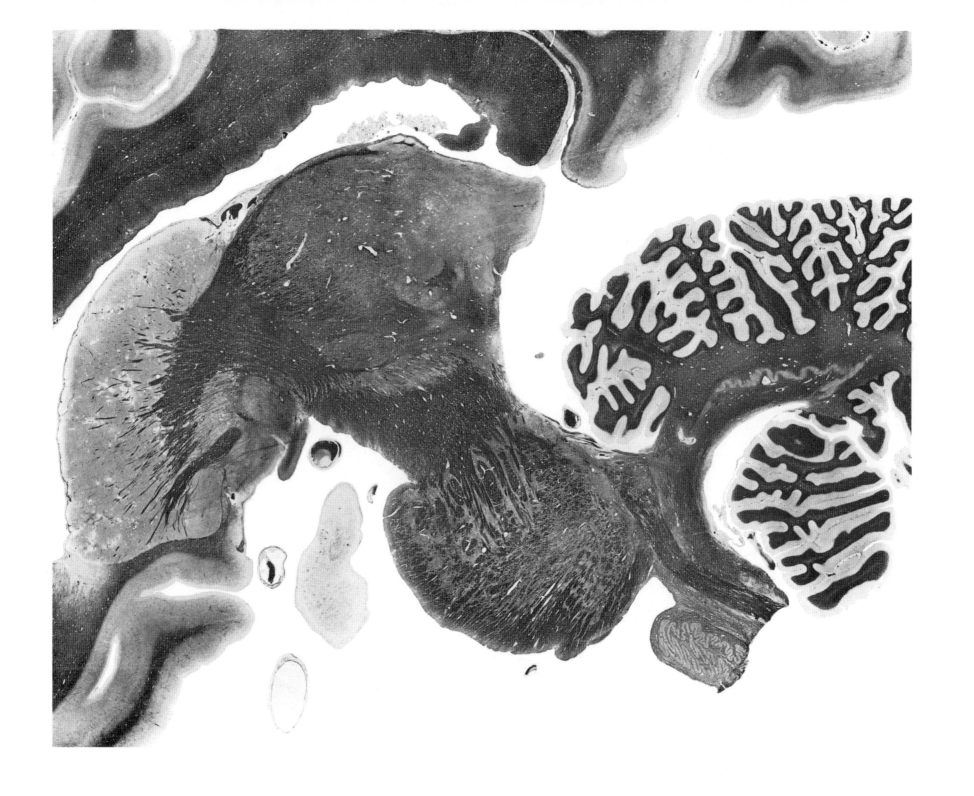

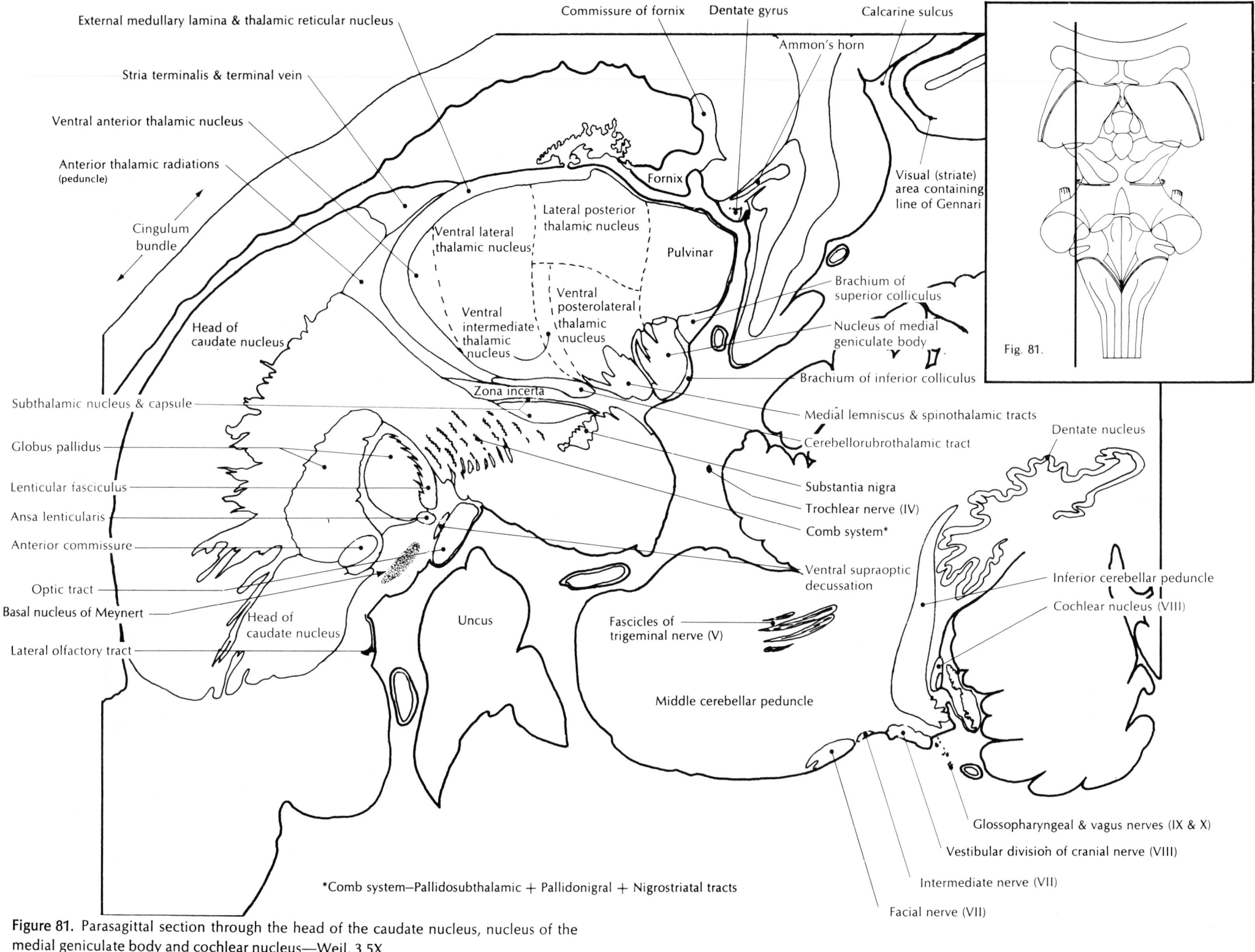

External medullary lamina & thalamic reticular nucleus

Stria terminalis & terminal vein

Ventral anterior thalamic nucleus

Anterior thalamic radiations (peduncle)

Cingulum bundle

Head of caudate nucleus

Subthalamic nucleus & capsule

Globus pallidus

Lenticular fasciculus

Ansa lenticularis

Anterior commissure

Optic tract

Basal nucleus of Meynert

Head of caudate nucleus

Lateral olfactory tract

Commissure of fornix

Dentate gyrus

Calcarine sulcus

Ammon's horn

Fornix

Visual (striate) area containing line of Gennari

Lateral posterior thalamic nucleus

Ventral lateral thalamic nucleus

Pulvinar

Ventral intermediate thalamic nucleus

Ventral posterolateral thalamic nucleus

Brachium of superior colliculus

Nucleus of medial geniculate body

Zona incerta

Brachium of inferior colliculus

Medial lemniscus & spinothalamic tracts

Cerebellorubrothalamic tract

Substantia nigra

Trochlear nerve (IV)

Comb system*

Ventral supraoptic decussation

Uncus

Fascicles of trigeminal nerve (V)

Middle cerebellar peduncle

Dentate nucleus

Inferior cerebellar peduncle

Cochlear nucleus (VIII)

Glossopharyngeal & vagus nerves (IX & X)

Vestibular division of cranial nerve (VIII)

Intermediate nerve (VII)

Facial nerve (VII)

Fig. 81.

*Comb system—Pallidosubthalamic + Pallidonigral + Nigrostriatal tracts

Figure 81. Parasagittal section through the head of the caudate nucleus, nucleus of the medial geniculate body and cochlear nucleus—Weil, 3.5X

162

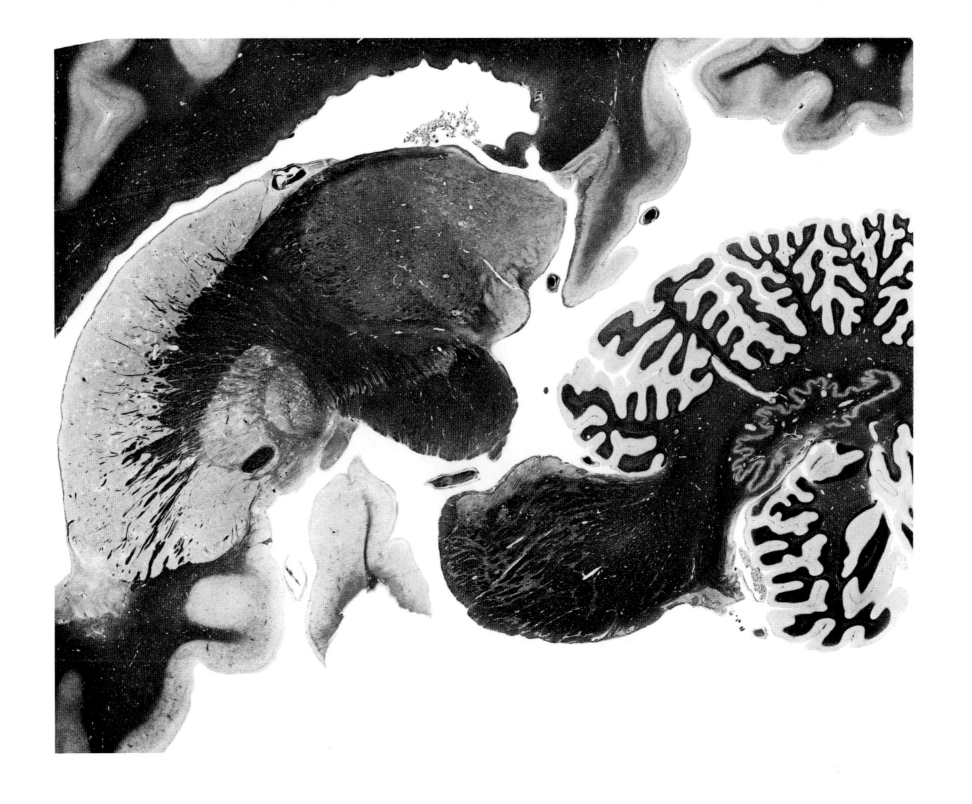

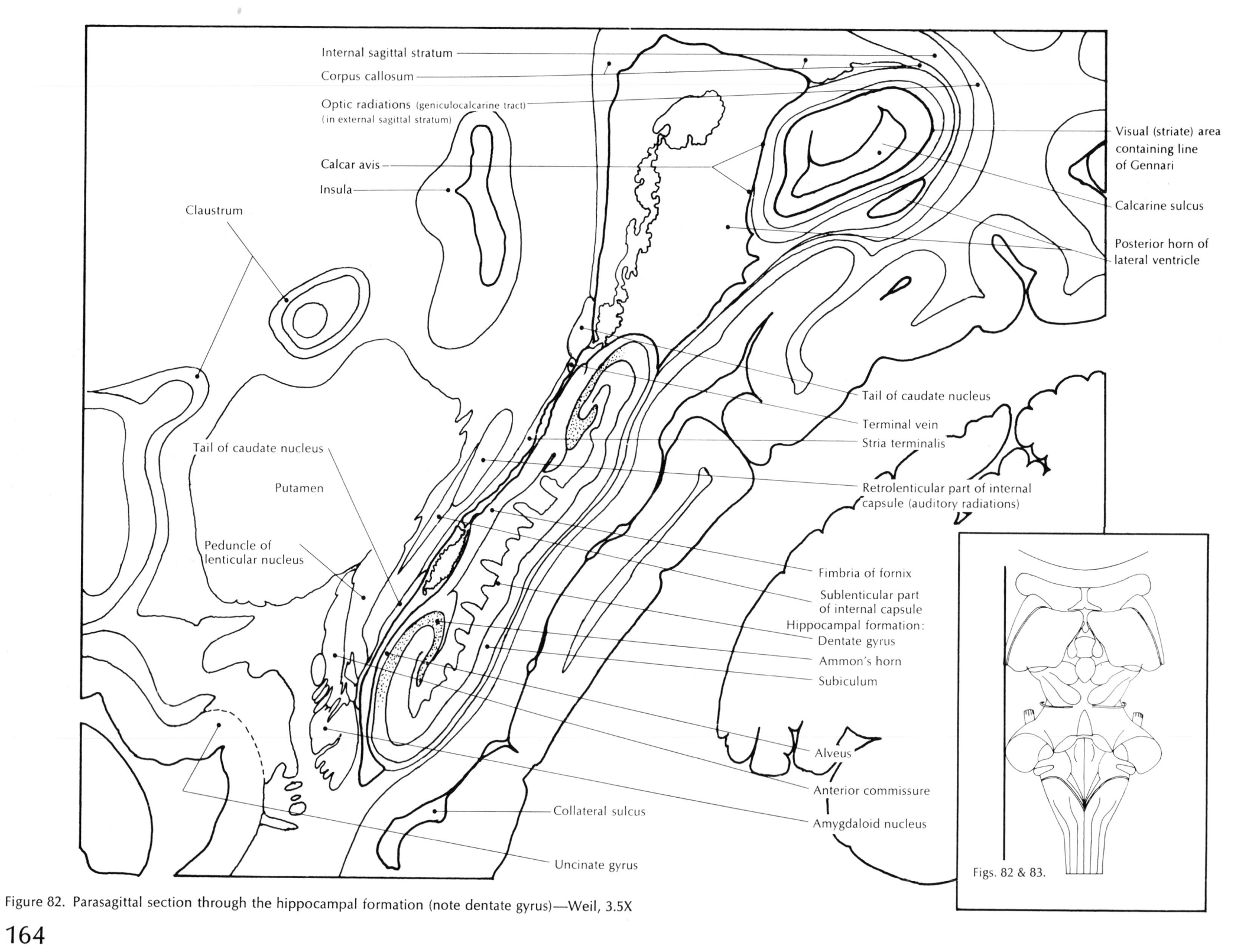

Internal sagittal stratum

Corpus callosum

Optic radiations (geniculocalcarine tract) (in external sagittal stratum)

Calcar avis

Insula

Claustrum

Tail of caudate nucleus

Putamen

Peduncle of lenticular nucleus

Visual (striate) area containing line of Gennari

Calcarine sulcus

Posterior horn of lateral ventricle

Tail of caudate nucleus

Terminal vein

Stria terminalis

Retrolenticular part of internal capsule (auditory radiations)

Fimbria of fornix

Sublenticular part of internal capsule

Hippocampal formation:
Dentate gyrus

Ammon's horn

Subiculum

Alveus

Anterior commissure

Amygdaloid nucleus

Collateral sulcus

Uncinate gyrus

Figs. 82 & 83.

Figure 82. Parasagittal section through the hippocampal formation (note dentate gyrus)—Weil, 3.5X

164

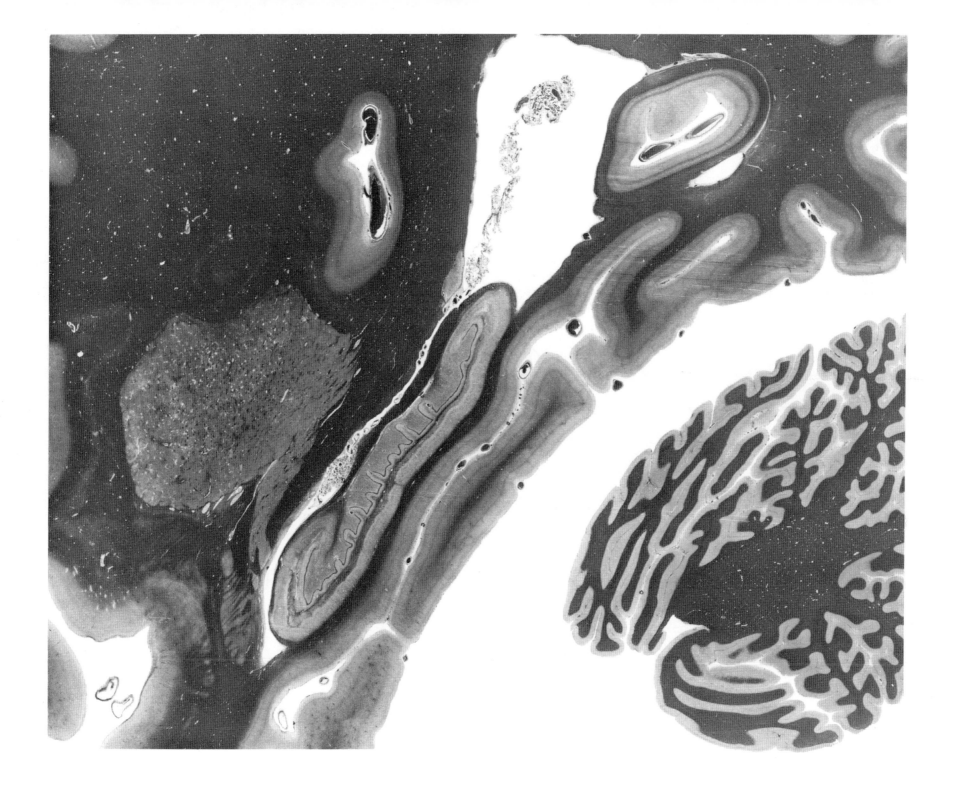

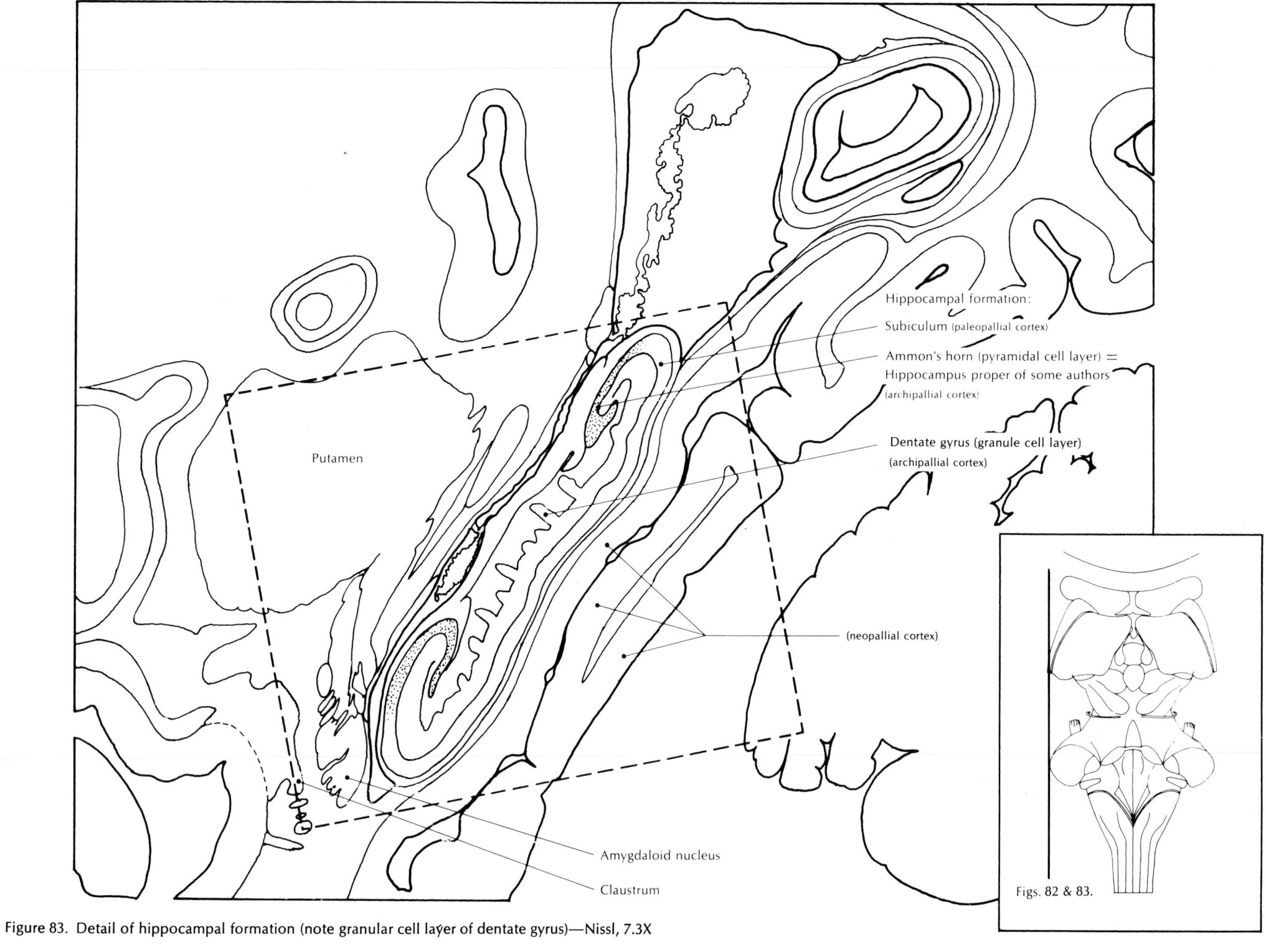

Hippocampal formation:

Subiculum (paleopallial cortex)

Ammon's horn (pyramidal cell layer) =
Hippocampus proper of some authors
(archipallial cortex)

Dentate gyrus (granule cell layer)
(archipallial cortex)

Putamen

(neopallial cortex)

Amygdaloid nucleus

Claustrum

Figs. 82 & 83.

Figure 83. Detail of hippocampal formation (note granular cell layer of dentate gyrus)—Nissl, 7.3X

166

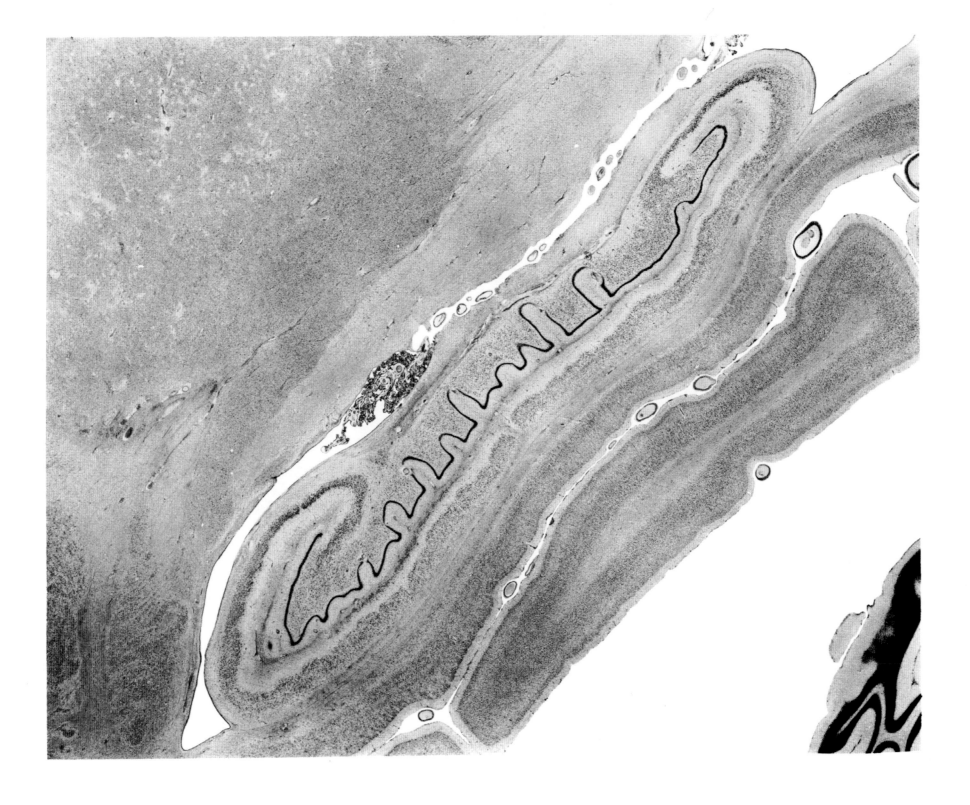

CYTOARCHITECTURE OF THE CEREBRAL CORTEX

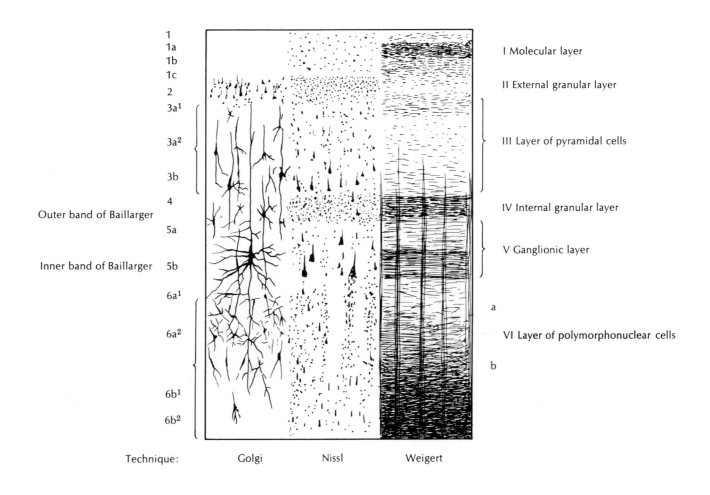

1
1a
1b
1c
2
3a¹
3a²
3b
4

Outer band of Baillarger   5a

Inner band of Baillarger   5b

6a¹

6a²

6b¹

6b²

I Molecular layer

II External granular layer

III Layer of pyramidal cells

IV Internal granular layer

V Ganglionic layer

a

VI Layer of polymorphonuclear cells

b

Technique: Golgi   Nissl   Weigert

Figure 84. Diagram of cerebral cortex architecture. In area 17 (primary visual cortex) the outer line of Baillarger is termed the line of Gennari and is visible to the naked eye. (From Brodmann)

169

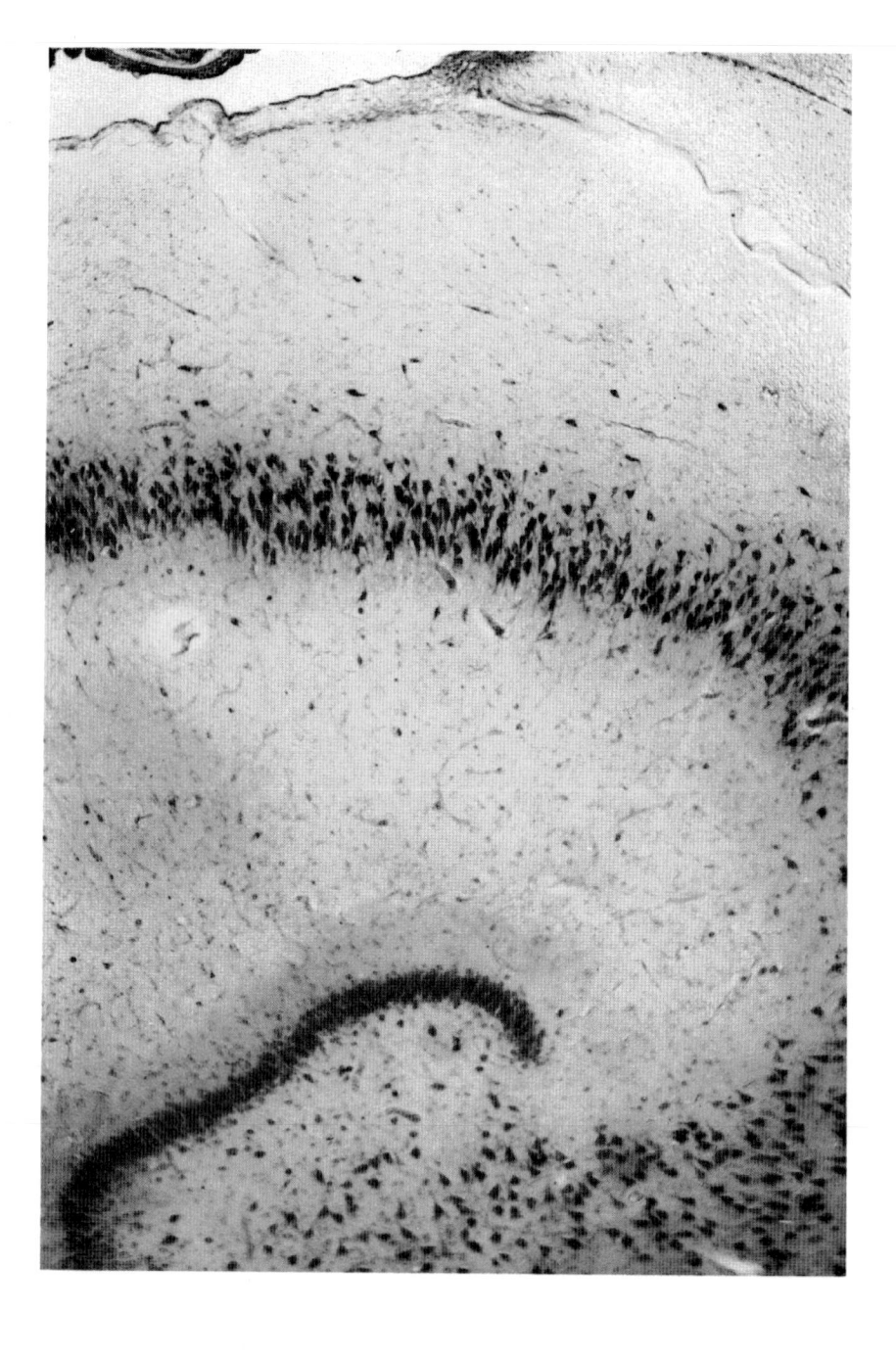

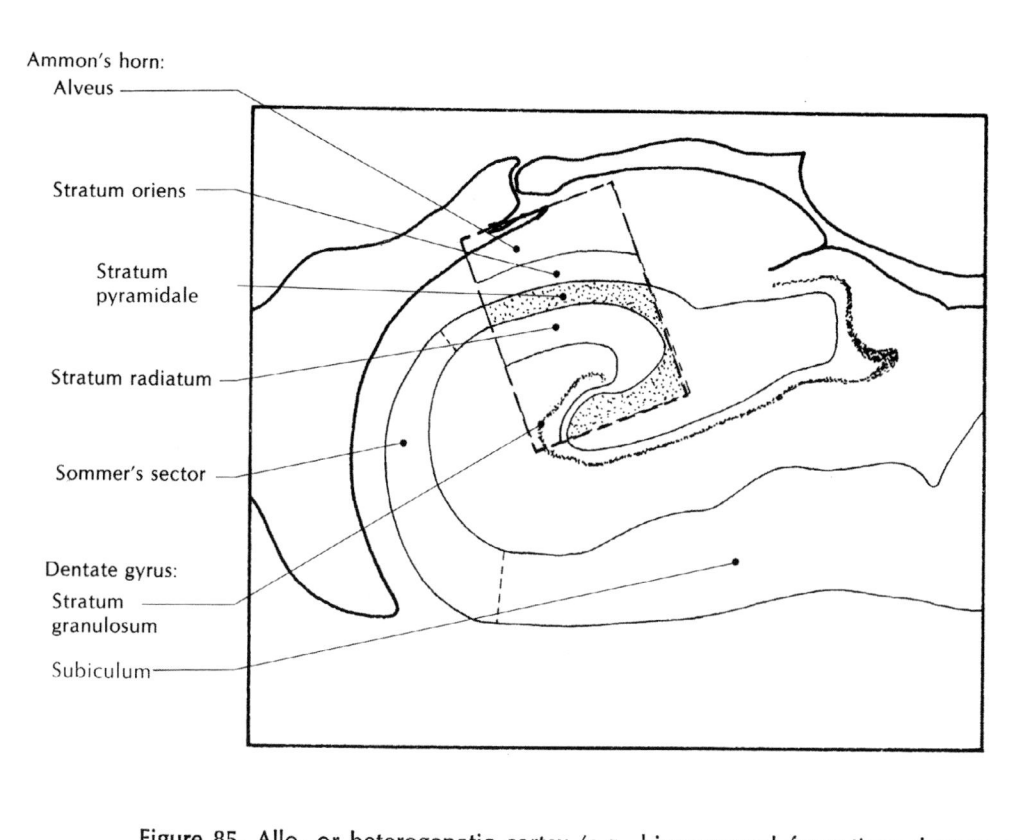

Ammon's horn:
Alveus

Stratum oriens

Stratum pyramidale

Stratum radiatum

Sommer's sector

Dentate gyrus:
Stratum granulosum

Subiculum

Figure 85. Allo- or heterogenetic cortex (e.g., hippocampal formation: dentate gyrus, Ammon's horn, and subiculum). Photograph of pyramidal cell layer of Ammon's horn and granule cell layer of dentate gyrus—Nissl, 75×. Drawing of transverse section of hippocampal formation indicating layers or strata of Ammon's horn. Sommer's sector is the cellular area of Ammon's horn most sensitive to anoxia

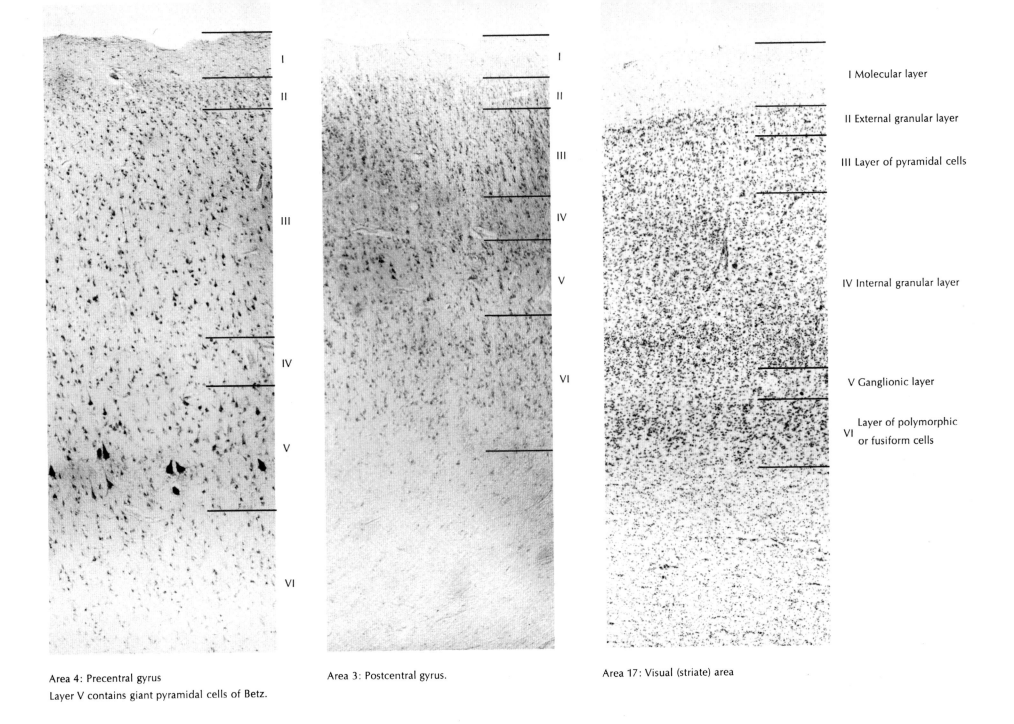

I Molecular layer

II External granular layer

III Layer of pyramidal cells

IV Internal granular layer

V Ganglionic layer

VI Layer of polymorphic or fusiform cells

Area 4: Precentral gyrus
Layer V contains giant pyramidal cells of Betz.

Area 3: Postcentral gyrus.

Area 17: Visual (striate) area

Figure 86. Iso- or homogenetic cortex (e.g., the six-layered cortex of the entire neopallium)—Nissl, 65X

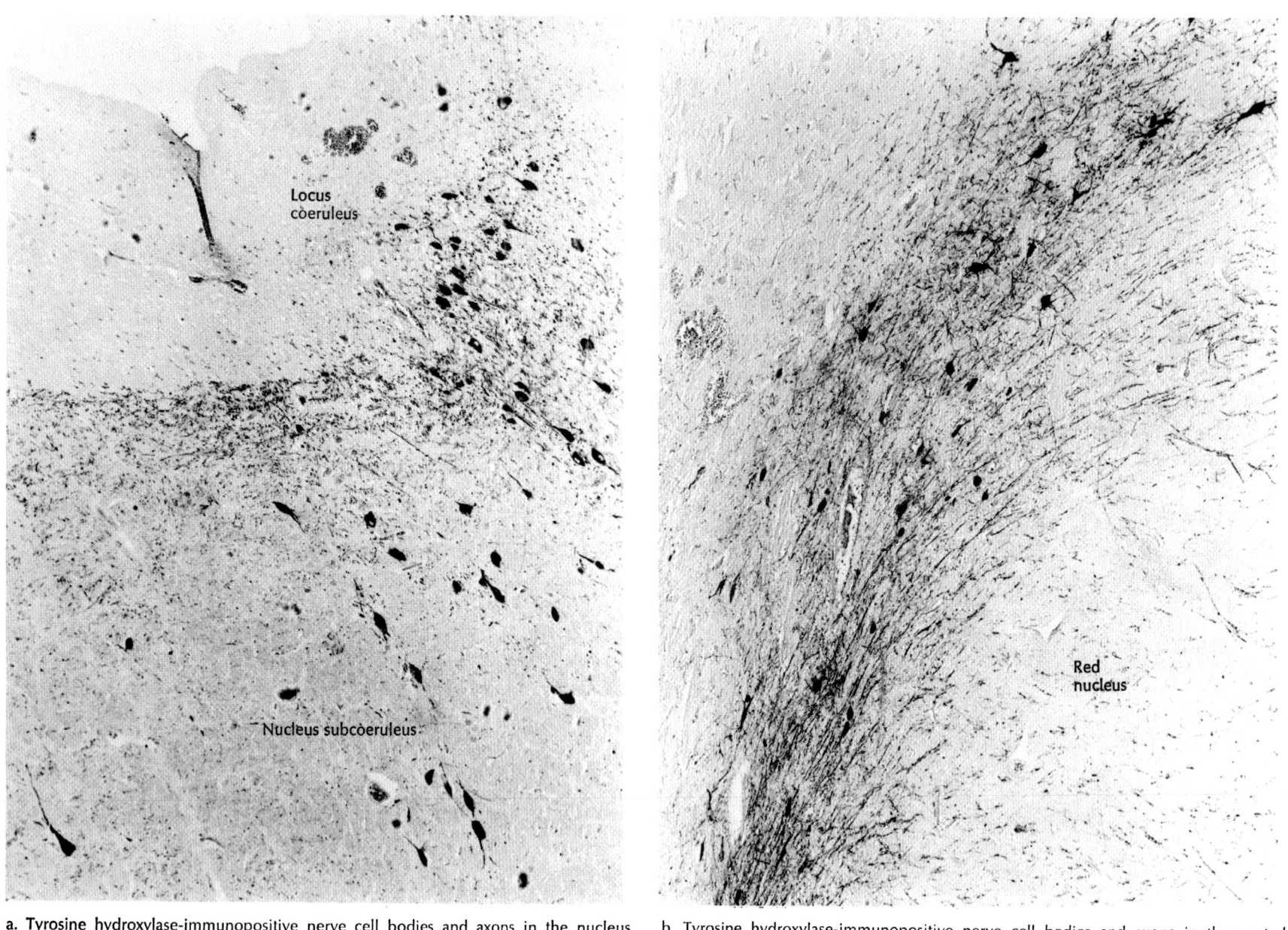

a. Tyrosine hydroxylase-immunopositive nerve cell bodies and axons in the nucleus of locus coeruleus and nucleus subcoeruleus. The immunopositive nerve cells in this location are mostly noradrenergic

b. Tyrosine hydroxylase-immunopositive nerve cell bodies and axons in the ventral tegmental area fan out medial and dorsomedial to the red nucleus. Most, if not all, of these nerve cell bodies and axons are dopaminergic.

Figure 87. Examples of peroxidase-immunohistochemical localization of tyrosine hydroxylase in the human central nervous system. Photographs were generously provided by Dr. John Pearson, New York University (Pearson et al., 1983)

CHEMOARCHITECTURAL STRUCTURE OF THE HUMAN CNS: INTRODUCTION

A variety of histochemical and immunohistochemical techniques have emerged during the past 20 years which have made it possible to chemically define individual nerve cells in terms of putative neurotransmitters and neuromodulators. The goal of this section is to correlate the distribution of some chemically defined nerve cells with classically defined neuroanatomical boundaries in the human Central Nervous System. This analysis comes with three caveats. First, the chemical definition of neurons in the human CNS is derived largely from animal studies; however, the results of the relatively few studies in human brain tissue have been similar to those from animals (for reviews, see Angevine and Cotman, 1981; Nieuwenhuys, 1985). The catecholamine systems (epinephrine, norepinephrine, and dopamine) have been mapped in human brain with antibodies to tyrosine hydroxylase (Pearson et al., 1983). One of the by-products of catecholamine metabolism in the CNS is neuromelanin, which accumulates in nerve cell bodies. The distribution of neuromelanin-containing neurons in the brain stem has been mapped (Bogerts, 1981; Saper and Petito, 1982), and their locations correspond well with the distribution of tyrosine hydroxylase-containing nerve cell bodies (Pearson et al., 1983) and with the distribution of catecholamine species, as determined by fluorescent histochemical techniques (Nobin and Björklund, 1973). The second caveat is that the neuroanatomical boundaries of CNS nuclei, which relate to many of the chemical findings, are not well defined or agreed upon. This is particularly true in the brain stem. The Olszewski and Baxter (1954) atlas of the human brain stem is used by most researchers as a starting point because of its cellular and topographical details. However, it has deficiencies. In particular, raphe nuclei are poorly described. Nevertheless, we have adhered strictly to the Olszewski and Baxter atlas, supplemented where necessary with newer neuroanatomical definitions. With regard to raphe nuclei, the nuclear boundaries in the human brain stem described by Braak (1970) are used. A third caveat is that neurons with specific chemical characteristics do not respect neuroanatomically defined boundaries and, furthermore, many neurons appear to contain more than one putative neurotransmitter.

It is not the purpose of this edition of the atlas to provide a detailed review of all known chemical-neuroanatomical correlations. The books by Angevine and Cotman (1981) and by Nieuwenhuys (1985) provide excellent overviews of this subject. Here we will outline and show the relationship of selected neurotransmitters with neuroanatomical structures. Five neurotransmitters have been selected because they have been studied extensively and because of their physiological and clinical importance. In this section, the location of adrenaline, noradrenaline, dopamine, and serotonin nerve cell bodies and pathways are emphasized. The distribution of acetylcholine nerve cells is outlined in Table 1. The important basal forebrain cholinergic system (basal nucleus of Meynert and nucleus of the diagonal band of Broca) is presented in figures in other sections of the atlas. The key publications used to construct the chemical correlations are listed below.

Selected References

Angevine, J. Jr., Cotman, C. W. *Principles of Neuroanatomy.* Oxford University Press, New York, 1981.

Bogerts, B. A brainstem atlas of catecholaminergic neurons in man, using melanin as a natural marker. J. Comp. Neurol. 197: 63–80 (1981).

Braak, H. Über die Kerngebiete des menschlichen Hirnstammes. II. Die Raphekerne. Z. Zellforsch. 107: 123–141 (1970).

Dahlström, A., Fuxe, K. Evidence for the existence of monoamine-containing neurons in the central nervous system. I. Demonstration of monoamines in the cell bodies of brain stem neurons. Acta Physiol. Scand. 62 (Suppl. 232): 1–55 (1964).

Dahlström, A., Fuxe, K. Evidence for the existence of monoamine neurons in the central nervous system. II. Experimentally induced changes in the intraneuronal amine levels of bulbospinal neuron systems. Acta Physiol. Scand. 64 (Suppl. 247): 1–36 (1965).

Felten, D. L., Sladek, J. R. Jr. Monoamine distribution in primate brain. V. Monoaminergic nuclei: Anatomy, pathways and local organization. Brain Res. Bull. 10: 171–284 (1983).

Hedreen, J. C., Struble, R. G., Whitehouse, P. J., Price, D. L. Topography of the magnocellular basal forebrain system in human brain. J. Neuropathol. Exp. Neurol. 43: 1–21 (1984).

Jones, B. E., Friedman, L. Atlas of catecholamine perikarya, varicosities and pathways in the brainstem of the cat. J. Comp. Neurol. 215: 382–396 (1983).

Kimura, H., McGeer, P. L., Peng, J. H., McGeer, E. G. The central cholinergic system studied by choline acetyltransferase immunohistochemistry in the cat. J. Comp. Neurol. 200: 151–201 (1981).

Mesulam, M.-M., Mufson, E. J., Levey, A. I., Wainer, B. H. Cholinergic innervation of cortex by the basal forebrain: Cytochemistry and cortical connections of the septal area, diagonal band nuclei, nucleus basalis (substantia innominata), and hypothalamus in the rhesus monkey. J. Comp. Neurol. 214: 170–197 (1983).

Mesulam, M.-M., Mufson, E. J., Levey, A. I., Wainer, B. H. Atlas of cholinergic neurons in the forebrain and upper brainstem of the macaque based on monoclonal choline acetyltransferase immunohistochemistry and acetylcholinesterase histochemistry. Neuroscience 12: 669–686 (1984).

Moore, R. Y., Bloom, F. E. Central catecholamine neuron systems: Anatomy and physiology of the dopamine systems. Ann. Rev. Neurosci. 1: 129–169 (1978).

Moore, R. Y., Bloom, F. E. Central catecholamine neuron systems: Anatomy and physiology of the norepinephrine and epinephrine systems. Ann. Rev. Neurosci. 2: 113–168 (1979).

Moore, R. Y., Halaris, A. E., Jones, B. E. Serotonin neurons of the midbrain raphe: Ascending projections. J. Comp. Neurol. 180: 417–438 (1978).

Nieuwenhuys, R. *Chemoarchitecture of the Brain.* Springer-Verlag, Berlin, 1985.

Nobin, A., Björklund, A. Topography of the monoamine neuron systems in the human brain as revealed in fetuses. Acta Physiol. Scand. (Suppl. 388): 1–40 (1973).

Olszewski, J., Baxter, D. *Cytoarchitecture of the Human Brain Stem.* J. B. Lippincott Co., Philadelphia, 1954.

Pearson, J., Goldstein, M., Markey, K., Brandeis, L. Human brainstem catecholamine neuronal anatomy as indicated by immunocytochemistry with antibodies to tyrosine hydroxylase. Neuroscience 8: 3–32 (1983).

Perry, R. H., Candy, J. M., Perry, E. K., Thompson, J., Oakley, A. E. The substantia innominata and adjacent regions in the human brain: Histochemical and biochemical observations. J. Anat. 138: 713–732 (1984).

Riley, H. A. *An Atlas of the Basal Ganglia, Brain Stem and Spinal Cord, Based on Myelin-stained Material.* Williams & Wilkins Co., Baltimore, MD, 1943.

Saper, C. B., Chelimsky, T. C. A cytoarchitectonic and histochemical study of nucleus basalis and associated cell groups in the normal human brain. Neuroscience 13: 1023–1037 (1984).

Saper, C. B., Petito, C. K. Correspondence of melanin-pigmented neurons in human brain with A1–A14 catecholamine cell groups. Brain 105: 87–101 (1982).

Steinbusch, H. W. M. Distribution of serotonin-immunoreactivity in the central nervous system of the rat—cell bodies and terminals. Neuroscience 6: 557–618 (1981).

Taber, E., Brodal, A., Walberg, F. The raphe nuclei of the brain stem in the cat. I. Normal topography and cytoarchitecture and general discussion. J. Comp. Neurol. 114: 161–187 (1960).

Veening, J. G., Swanson, L. W., Cowan, W. M., Nieuwenhuys, R., Geeraedts, L. M. G. The medial forebrain bundle of the rat. II. An autoradiographic study of the topography of the major descending and ascending components. J. Comp. Neurol. 206: 82–108 (1982).

Table 1. *The Cholinergic System*

Nuclei	Pathways
1. Alpha and gamma motoneurons	
a. spinal cord (anterior horn cells)	ventral nerve roots
b. brain stem (cranial nerve nuclei)	cranial nerves
2. Preganglionic autonomic neurons	
a. spinal cord (intermediomedial and lateral cell columns)	ventral nerve roots
b. brain stem (cranial nerve nuclei)	cranial nerves
3. Periolivary nuclei surrounding the superior olivary complex in the caudal pons	olivocochlear fasciculus
4. Lateral reticular formation of the rostral pons (lateral and medial parabrachial nucleus and pedunculopontine nucleus)	dorsal tegemental pathway in the region of the catecholamine pathway
5. Basal forebrain cholinergic system (subdivisions of Mesulam [1983, 1984])	
a. CH 1: medial septal nuclei (10% cholinergic)	stria medullaris of thalamus and habenulopeduncular tract
b. CH 2: verticle limb of the nucleus of the diagonal band of Broca (70% cholinergic)	
c. CH 3: horizontal limb of the nucleus of the diagonal band of Broca (1% cholinergic)	
d. CH 4: nucleus basalis of Meynert (the substantia innominata) (90% cholinergic)	diffuse, topographically organized projections to the cerebral cortex
6. Local circuits (interneurons)	
a. caudate nucleus, nucleus accumbens, and putamen (1% cholinergic)	
b. cerebral cortex	

Table 2. *The Dopaminergic System*
(subdivisions of Dahlström and Fuxe [1964, 1965])

Nuclei	Pathways
A. *Midbrain*	There are two main dopaminergic pathways:
1. Group A8: located in the lateral tegmentum at inferior colliculus levels (region of nucleus paralemniscalis)	1. *Mesostriatal system:* Arises from A8, A9, and A10. Its fibers gather in the ventral tegmental area and enter the dorsal part of the lateral hypothalamus lateral to the medial forebrain bundle. Its fibers cross the posterior limb of the internal capsule (comb fibers) to enter the caudate and putamen.
2. Group A9: pars compacta of substantia nigra	
3. Group A10: unpaired midline aggregates in the ventral tegmental area at superior colliculus levels	
B. *Diencephalon*	
1. Group A11: caudal hypothalamus surrounding mamillothalamic tract	2. *Mesolimbic system:* Arises from A10 and the most medial part of substantia nigra. Its fibers ascend with the medial forebrain bundle in the lateral hypothalamus and project to basal forebrain structures, including the olfactory bulb, anterior perforated substance, lateral septal nucleus, bed nucleus of the stria medullaris, and the amygdala.
2. Group A12: region of infundibulum	
3. Group A13: caudomedial zona incerta	
C. *Telencephalon* Olfactory bulb	

Table 3. *The Adrenergic System*
(subdivisions of Dahlström and Fuxe [1964, 1965])

Small Clusters of Neurons Located Exclusively in the Medulla	
1. Group C1: located between the inferior olivary nucleus and the nucleus reticularis lateralis (an unnamed region)	Project to both the spinal cord and hypothalamus
2. Group 2: located partly within and partly adjacent to the nucleus solitarius	
3. Group C3: scattered neurons within the medial longitundinal fasciculus	

Table 4. *The Noradrenergic System*
(subdivisions of Dahlström and Fuxe [1964, 1965])

1. Group A1*: surrounds nucleus reticularis lateralis and extends dorsomedially into nucleus medullae oblongatae centralis
2. Group A2: located in nucleus solitarius and the dorsal efferent nucleus of the vagus
3. Group A3: not present in primates
4. Group A4: located subependymally adjacent to the superior cerebellar peduncle
5. Group A5*: located in nucleus parvocellularis immediately dorsal to the facial nucleus and the superior olivary complex in the caudal pons
6. Group A6: nucleus of locus coeruleus
7. Group A7*: located in the ventral part of nucleus subcoeruleus in the mid-third of the pons and in nucleus parabrachialis in the rostral third of the pons

Axons from noradrenergic neurons gather together in the dorsal lateral tegmentum of the brain stem to form the *catecholamine pathway*. Two distinct bundles, the dorsal and ventral catecholamine, have been described in some animals; however, the two divisions merge with each, forming a common bundle. It is both an ascending and a descending system, and is partially located in the *central tegmental tract*.

Another group of noradrenergic axons joins the *dorsal longitudinal fasciculus* in the periaqueductal gray.

In the hypothalamus, ascending noradrenergic axons in the main catecholamine pathway join the *medial forebrain bundle*.

* **Groups A1, A5, and A7** form a caudal-to-rostral column of noradrenergic cells in the lateral reticular formation.

Table 5. *The Serotonergic System*
(subdivisions of Dahlström and Fuxe [1964, 1965])

The serotonin system is mainly within the boundaries of the brain stem raphe nuclei, although it is not congruent with it. In particular, in the pons, lateral winglike expansions occur. The raphe is not exclusively serotonergic; rather, it is a multiple-transmitter complex that includes dopamine, noradrenaline, gamma-aminobutyric acid (GABA), substance P, vasoactive intestinal peptide (VIP), cholecystokinin, enkephalins, and thyrotropin-releasing hormone (TRH). The serotonergic system of projections is the most widely and diffusely distributed of the central nervous system.

1. Group B1: nucleus raphe pallidus
2. Group B2: nucleus raphe obscurus
3. Group B3: nucleus raphe magnus and an extension into the trapezoid body
4. Group B4: dorsal to nucleus prepositus
5. Group B5: nucleus raphe pontis
6. Groups B6 and B8: superior central nucleus and lateral extensions in the rostral pons that intermingle with noradrenergic cells of the locus coeruleus, nucleus subcoeruleus, and nucleus parabrachialis
7. Group B7: nucleus raphe dorsalis in the periaqueductal gray of the rostral pons and inferior colliculus level of the midbrain
8. Group B9: a small serotonergic population in the region of the nucleus pedunculopontis of the caudal midbrain

1. The *dorsal* and *ventral serotonin pathways* are the two main ascending and descending serotonergic pathways in the brain stem. Their ascending components join the *medial forebrain* bundle in the hypothalamus.
2. Some serotonergic axons also join the *dorsal longitudinal fasciculus* in the periaqueductal gray.
3. *Raphe-spinal* projections arise from nucleus raphe magnus, pallidus, and obscurus.
4. *Raphe-cerebellar* projections arise primarily from nucleus raphe pontis and obscurus and enter the cerebellum via the middle cerebellar peduncle.
5. The *supraependymal serotonin plexus* arises primarily from nucleus raphe dorsalis.

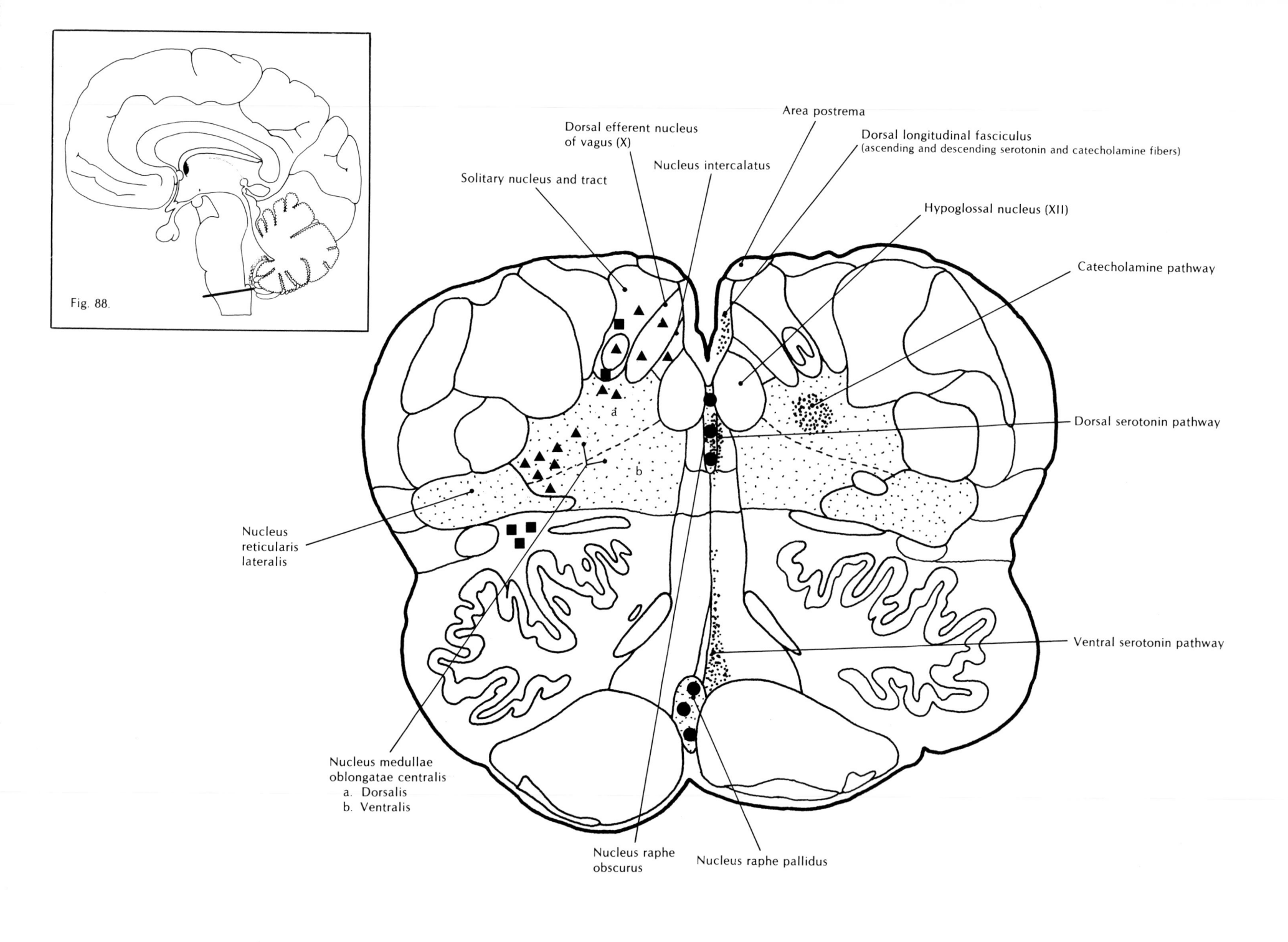

Figure 88. Medulla: Transition from closed to open medullas (see also Fig. 43). Squares, adrenergic neurons; triangles, noradrenergic; circles, serotonergic

176

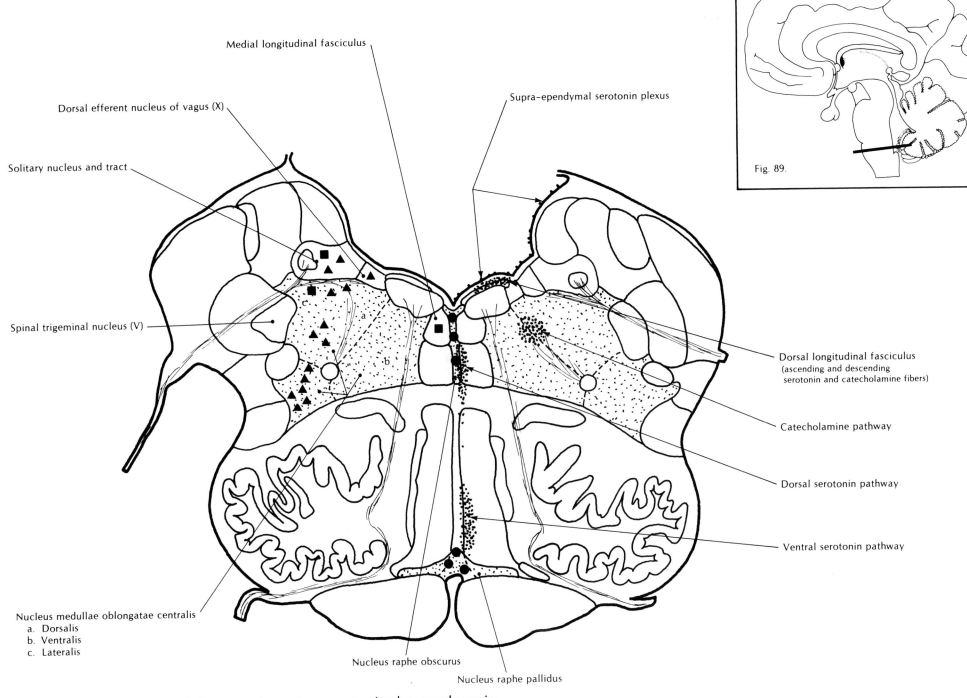

Medial longitudinal fasciculus

Dorsal efferent nucleus of vagus (X)

Solitary nucleus and tract

Supra-ependymal serotonin plexus

Fig. 89.

Spinal trigeminal nucleus (V)

Dorsal longitudinal fasciculus
(ascending and descending
serotonin and catecholamine fibers)

Catecholamine pathway

Dorsal serotonin pathway

Ventral serotonin pathway

Nucleus medullae oblongatae centralis
  a. Dorsalis
  b. Ventralis
  c. Lateralis

Nucleus raphe obscurus

Nucleus raphe pallidus

Figure 89. Open medulla (see also Fig. 44). Squares, adrenergic neurons; triangles, noradrenergic; circles, serotonergic

177

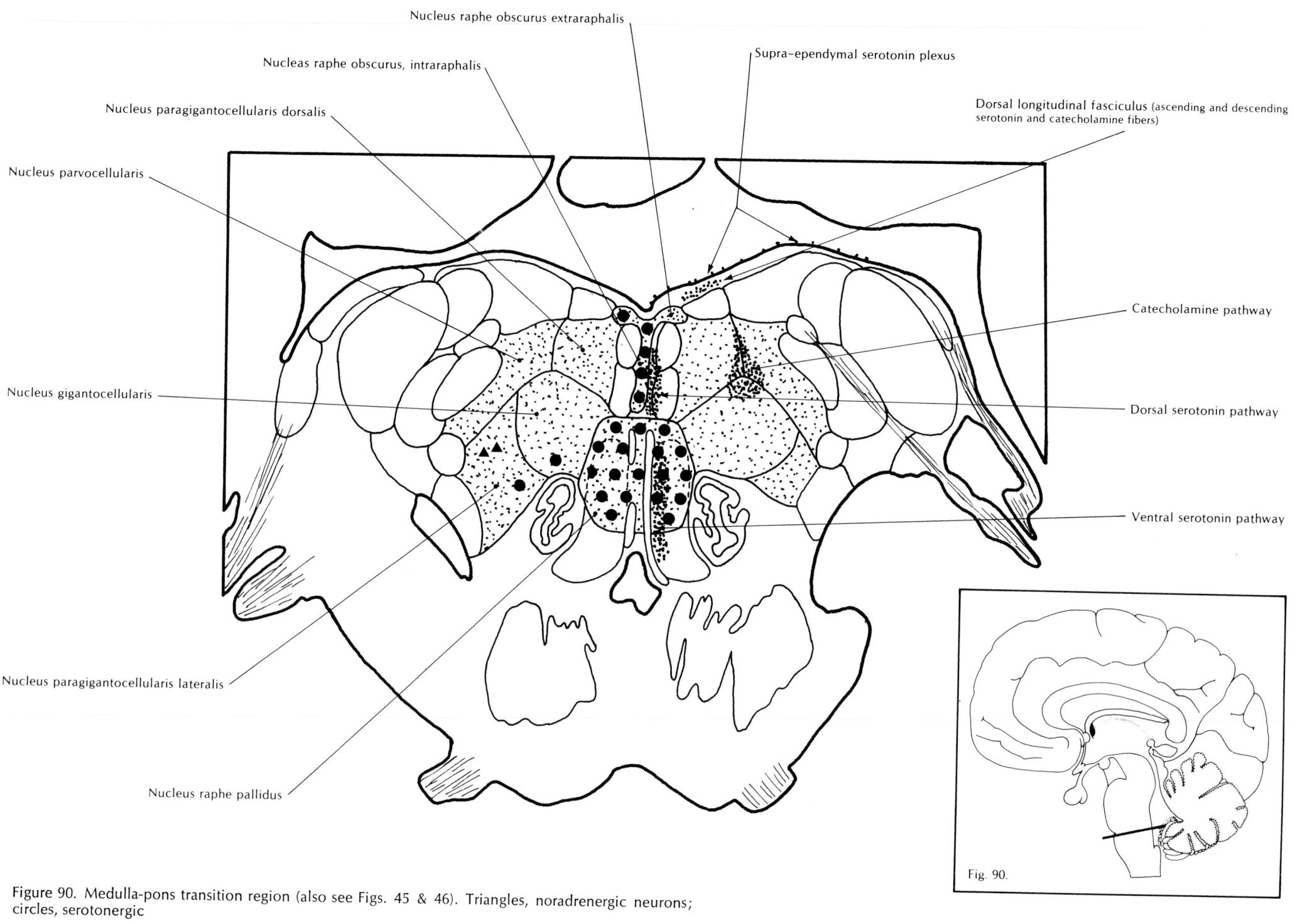

Nucleus raphe obscurus extraraphalis

Nucleas raphe obscurus, intraraphalis

Supra-ependymal serotonin plexus

Nucleus paragigantocellularis dorsalis

Dorsal longitudinal fasciculus (ascending and descending serotonin and catecholamine fibers)

Nucleus parvocellularis

Catecholamine pathway

Nucleus gigantocellularis

Dorsal serotonin pathway

Ventral serotonin pathway

Nucleus paragigantocellularis lateralis

Nucleus raphe pallidus

Fig. 90.

Figure 90. Medulla-pons transition region (also see Figs. 45 & 46). Triangles, noradrenergic neurons; circles, serotonergic

178

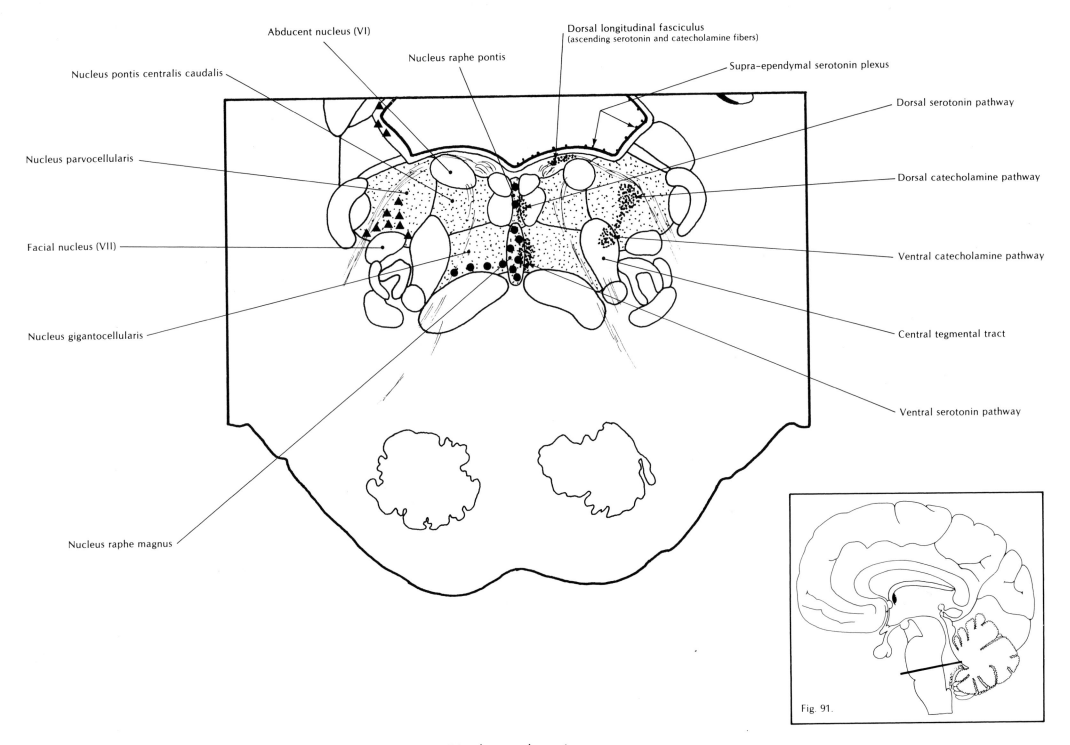

Figure 91. Pons: Level of cranial nerve nuclei VI and VII (also see Fig. 48). Triangles, noradrenergic neurons; circles, serotonergic

179

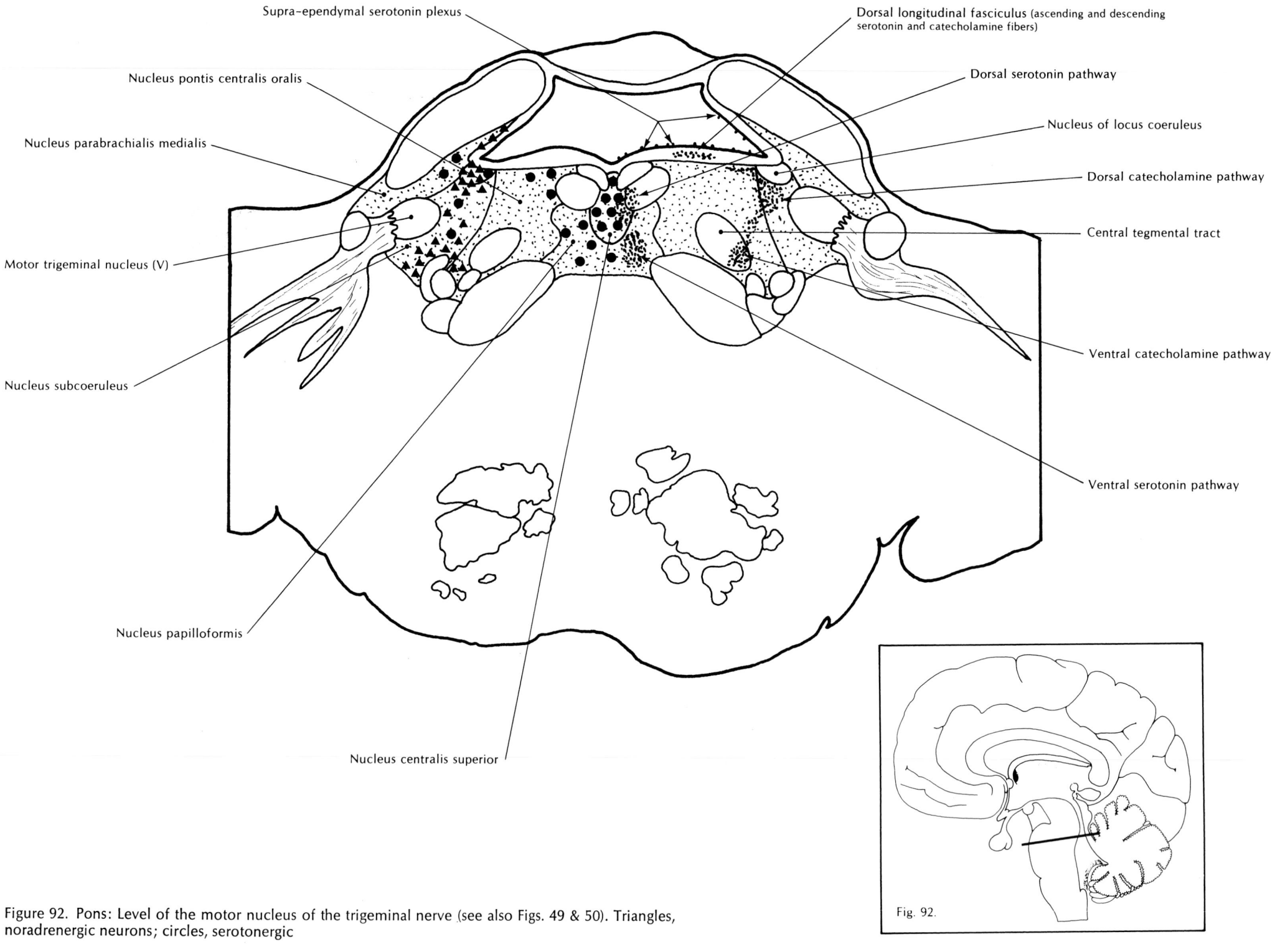

Supra-ependymal serotonin plexus

Dorsal longitudinal fasciculus (ascending and descending serotonin and catecholamine fibers)

Nucleus pontis centralis oralis

Dorsal serotonin pathway

Nucleus parabrachialis medialis

Nucleus of locus coeruleus

Dorsal catecholamine pathway

Motor trigeminal nucleus (V)

Central tegmental tract

Nucleus subcoeruleus

Ventral catecholamine pathway

Ventral serotonin pathway

Nucleus papilloformis

Nucleus centralis superior

Fig. 92.

Figure 92. Pons: Level of the motor nucleus of the trigeminal nerve (see also Figs. 49 & 50). Triangles, noradrenergic neurons; circles, serotonergic

180

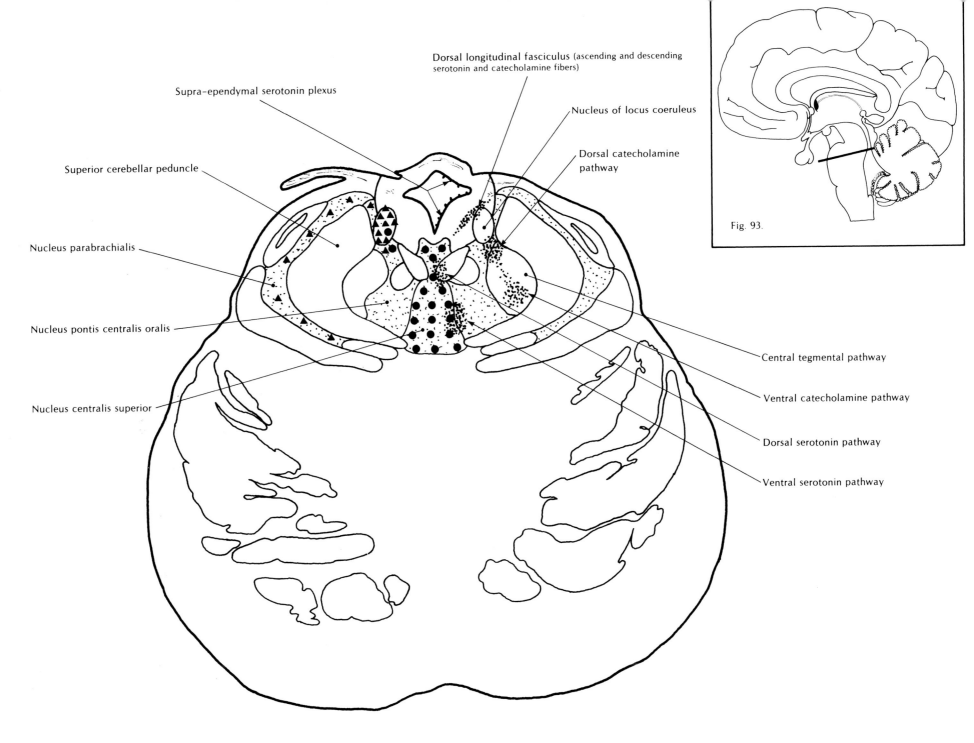

Figure 93. Pons: Isthmus region (see also Fig. 51). Triangles, noradrenergic neurons; circles, serotonergic

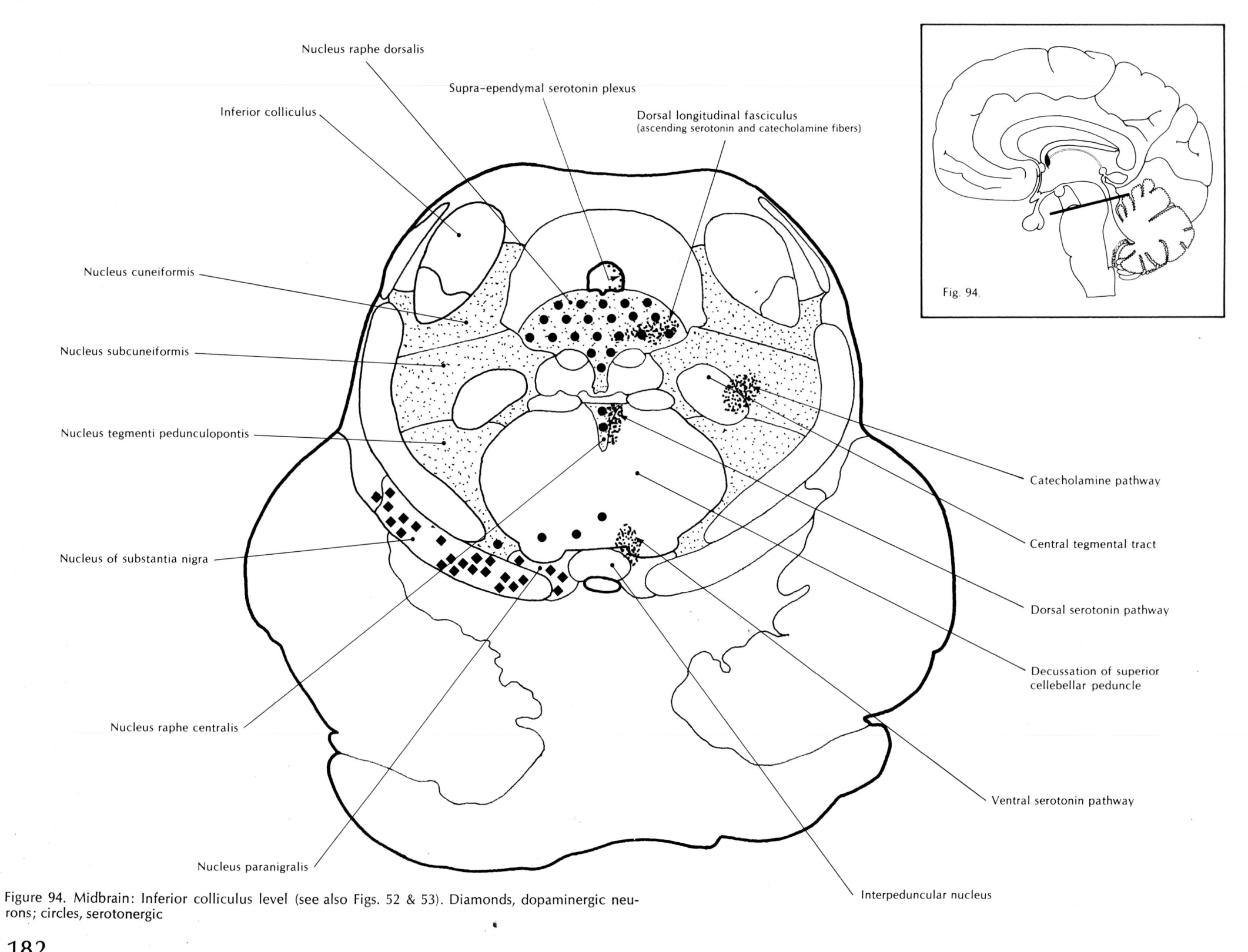

Nucleus raphe dorsalis

Supra-ependymal serotonin plexus

Inferior colliculus

Dorsal longitudinal fasciculus
(ascending serotonin and catecholamine fibers)

Nucleus cuneiformis

Nucleus subcuneiformis

Nucleus tegmenti pedunculopontis

Nucleus of substantia nigra

Catecholamine pathway

Central tegmental tract

Dorsal serotonin pathway

Decussation of superior
cellebellar peduncle

Nucleus raphe centralis

Ventral serotonin pathway

Nucleus paranigralis

Interpeduncular nucleus

Fig. 94.

Figure 94. Midbrain: Inferior colliculus level (see also Figs. 52 & 53). Diamonds, dopaminergic neurons; circles, serotonergic

182

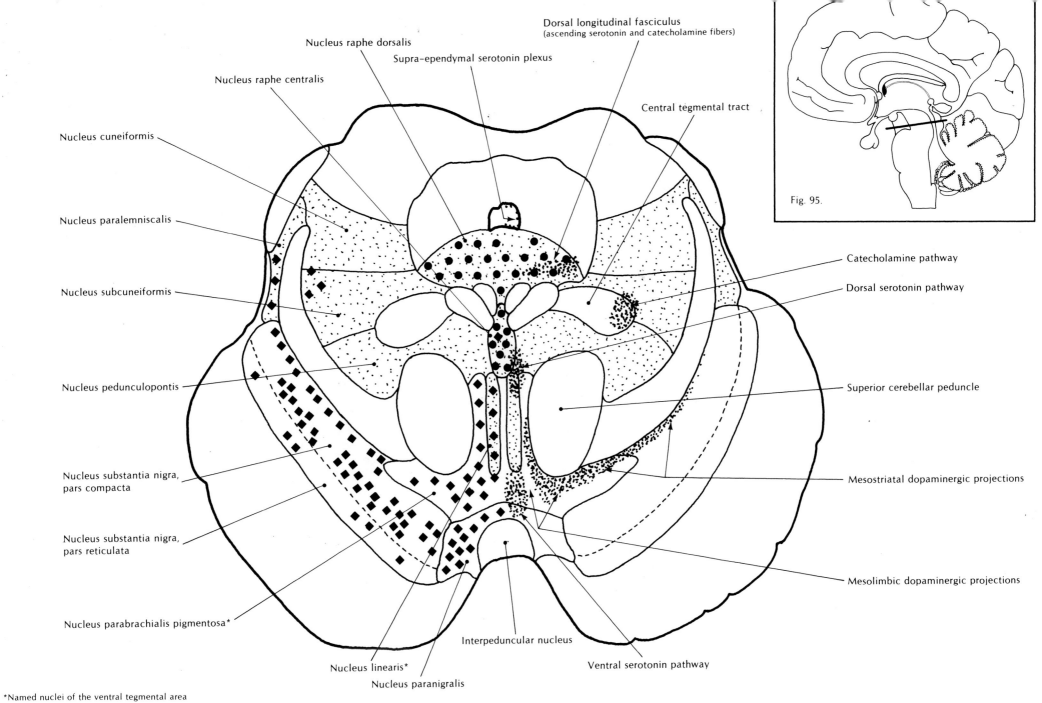

Nucleus cuneiformis

Nucleus paralemniscalis

Nucleus subcuneiformis

Nucleus pedunculopontis

Nucleus substantia nigra, pars compacta

Nucleus substantia nigra, pars reticulata

Nucleus parabrachialis pigmentosa*

Nucleus raphe centralis

Nucleus raphe dorsalis

Supra-ependymal serotonin plexus

Dorsal longitudinal fasciculus (ascending serotonin and catecholamine fibers)

Central tegmental tract

Fig. 95.

Catecholamine pathway

Dorsal serotonin pathway

Superior cerebellar peduncle

Mesostriatal dopaminergic projections

Mesolimbic dopaminergic projections

Interpeduncular nucleus

Ventral serotonin pathway

Nucleus linearis*

Nucleus paranigralis

*Named nuclei of the ventral tegmental area

Figure 95. Midbrain: Level between inferior and superior colliculi. Diamonds, dopaminergic neurons; circles, serotonergic

183

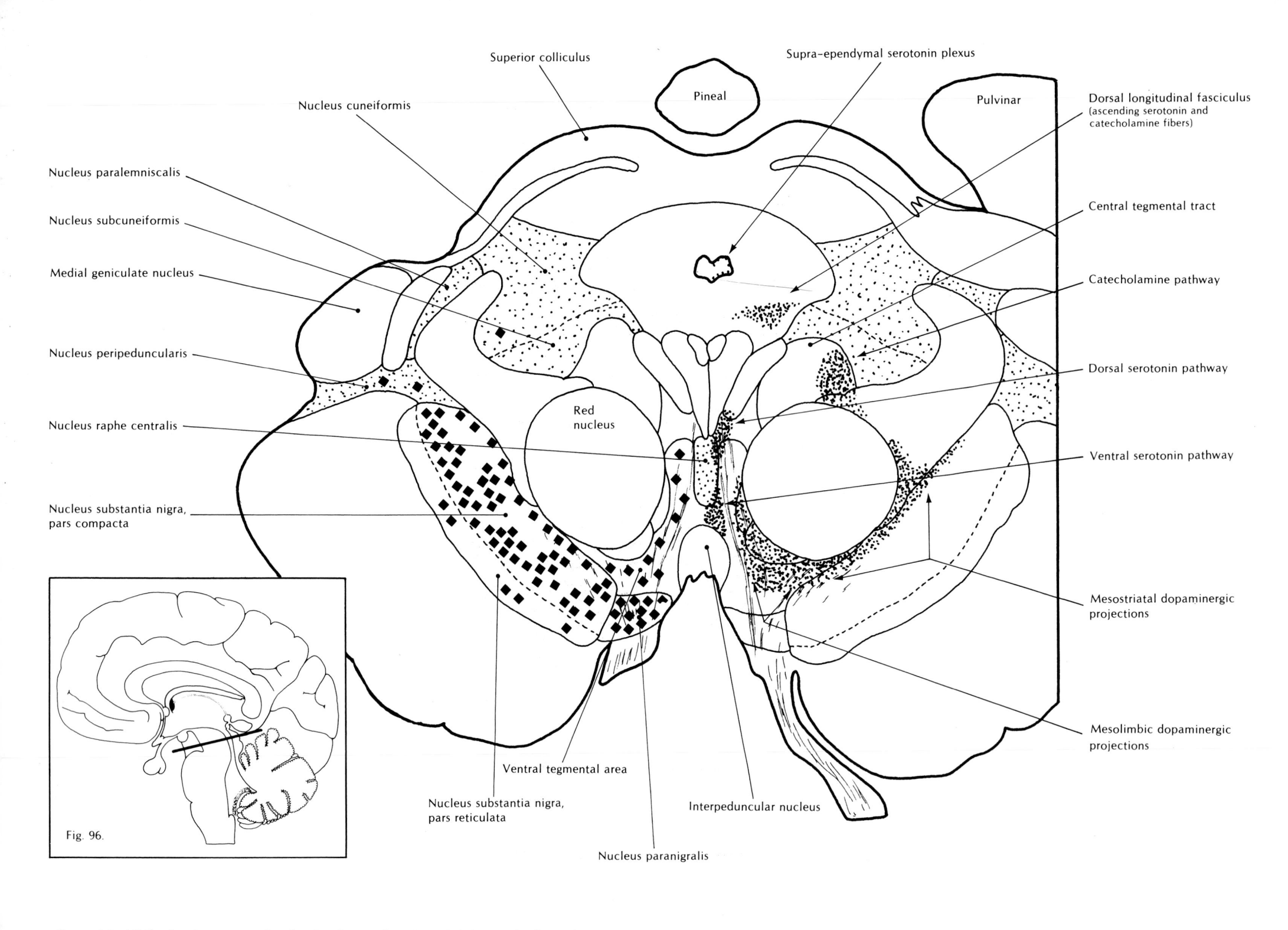

Figure 96. Midbrain: Superior colliculus level (see also Fig. 54). Diamonds, dopaminergic neurons

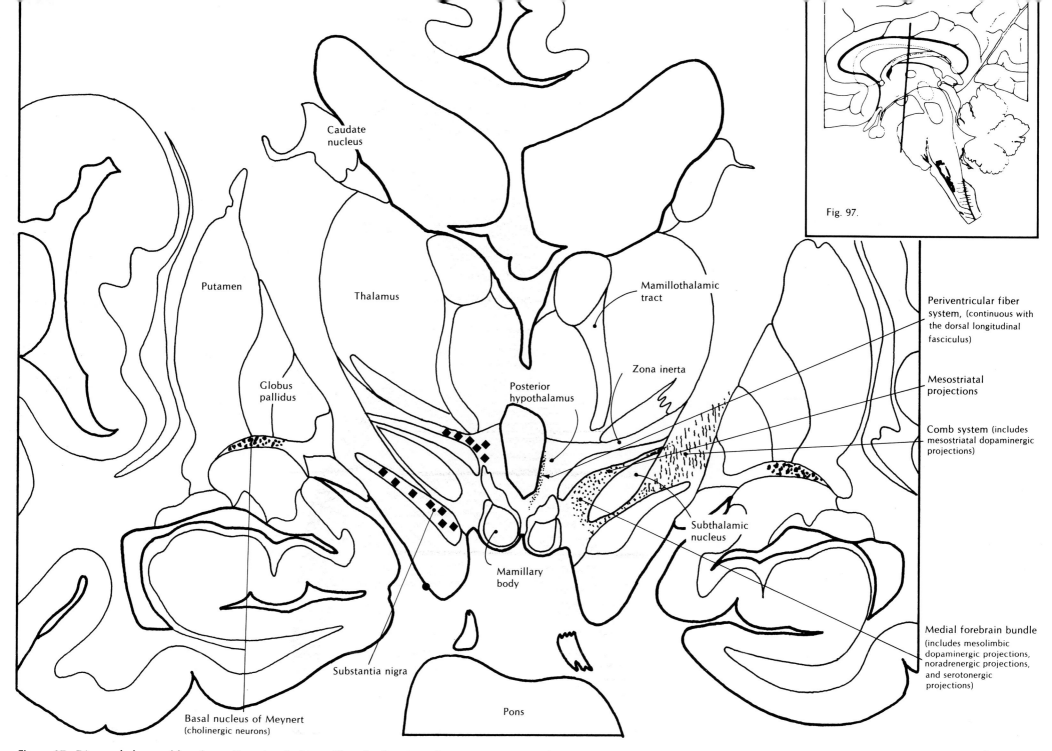

Figure 97. Diencephalon and basal ganglia at level of mamillary bodies (see also Fig. 67). Diamonds, dopaminergic neurons

185

THE VASCULAR STRUCTURE OF THE BRAIN: ANATOMY AND ANGIOGRAPHY

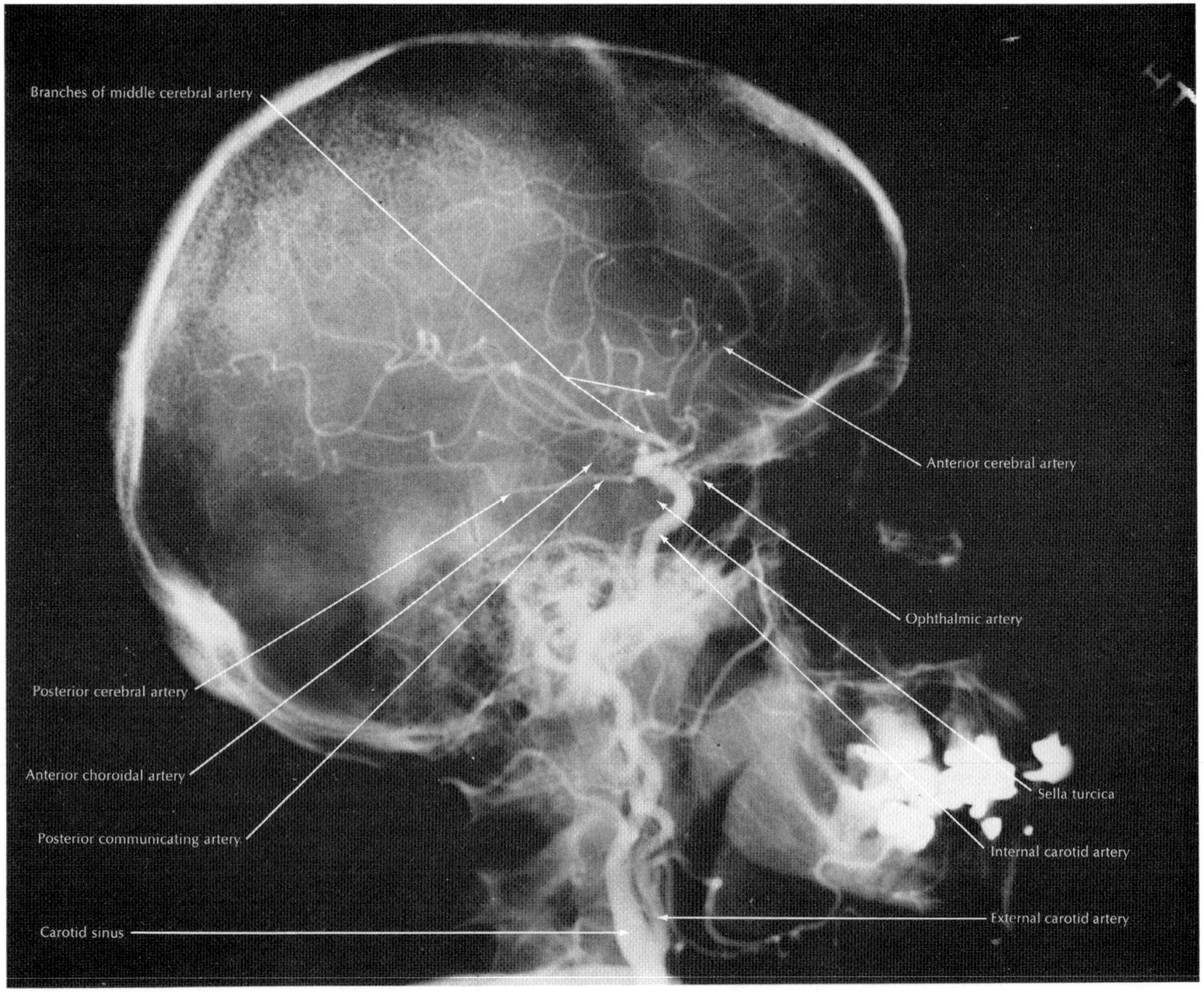

Figure 98. The major cerebral arteries, carotid angiography lateral projection

REMARKS ON BRAIN VASCULAR STRUCTURE

The drawings and angiograms on the following pages were chosen to demonstrate the most common vascular patterns. Individual variations in the venous pattern are quite common whereas the arterial pattern is more predictable. For further details the following references may be helpful.

1. Duvernoy, Henri M. *The Superficial Veins of the Human Brain, Veins of the Brain Stem and of the Base of the Brain*. Springer-Verlag, Berlin, Heidelberg, New York, 1975.
2. George, Ajax E. A Systematic approach to the interpretation of posterior fossa angiography. Radiologic Clinics of North America XII (no. 2): 371–400 (1974).
3. Huang, Y. P., Wolf, B. S. The vein of the lateral recess of the fourth ventricle and its tributaries. Amer. J. Roentgenol. 101: 1–21 (1967).
4. Taveras, Juan M., Wood, Ernest H. *Diagnostic Neuroradiology*. The Williams & Wilkins Co., Baltimore, 1964.

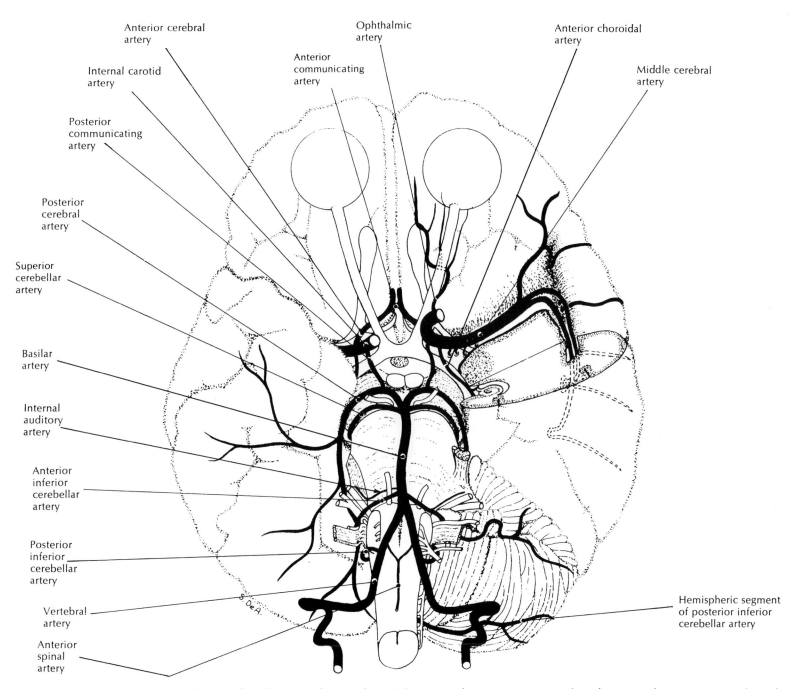

Anterior cerebral
artery

Internal carotid
artery

Posterior
communicating
artery

Posterior
cerebral
artery

Superior
cerebellar
artery

Basilar
artery

Internal
auditory
artery

Anterior
inferior
cerebellar
artery

Posterior
inferior
cerebellar
artery

Vertebral
artery

Anterior
spinal
artery

Ophthalmic
artery

Anterior
communicating
artery

Anterior choroidal
artery

Middle cerebral
artery

Hemispheric segment
of posterior inferior
cerebellar artery

Figure 99. The circle of Willis and major branches of the vertebral-basilar and internal carotid arteries. The recurrent artery of Heubner, not shown, originates from the anterior cerebral artery and courses posterolaterally to enter the anterior perforated substance and supply the anteromedial portion of the basal ganglia and part of the anterior limb of the internal capsule

187

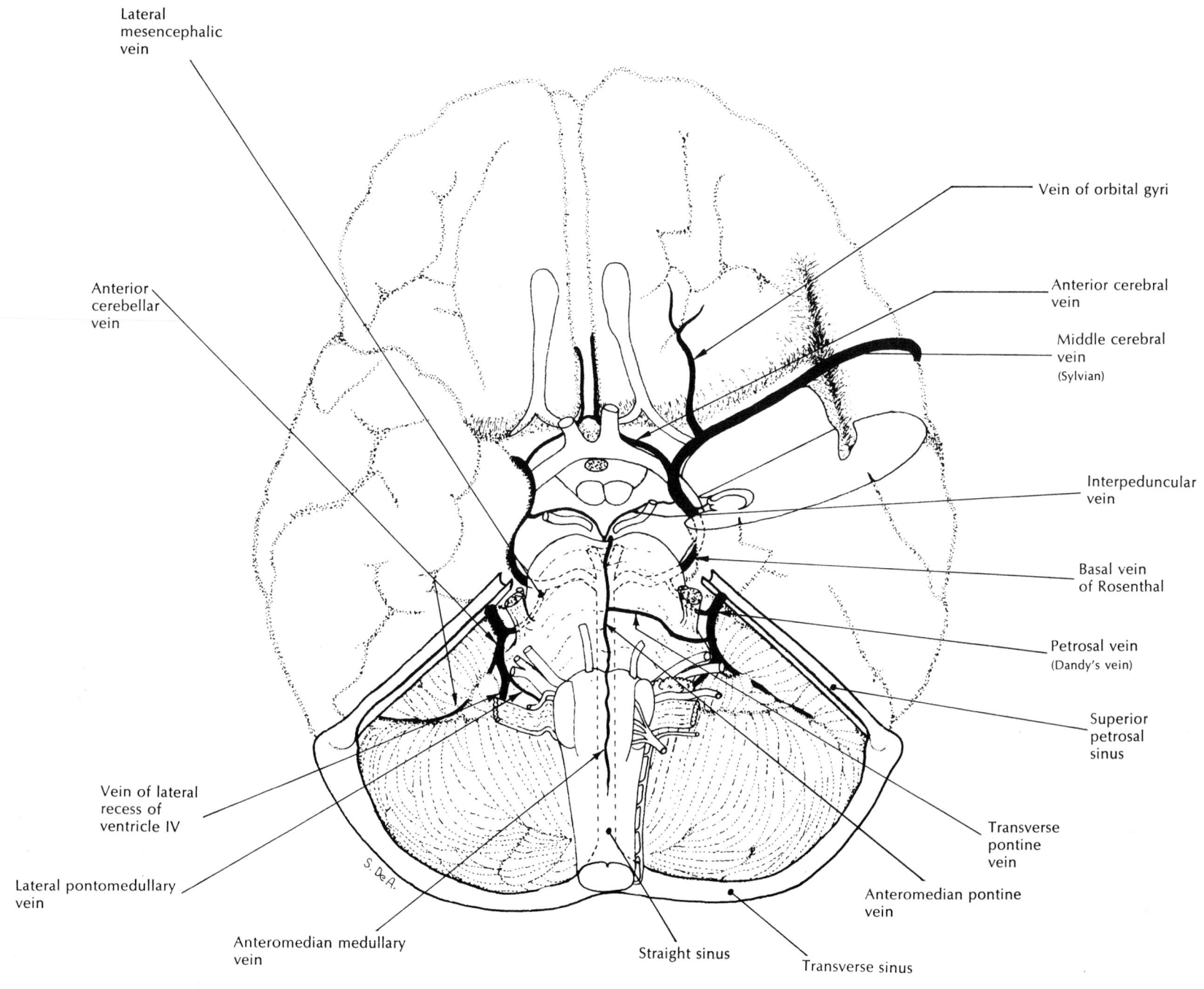

Lateral
mesencephalic
vein

Anterior
cerebellar
vein

Vein of orbital gyri

Anterior cerebral
vein

Middle cerebral
vein
(Sylvian)

Interpeduncular
vein

Basal vein
of Rosenthal

Petrosal vein
(Dandy's vein)

Superior
petrosal
sinus

Vein of lateral
recess of
ventricle IV

Transverse
pontine
vein

Lateral pontomedullary
vein

Anteromedian pontine
vein

Anteromedian medullary
vein

Straight sinus

Transverse sinus

S. De A.

Figure 100. Major superficial veins, basal view

188

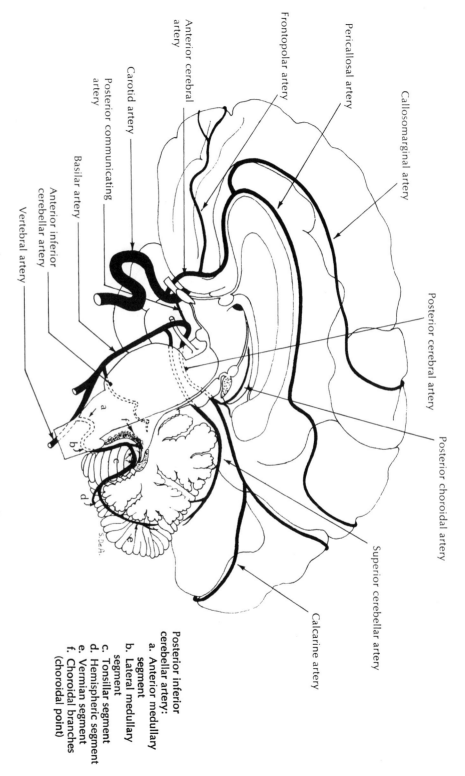

Figure 101. Arteries viewed from the medial surface of the brain

Anterior cerebral artery

Frontopolar artery

Pericallosal artery

Callosomarginal artery

Posterior choroidal artery

Superior cerebellar artery

Calcarine artery

Posterior cerebral artery

Carotid artery

Posterior communicating artery

Basilar artery

Anterior inferior cerebellar artery

Vertebral artery

Posterior inferior cerebellar artery:
a. Anterior medullary segment
b. Lateral medullary segment
c. Tonsillar segment
d. Hemispheric segment
e. Vermian segment
f. Choroidal branches (choroidal point)

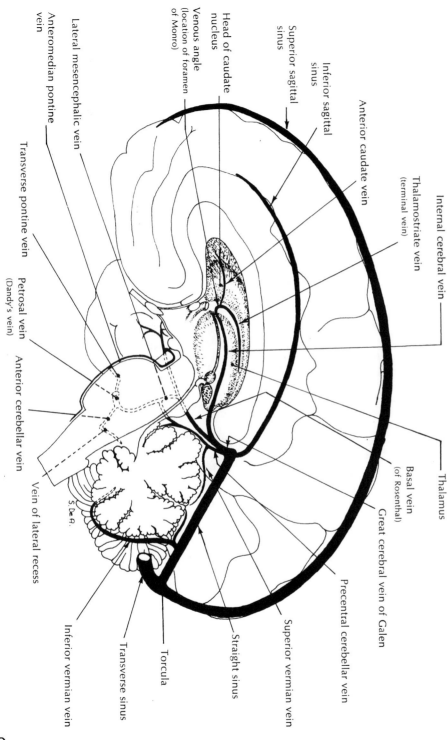

Figure 102. Major superficial veins viewed from the medial surface of the brain

Head of caudate nucleus

Venous angle (location of foramen of Monro)

Anterior caudate vein

Superior sagittal sinus

Inferior sagittal sinus

Thalamostriate vein (terminal vein)

Internal cerebral vein

Thalamus

Basal vein (of Rosenthal)

Great cerebral vein of Galen

Precentral cerebellar vein

Superior vermian vein

Straight sinus

Torcula

Transverse sinus

Inferior vermian vein

Anterior cerebellar vein

Vein of lateral recess

Petrosal vein (Dandy's vein)

Transverse pontine vein

Lateral mesencephalic vein

Anteromedian pontine vein

S.D.P.

189

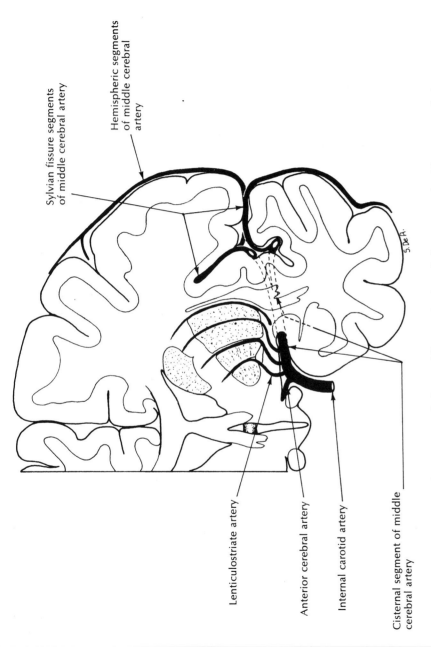

Sylvian fissure segments of middle cerebral artery

Hemispheric segments of middle cerebral artery

S. De A.

Lenticulostriate artery

Anterior cerebral artery

Internal carotid artery

Cisternal segment of middle cerebral artery

Figure 103. The course of the middle cerebral and the reversed "S" course of the lenticulostriate arteries seen in a coronal brain section

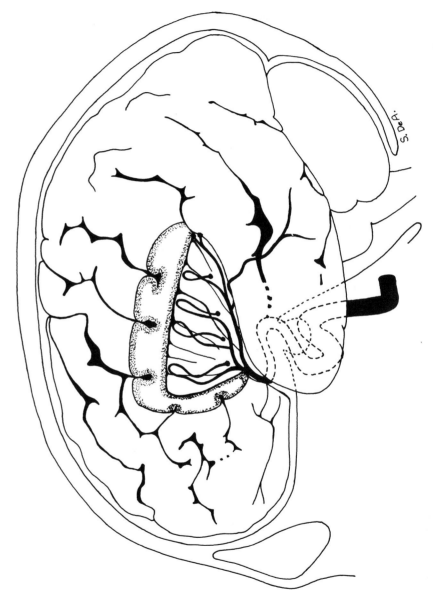

S. De A.

Figure 104. The sylvian triangle. Frontal and parietal opercula of the sylvian fissure have been removed to demonstrate how branches of the middle cerebral artery are distributed over the surface of the insula and form the sylvian triangle. The dots at the end of the arteries indicate their exit from the sylvian fissure

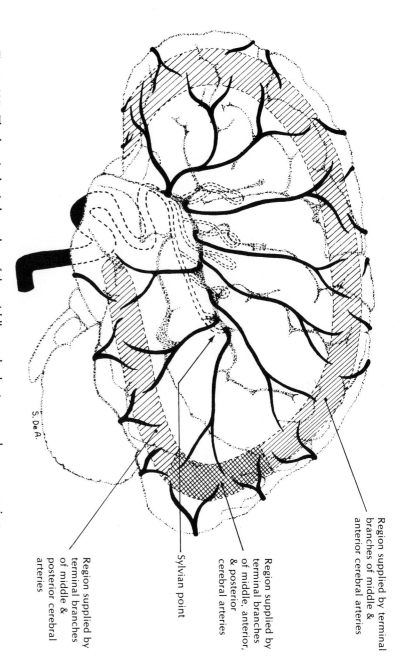

Figure 105. The hemispheric branches of the middle cerebral artery are shown emerging from the sylvian fissure. Their distribution over the insula (the sylvian triangle) is included. The last or most posterior branch to leave the fissure is the sylvian point

S. De A.

Region supplied by terminal branches of middle & anterior cerebral arteries

Region supplied by terminal branches of middle, anterior, & posterior cerebral arteries

Sylvian point

Region supplied by terminal branches of middle & posterior cerebral arteries

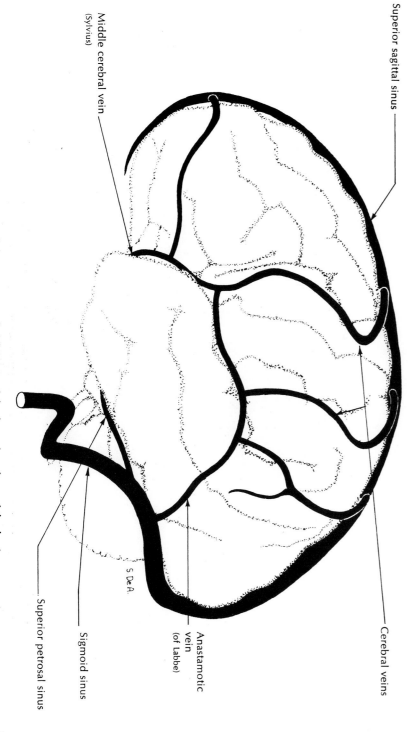

Figure 106. The major superficial veins of the lateral surface of the brain

Superior sagittal sinus

Middle cerebral vein (Sylvius)

S. De A.

Cerebral veins

Anastamotic vein (of Labbe)

Sigmoid sinus

Superior petrosal sinus

191

Artery(ies) (Figs. 107 & 108)

2. Callosomarginal

3. Carotid, internal

4. Carotid, internal, intracavernous segment

8. Cerebral, anterior

9. Cerebral, middle
   a. temporoparietal branch

11. Choroidal, anterior

13. Communicating, posterior

15. Lenticulostriate

16. Ophthalmic

17. Pericallosal

18. Sylvian point

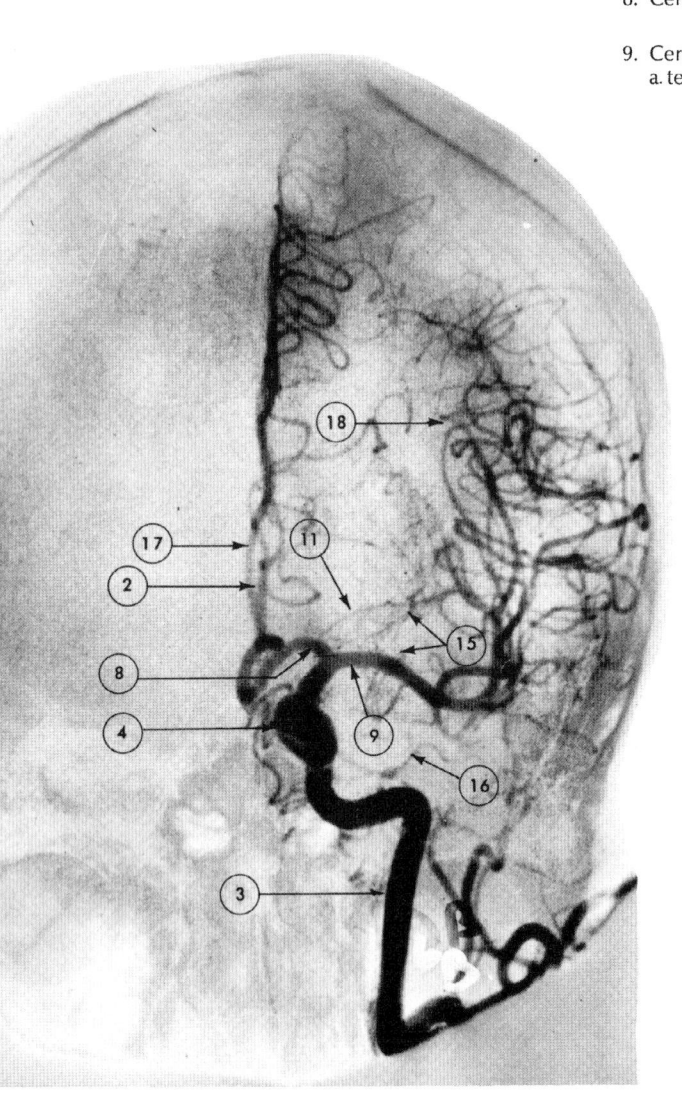

Figure 107. Internal carotid artery angiogram, arterial phase, frontal projection. The direction of the X-ray beam is indicated by the large arrow to Figure 108

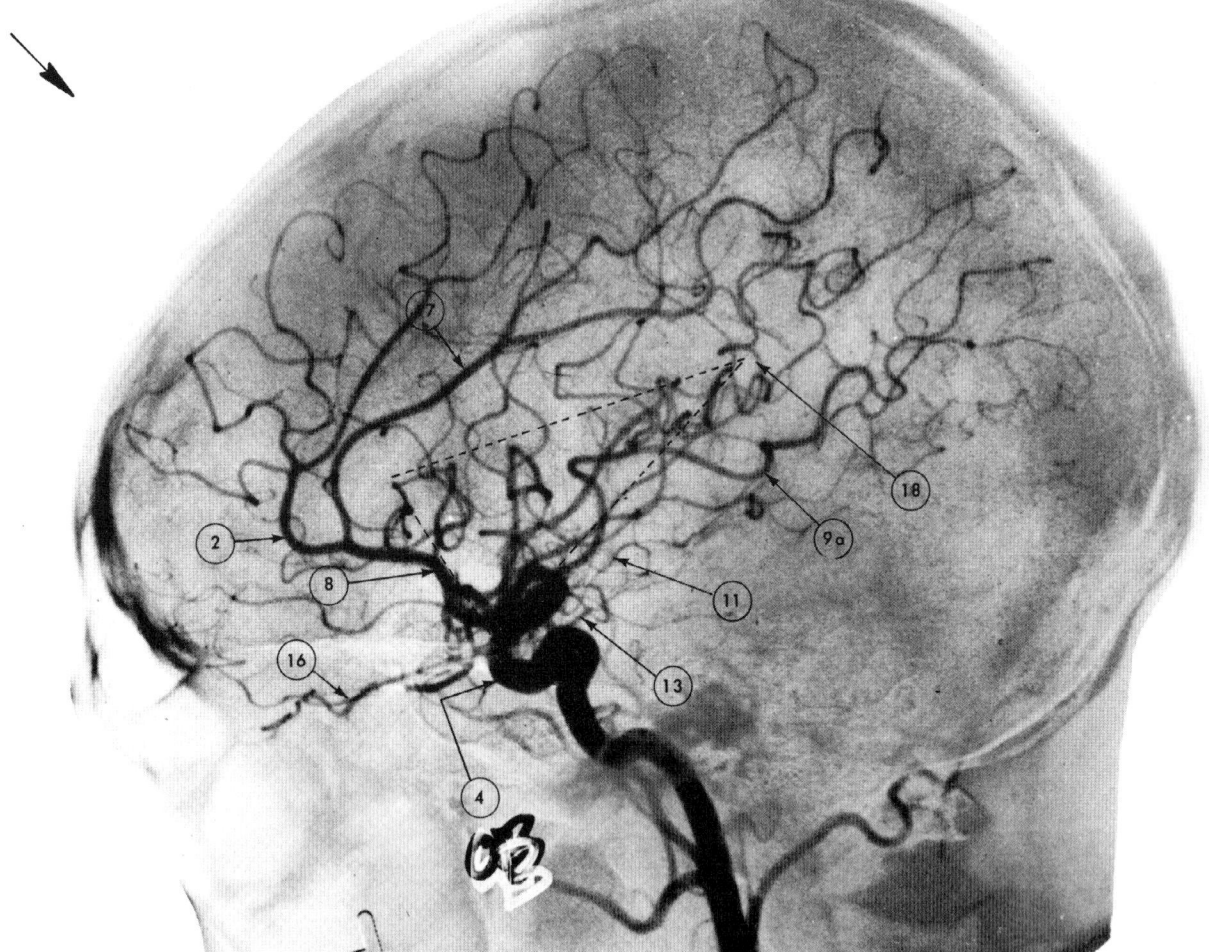

Figure 108. Internal carotid artery angiogram, arterial phase, lateral projection. The Sylvian triangle is demarcated by the dotted line. The small arrows mark the exit of branches of the middle cerebral artery from the Sylvian fissure

192

Vein(s) (Figs. 109 & 110)

1. Anastamotic (of Labbe)

2. Basal (of Rosenthal)

6. Cerebral, anterior temporal

7. Cerebral, hemispheric branches

8. Cerebral, internal

10. Great cerebral (of Galen)

17. Sinus, inferior sagittal

19. Sinus, straight

21. Sinus, superior sagittal

23. Sinus, transverse

24. Thalamostriate (terminal)

25. Venous angle (location of foramen of Monro)

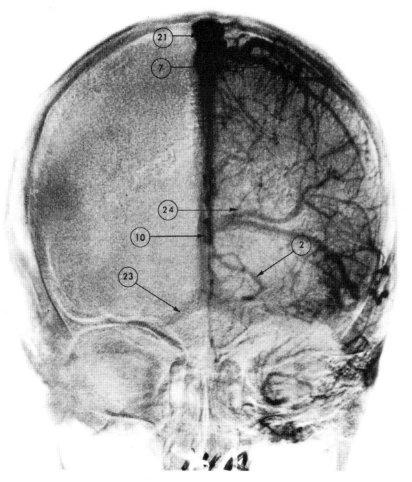

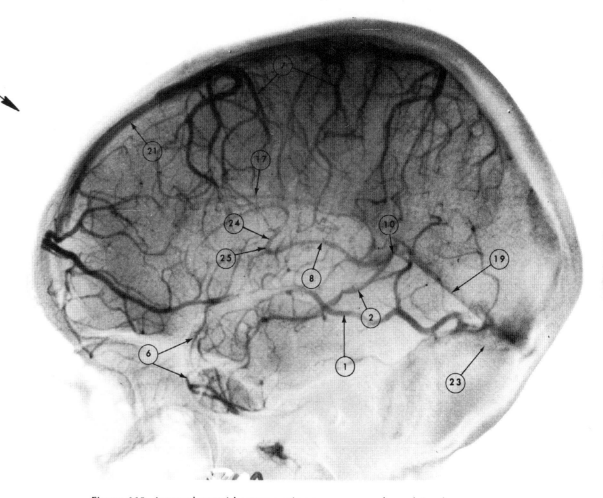

Figure 109. Internal carotid artery angiogram, venous phase, frontal projection. The direction of the X-ray beam is indicated by the large arrow to Figure 110

Figure 110. Internal carotid artery angiogram, venous phase, lateral projection

Artery(ies) (Figs. 111 & 112)

ST. Sella turcica

1. Basilar

5. Cerebellar, anterior inferior (AICA)

6. Cerebellar, posterior inferior (PICA)
   a. Hemispheric segment
   b. Lateral medullary segment
   c. Vermian segment

7. Cerebellar, superior
   a. Hemispheric branches

10. Cerebral, posterior
   a. Parietooccipital branches

12. Choroidal, posterior

19. Vertebral

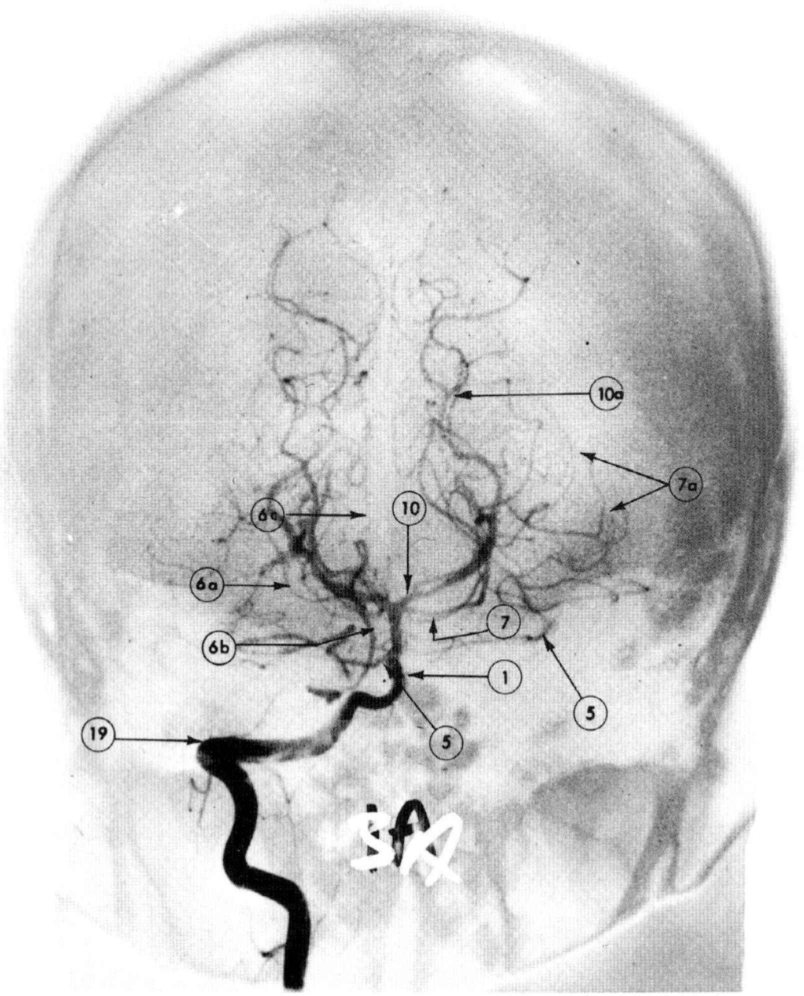

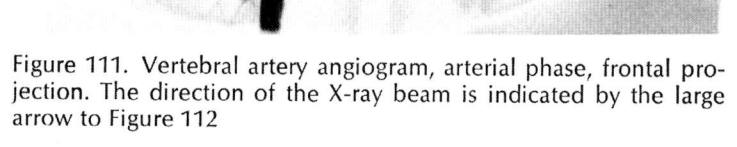

Figure 111. Vertebral artery angiogram, arterial phase, frontal projection. The direction of the X-ray beam is indicated by the large arrow to Figure 112

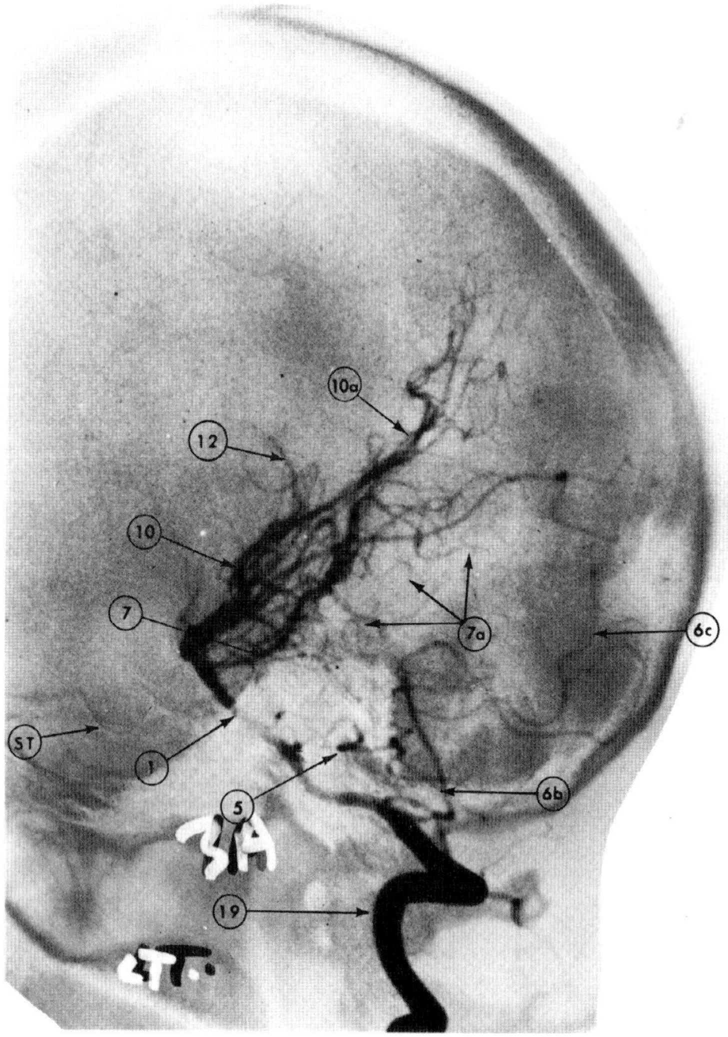

Figure 112. Vertebral artery angiogram, arterial phase, lateral projection

Vein(s) (Figs. 113 & 114)

ST. Sella turcica

3. Cerebellar, anterior

4. Cerebellar, hemispheric

5. Cerebellar, precentral

8. Cerebral, internal

10. Great cerebral (of Galen)

11. Jugular, internal

12. Of lateral recess of ventriclue IV*

13. Mesencephalic, lateral

14. Mesencephalic, posterior (infratentorial analog of basal vein of Rosenthal)

15. Petrosal (of Dandy)

16. Pontine, anteromedian

18. Sinus, sigmoid

19. Sinus, straight

20. Sinus, superior petrosal

21. Sinus, superior sagittal

22. Sinus, torcula

23. Sinus, transverse

26. Vermian, inferior

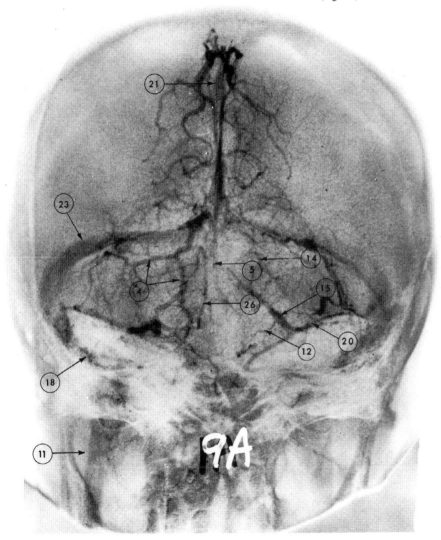

Figure 113. Vertebral artery angiogram, venous phase, frontal projection. The direction of the X-ray beam is indicated by the large arrow to Figure 114

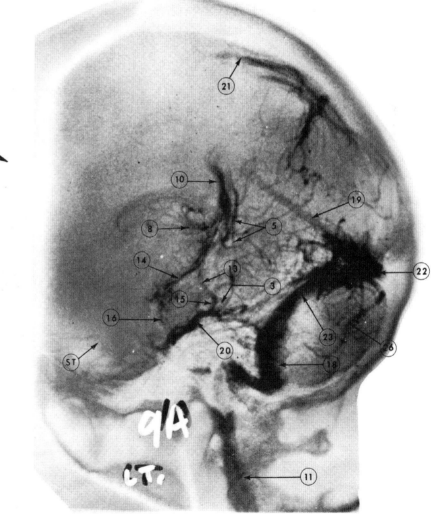

Figure 114. Vertebral artery angiogram, venous phase, lateral projection

* The vein of the lateral recess of ventricle IV, a branch of the anterior cerebellar vein, is sometimes prominent radiologically

INDEX

Pages on which the main or the most illustrative examples of structures are located are shown in *italics*.

200

201